Office Orthopedics
for Primary Care:
Treatment

Office Orthopedics
for Primary Care:
Treatment

THIRD EDITION

BRUCE CARL ANDERSON, MD
Clinical Associate Professor of Medicine
Oregon Health Sciences University
Portland, Oregon

Director, Medical Orthopedic Department
Sunnyside Medical Center
Portland, Oregon

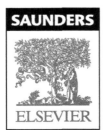

SAUNDERS

ELSEVIER

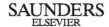

SAUNDERS
ELSEVIER

1600 John F. Kennedy Blvd.
Ste 1800
Philadelphia, PA 19103-2899

OFFICE ORTHOPEDICS FOR PRIMARY CARE: TREATMENT ISBN 1-4160-2206-6
Copyright © 2006, 1999, 1995 by Elsevier Inc.

Notice

Library of Congress Cataloging-in-Publication Data

Anderson, Bruce Carl.
   Office orthopedics for primary care: treatment / Bruce Carl Anderson.—3rd ed.
   ISBN 1-4160-2206-6
     1. Orthopedics. 2. Primary care (Medicine) I. Title.
   RD732.A53 2006
   616.7—dc22

                       2005046537

Acquisitions Editor: Rolla Couchman
Developmental Editor: Matthew Ray
Publishing Services Manager: Frank Polizzano
Project Manager: Lee Ann Draud
Design Direction: Karen O'Keefe Owens

Printed in the United States of America

Transferred to Digital Printing, 2015

To the pioneering work of
P. Hume Kendall of the Department of Physical Medicine,
Guy's Hospital, London, England
and
Joseph L. Hollander of the Arthritis Section,
Department of Medicine, Hospital of the University of Pennsylvania,
Philadelphia, Pennsylvania

PREFACE

Over the last 60 years, corticosteroids have been used to treat acute and chronic inflammation of a wide variety of diseases. Cortisone was originally identified and subsequently purified from animal adrenal glands in the 1930s. Fifteen years later, cortisone and hydrocortisone were synthesized from bile acids, setting the stage for the clinical application of the glucocorticoid hormone in the late 1940s. Injectable hydrocortisone was originally used by the rheumatology group at the Mayo Clinic to treat patients suffering from the acute and chronic inflammation of rheumatoid arthritis. Soon thereafter, having documented hydrocortisone's dramatic benefit in this select group of patients, the novel treatment was extended to the treatment of other arthritic conditions and eventually to local orthopedic conditions. Over the next 30 years, hydrocortisone and its derivatives (triamcinolone, methylprednisolone, dexamethasone, and betamethasone) were used to treat the entire gamut of conditions characterized by acute and chronic inflammation, from the mildly inflammatory osteoarthritis and focal tendinitis to the intensely inflammatory gout and systemic lupus erythematosus. Percy Julian—a black educator born in Alabama—is credited with the synthesis of cortisone from soy beans in the 1950s.

The Mayo Clinic pioneered the use of cortisone as an effective anti-inflammatory medication in the late 1940s and early 1950s. Kendall, Henoch, and Slocumb first administered cortisone by daily injection to patients with rheumatoid arthritis. Their results (Mayo Clin Proc 24:181, 1949), along with those of the studies later published by Hollander, Brown, Frain, Udell, and Jessar (JAMA 147:1629-1635, 1951; J Bone Joint Surg Am 35A:983-990, 1953;Am J Med 15:656-665, 1953), were so significant that cortisone was originally proclaimed as a "cure for arthritis." Because of its early success with arthritic patients, injectable cortisone was also pursued as a possible anti-inflammatory treatment for a variety of local orthopedic conditions. Kendall, Lapidus, and others published studies in the late 1950s and early 1960s demonstrating cortisone's remarkable ability to arrest the persistent inflammation of tendinitis, bursitis, and other local musculoskeletal conditions (Industr Med Surg 26:234-244, 1957; BMJ 1:1500-1501, 1955;Ann Phys Med 6:287-294, 1962; BMJ 1:1277-1278, 1956).

These initial studies were summarized in publications and editorials in the early 1960s. Hollander published his 10-year experience in 1961. His research group performed 100,000 intra-articular injections with a remarkable safety profile; only a 1 in 10,000 risk of postinjection infection was noted (Bull Rheum Dis 11:239-240, 1961). Kendall came to the same conclusion, having analyzed 6700 injections over a 3-year period between March 1954 and March 1957. *"Because it exerts a powerful local action and does not appear to give rise to any general hormonal effects, hydrocortisone by local injection has proved of great value in the treatment of isolated joint and soft-tissue disease."* And *"It is considered that the over-all incidence and morbidity of the side-effects following the local use of hydrocortisone are so low as not to constitute a contraindication to this method of treatment."* (Ann Phys Med 4:170-175, 1961).

Yet this early enthusiasm about the clinical application of cortisone for arthritis and local musculoskeletal conditions was short lived. Through the 1960s and 1970s a series of publications appeared that emphasized the serious side effects that occurred when large doses of cortisone were given over prolonged periods of time. In addition, a number of reports—nearly all single-case reports or anecdotal series of five patients or fewer—showed that local injection of tendons and other soft tissue conditions were not without hazard. Local cortisone injection was implicated in postinjection tendon rupture, postinjection atrophy of tissue, and postinjection avascular necrosis of the hip. The constant stream of negative reports had the net effect of overshadowing the extensive research published by Kendall and Hollander from the 1950s and cast a dark cloud over the use of cortisone, especially local injection of cortisone, over the next 2 decades.

Thirty-five studies were published through the 1960s and 1970s, all of which intimated a direct relationship between the injection of cortisone and the reported adverse clinical outcome. However, a closer analysis of these case reports suggests that other factors may have been equally important in affecting the outcome. For example, a review of the 23 case reports on postinjection tendon rupture, representing 50 combined patients (the largest published series of 5 patients was published in the *Western Journal of Medicine*), shows that half of these 50 patients were taking systemic steroids at the time of injection. More than half of these patients had an underlying connective tissue disease, mostly rheumatoid arthritis and systemic lupus erythematosus. In addition, details of the procedures and rehabilitation methods were not disclosed in detail in these reports. None of the studies provided information assessing the severity of the condition. None provided radiographic studies to determine whether degenerative changes or partial tears were present. None of the studies supplied details of the exact method of injection, whether peritendinous, intratendinous, and so forth. Lastly, none of the 23 publications provided any detail of the management of the patient following the injection, either to what degree the joint was protected after the injection or the specific rehabilitation exercises required for recovery.

Interestingly, only four tendons were described in these reports, including the Achilles, patellar, biceps, and rotator cuff tendons (the four largest tendons under the greatest degree of tension and, more important, the tendons that undergo a slow degenerative process [mucinoid degenerative thinning] when exposed to chronic inflammation, contributing directly to the well-known fact of traumatic rupture). This is in sharp contrast to the tendons that were not described, namely, the gluteus medius tendon at the hip and the intermediate or small tendons of the distal extremities. This disparity begs the question whether the injection of cortisone or the chronic inflammation and degenerative processes were more important in the process of tendon disruption.

The relationship of corticosteroid injection to avascular necrosis of the hip is even more tenuous. Only one publication alleges a relationship of local injection to avascular necrosis of the hip (Am J Med 77:1119-1120, 1984). In this case report, the patient had been treated with multiple injections over an 18-year period. The patient had received at least 200 injections of methylprednisolone at weekly intervals at the trochanteric bursa, upper neck, and olecranon bursa. At the time this patient suffered the acute vascular event, he was frankly cushingoid. Since systemic steroids are a well-known cause of avascular necrosis, the validity of the causal relationship between single injection and avascular necrosis of the hip seems doubtful. Three publications described local subcutaneous atrophy following injection of corticosteroids (Ann Intern Med 65:1008-1019, 1966; BMJ 3:600, 1967; J Bone Joint Surg Am 61A:627-628, 1979). These all occurred in superficial areas—hand, forearm, and anterior knee. British researcher Ann Beardwell commented, *"Though local atrophy cannot be regarded as a serious complication of corticosteroid therapy, it is unsightly and may persist for several years."*

Certainly, local corticosteroid injection is not without potential problems. However, adverse outcomes can be minimized by thoroughly assessing the patient, screening patients who are at higher risk for infection or tendon rupture, performing a standardized method of injection, prescribing individualized postinjection aftercare instructions, and adjusting recovery exercises based on close follow-up examinations. The development of ever-improving technical skill is extremely important in ensuring a favorable response.

This expanded third edition has emphasized a comprehensive approach to the evaluation and treatment of each individual orthopedic and arthritic condition. When more than one technique of injection is possible, the safest approach and the ease of administration have been chosen. The "step-care" treatment protocols; the specific postinjection management guidelines; the physical therapy exercise instruction sheets; the illustrations of the various braces, casts, and supports; and the detailed descriptions of local injection techniques allow the clinician to effectively "office manage" 90% to 95% of the outpatient medical orthopedic problems while minimizing adverse outcomes. Treatment guidelines provide details on specific restrictions. The length of time for immobilization is both efficacious and practical. The appropriate timing and anatomic details of local injection and the extremely important post-treatment rehabilitation exercises are included. Although local corticosteroid injection has been emphasized, this book was not intended to be simply an "injection manual." Injection of corticosteroids can be exceedingly helpful in assessing and reducing the local inflammatory reaction to tissue injury. However, it must not take the place of simpler, less invasive treatments. In any given patient, the anti-inflammatory effects of injection are as important as restricting use by immobilization and the physical therapy exercises of stretching and toning. Treatment must be individualized for each patient.

There are as many ways to accomplish the same treatment goals in the field of musculoskeletal medicine as there are conditions. Differences in technique and approach are widespread in this overlooked field of medicine. I hope this book can serve as a starting point for those interested in expanding their expertise in the treatment of musculoskeletal disease in outpatients. In addition, I hope that the information contained herein can bridge the gaps among the disciplines of rheumatology, orthopedics, neurology, and physiatry.

Kendall summarized his opinion on the use of corticosteroid injection for local orthopedic conditions by saying, *"It is perhaps surprising that an empirical treatment such as local corticosteroid injection therapy has received wide acceptance for the treatment of all the rheumatic diseases. Nevertheless, as an adjunct to the over-all management of these conditions it is now firmly established and is invaluable. Perhaps the greatest credit for this can be given to the safety factor: side-effects are so unusual that even should injection prove of no value the physician may feel secure that harm will seldom result."* After 27 years of clinical practice and residency teaching and the administration of more than 50,000 local corticosteroid injections, I agree with his conclusions. However, I would add that local corticosteroid injection for local musculoskeletal conditions is one of the most predictably successful treatments to reduce and arrest the body's exaggerated inflammatory response to injury only when combined with specific periods of rest, selective use of immobilization, and sequential recovery physical therapy exercises.

Fortunately, the pessimism of the 1960s and 1970s is fading, in large part because of the number of clinical studies that have been published over the last 10 to 15 years. Clinicians and researchers of the late 20th and early 21st centuries have taken Hollander's and Kendall's opinions to heart and have reinvestigated the utility of local corticosteroid injection. Longitudinal outcome studies and controlled, double-blind studies evaluating the efficacy of corticosteroids have been published in such diverse areas as cervical and lumbar radiculopathy, carpal tunnel, rotator cuff tendinitis, frozen shoulder, lateral epicondylitis, olecranon bursitis, trigger finger, de Quervain's tenosynovitis, trochanteric bursitis, Morton's neuroma, and gout. Studies reporting on these and other topics are tabulated in the reference section of the book.

Bruce Carl Anderson, MD

ACKNOWLEDGMENTS

This book represents the outgrowth of 27 years of post-residency education and clinical experience, including more than 50,000 local procedures, that would not have been possible without the support and encouragement from many sources. I wish to thank all the members of the departments of medicine, family practice, physiatry, neurosurgery, and surgical orthopedics at the Sunnyside Medical Center, especially Dr. Ian MacMillan of the Department of Medicine for his support and assistance in developing the medical orthopedic department, and the surgeons of the Department of Orthopedics, Dr. Steven Ebner, Dr. Edward Stark, and Dr. Stephen Groman, for their stimulating feedback. I also wish to thank my extremely capable physician assistant, Linda Onheiber, for her steady contributions to the medical orthopedic department and all the medical residents of the graduating classes of 2003 and 2004 at Oregon Health Sciences University, Eastmoreland Hospital, Legacy Emanuel Hospital, and the Sisters of Providence teaching hospitals for their constant encouragement, contributions, and critical appraisal of the content of the book. I also wish to thank the medical directors of the various Portland, Oregon, teaching hospitals for their support, namely, Dr. Nancy Loeb at Providence St. Vincent Medical Center, Dr. Steven Jones at Legacy Emanuel Hospital, and Dr. Don Girard at the Oregon Health Sciences University. Lastly, I wish to thank Dr. David Gilbert, director emeritus of the Providence Portland Medical Center—my internal medicine residency director—for his stimulation to excellence, his encouragement to examine ever deeper into clinical problems, and his support and inspiration in my return to clinical research.

Bruce Carl Anderson, MD

CONTENTS

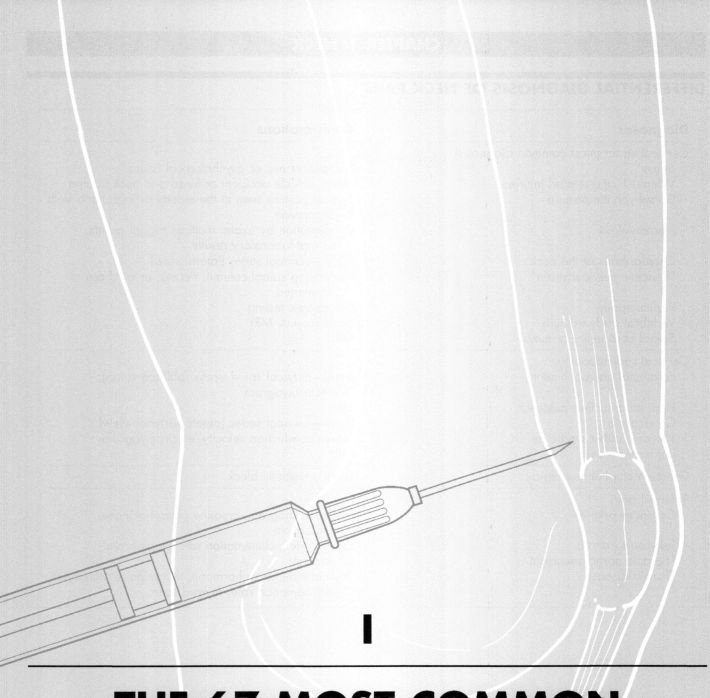

I

THE 67 MOST COMMON OUTPATIENT ORTHOPEDIC CONDITIONS

DIFFERENTIAL DIAGNOSIS OF NECK PAIN

Diagnoses	Confirmations
Cervical strain (most common diagnosis)	
Stress	Socioeconomic or psychological issues
Whiplash and related injuries	Motor vehicle accident or head and neck trauma
Dorsokyphotic posture	Typical posture seen in the elderly or in patients with depression
Fibromyalgia	Confirmation by exam: multiple trigger points; normal laboratory results
Osteoarthritis of the neck	X-ray—cervical series (lateral view)
"Reactive cervical strain"	Underlying spinal column, nerves, or cord are threatened
Radiculopathy	Neurologic testing
Vertebral body fracture	Bone scan or MRI
Spinal cord injury or tumor	MRI
Cervical radiculopathy	
Foraminal encroachment	X-ray—cervical spine x-rays (oblique views); electromyogram
Herniated nucleus pulposus	MRI
Cervical rib	X-ray—cervical series (anteroposterior view)
Thoracic outlet syndrome	Nerve conduction velocity/electromyogram
Epidural process	MRI
Greater occipital neuralgia	Local anesthetic block
Referred pain	
Coronary arteries	Electrocardiogram, creatine phosphokinase, angiogram
Takyasu's arteritis	Erythrocyte sedimentation rate, angiogram
Thoracic aortic aneurysm	Chest x-ray
Thyroid disease	Thyroid-stimulating hormone, thyroxine, erythrocyte sedimentation rate, thyroid scan

CERVICAL STRAIN

Enter the upper trapezius muscle at the point of maximum tenderness; the angle is perpendicular to the skin.

Needle: 1¹/₂-inch, 22-gauge
Depth: 1 to 1¹/₂ inches
Volume: 3 to 4 mL of anesthesia, 1 mL of D80, or both

NOTE: Lightly advance the needle to feel the outer fascia, then enter the body of the muscle. Triamcinolone should not be used because of the greater chance of atrophy of muscle or overlying subcutaneous tissue.

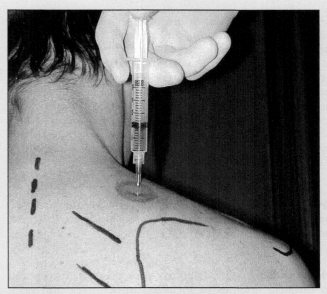

FIGURE 1-1. Trigger point injection of the paracervical or upper trapezial muscles.

DESCRIPTION   Cervical strain is an irritation and spasm of the cervical and upper back muscles. Physical and emotional stress, whiplash-like injuries, cervical arthritis, dorsokyphotic posture, and underlying abnormal cervical alignment are common causes. Spinal nerve or spinal cord irritation or injury is a much less common cause of cervical strain. The upper portion of the trapezius muscle and the levator scapulae, rhomboid major and minor, and long cervical muscles are most commonly affected. Symptoms are bilateral in most cases. Several names are used to describe this condition, depending on cause, the length of time symptoms have been present, and anatomic predominance: neck strain, whiplash, trapezial strain, wry neck, torticollis, fibromyalgia, and fibrositis.

SYMPTOMS   The patient complains of pain, stiffness, and tightness in the upper back or shoulder. The patient characteristically places the hand over the upper back or base of the neck and rubs the affected area when describing the symptoms.

"Oh, my aching neck."

"My neck is just a bunch of knots."

"My neck is so tight and tender."

"At the end of a hard day, my neck is so full of tension."

"My upper back feels like it has been tightened in a vise."

"My upper shoulder gets so stiff and tight."

"If I sleep wrong, I wake up with a stiff neck and then I get this horrendous headache."

EXAM   Each patient is examined for the degree of muscle spasm, for the specific points of irritation in the upper back and lower cervical muscles (referred to as *trigger points*), and for the extent of loss of normal neck range of motion.

EXAM SUMMARY

1. Trigger points (upper back, paracervical, and rhomboids)
2. Reduced ipsilateral rotation and contralateral bending of the neck, passively performed
3. Normal neurologic exam
4. No bony tenderness

(1) Trigger points are seen most frequently in the middle portion of the upper trapezius muscle, in the long cervical muscles at the base of the neck (at the C6-C7 vertebral level), and in the rhomboid muscles along the medial scapular border. The tenderness may be localized to a small, quarter-sized area or may affect a diffuse area of muscle in chronic cases. *(2)* The range of motion of the neck may be limited, correlating well with the degree of muscle spasm. As muscle spasm increases, greater loss of ipsilateral neck rotation and of contralateral neck bending is seen. (Normal rotation of the neck is 90 degrees; normal lateral bending is 45 degrees.) Flexion and extension of the neck are affected in extreme cases and in cases in which there is underlying arthritis. *(3)* In an uncomplicated case, the neurologic exam of the upper

extremities is normal. *(4)* Bony structures of the neck, shoulder, and upper back usually are not tender.

X-RAYS A cervical spine series (including postero-anterior, lateral, odontoid, and oblique views) is recommended. Mild to moderate cases of cervical strain show normal findings or nonspecific arthritic changes on x-rays. Changes specific for cervical strain are seen only in moderate to severe cases. The normal cervical lordotic curve can be replaced by a straightened or even a reversed curve. Loss of normal vertebral alignment is best evaluated on the lateral view of the neck. Severe torticollis may cause a lateral deviation of the cervical spine, which is best seen on the posteroanterior view of the neck.

SPECIAL TESTING MRI and electromyogram are used for cases complicated by persistent or moderate to severe radicular symptoms (p. 7).

DIAGNOSIS The diagnosis is based on a history and on physical findings of localized upper back and neck tenderness, the characteristic aggravation of symptoms by ipsilateral rotation and contralateral bending of the neck, and the absence of evidence of radiculopathy by history or exam. Plain x-rays of the cervical spine are used to assess the severity of the condition and to exclude underlying bony pathology. Regional anesthetic block into a trigger point may be helpful in complex cases to differentiate referred pain from cervical radiculopathy or subscapular bursitis.

TREATMENT The goals of treatment are to reduce muscle irritability and spasm and to re-establish the normal cervical lordosis. Ice applications, a muscle relaxant at night for 7 to 10 days, and physical therapy exercises are the treatments of choice.

STEP 1 Perform a thorough exam of the neck, measure the baseline range of motion of the neck, obtain routine cervical series *x-rays* if symptoms are severe or long-lasting, and consider ordering *MRI* if symptoms and signs of sensorimotor radiculopathy are present.

Suggest simple changes in lifestyle, including sitting straight with the shoulders held back, sleeping with the head and neck aligned with the body (a small pillow under the neck), driving with the arms slightly shrugged (arm rests), and avoiding straps over the shoulders.

Recommend ice applications to the base of the neck and upper back for temporary relief of pain and muscle spasm in acute cases.

Begin gentle stretching exercises that are to be performed daily, including shoulder rolls, scapular pinch, and neck stretches (p. 268).

Prescribe a muscle relaxant for nighttime use.

Recommend heat and massage for the upper back and the base of the neck (p. 267).

Discuss stress reduction and how stress contributes to symptoms.

Prescribe a nonsteroidal anti-inflammatory drug (NSAID) (e.g., ibuprofen [Advil, Motrin]) and note its secondary role (inflammation is not a prominent part of cervical strain).

STEP 2 (3 TO 4 WEEKS FOR PERSISTENT CASES) **Order x-rays of the neck.**

Prescribe therapeutic ultrasound for persistent strain.

Recommend deep massage for palliative care.

Prescribe gentle cervical traction, beginning at 5 lb for 5 to 10 minutes once a day (p. 245).

Prescribe a soft cervical collar or a soft Philadelphia collar to be worn during the day, especially when involved in physical work (p. 245).

STEP 3 (6 TO 8 WEEKS FOR CHRONIC CASES) **Perform trigger point injection with a local anesthetic. This can be combined with a long-acting corticosteroid.**

Prescribe a tricyclic antidepressant for long-term control of pain.

Consider referral to physical therapy for a transcutaneous electrical nerve stimulator unit or to a pain clinic for long-term control of refractory pain.

PHYSICAL THERAPY Physical therapy is fundamental in the treatment and prevention of cervical strain.

PHYSICAL THERAPY SUMMARY

1. Ice
2. Heat before stretching of the neck and upper back muscles
3. Deep-muscle massage
4. Therapeutic ultrasound
5. Gentle vertical cervical traction, performed manually or with a traction unit

Acute Period Heat, massage, and gentle stretching exercises are used to reduce muscular irritation. These exercises should be performed daily at home. *Heat and massage* to the upper back and to the base of the neck provide temporary relief of pain and spasm. These can be combined with a nighttime muscle relaxant for greater effects. *Stretching exercises* always are recommended to regain flexibility and to counteract muscular spasm. Heat and a muscle relaxant may enhance the effects of stretching. More advanced or protracted cases may need deep-pressure massage or *ultrasound treatment* from a licensed therapist.

Recovery and Rehabilitation Muscular stretching exercises and cervical traction are used to treat persistent or chronic cases. *Stretching exercises* must be continued three times a week to maintain neck flexibility. Chronic cases benefit from gentle *cervical traction,* beginning with a low weight of 5 to 10 lb for 5 minutes once or twice a day (p. 269). Severely irritated cervical muscles must be stretched cautiously. Traction can be irritating if applied too long, too frequently, or with too heavy a weight. The patient's tolerance to traction can be assessed by applying vertical traction in the office, using either manual traction or a cervical traction unit.

INJECTION TECHNIQUE   Local injection of anesthetic, corticosteroid, or both is used to treat the acute muscle spasms of torticollis and severe cervical strain and to assist in the management of the acute flare-up of fibromyalgia. At best, its use is adjunctive to the physical therapy exercises.

Positioning   The patient is placed in the sitting position with the shoulders back and the hands placed in the lap.

Surface Anatomy and Point of Entry   The midpoint of the superior trapezius is located halfway between the cervical spinous processes and the lateral aspect of the acromion. The muscles are located 1 inch lateral to the spinous processes.

Angle of Entry and Depth   The needle is inserted into the skin at a perpendicular angle. The depth is 1 to 1½ inches.

Anesthesia   Ethyl chloride is sprayed on the skin. Local anesthetic is placed at the outer fascial plane (1 mL) and in the belly of the muscle (0.5 mL with each puncture).

Technique   The success of injection depends on the accurate injection of the most seriously affected muscle. The point of maximum tenderness is palpated. The thick skin is punctured rapidly. While holding the syringe as lightly as possible, the needle is passed through the subcutaneous layer until the tissue resistance of the outer fascia is met, approximately ¾ to 1 inch in depth. (*Note:* The needle will not enter the muscle unless pressure is applied.) Holding the syringe as lightly as possible allows identification of the subtle tissue resistance of the outer fascial layer. Local anesthetic (1 to 2 mL) is injected just outside the muscle. With firm pressure, the needle is passed into the muscle belly an additional ¼ to ⅜ inch beyond the outer fascia. Often a "giving way" or "popping" is felt as the fascia is penetrated. With three separate punctures, 1 to 2 mL of anesthetic, corticosteroid, or both is injected into an area the size of a quarter. The second and third punctures are placed in a line that is perpendicular to the course of the muscle fibers. Treatments are restricted to three injections per year to avoid "woody atrophy" of the muscle or the psychological dependence on injection.

INJECTION AFTERCARE
1. *Rest* the neck for the first 3 days by avoiding direct pressure, neck rotation, and lateral bending.
2. Recommend a soft Philadelphia *collar* for 3 to 7 days for patients with severe symptoms.
3. Use *ice* (15 minutes every 4 to 6 hours), *acetaminophen (Tylenol ES)* (1000 mg twice a day), or both for postinjection soreness.

TRAPEZIUS MUSCLE INJECTION

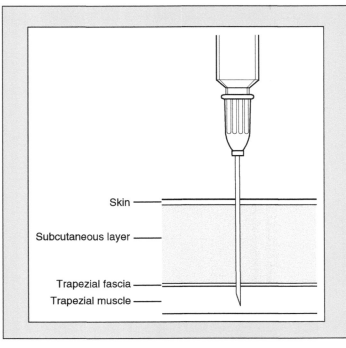

Skin
Subcutaneous layer
Trapezial fascia
Trapezial muscle

4. *Protect* the upper back and neck for 30 days by limiting neck rotation and lateral bending and by maintaining good posture.
5. Resume passively performed *rotation stretching exercises* at 2 to 3 weeks.
6. *Repeat* the injection at 6 weeks if overall improvement is less than 50%.
7. Obtain *plain x-rays* of the cervical spine to assess for the loss of normal cervical lordosis, the degree of underlying osteoarthritis, and the presence of significant foraminal encroachment disease (reduction of 50% of the area of the foramina is significant).
8. Order *MRI* to detect an underlying cervical disk disease if patients fail to respond over the course of 2 to 3 months (<5% of cases are chronic).

SURGICAL PROCEDURE   No surgical procedure is available.

PROGNOSIS   Cervical strain is a universal problem. Most episodes of cervical strain resolve completely with a combination of stress reduction, attention to posture, physical therapy, a short course of a muscle relaxant, and corticosteroid injection. Because the muscle spasm of cervical strain can represent a reaction to an underlying threat to the spinal column, cord, or nerve, however, any patient with recurrent or severe strain must be evaluated for underlying arthritis, disk disease, radiculopathy, and spinal stenosis. Patients suspected to have reactive cervical strain should have plain x-rays and MRI. Patients with diffuse muscular irritation of the cervical, thoracic, and lumbosacral spinal areas likely have fibromyalgia. These patients require a long-term management strategy incorporating all the principles of treatment for cervical strain.

CERVICAL RADICULOPATHY

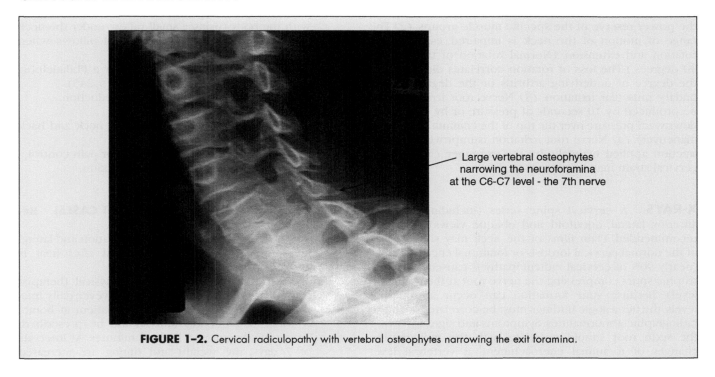

Large vertebral osteophytes narrowing the neuroforamina at the C6-C7 level - the 7th nerve

FIGURE 1-2. Cervical radiculopathy with vertebral osteophytes narrowing the exit foramina.

DESCRIPTION Cervical radiculopathy is an impairment of upper extremity neurologic function resulting from compression of spinal nerve, spinal cord, or both. Cervical arthritis with foraminal encroachment (90%) and a herniated nucleus pulposus (9%) are the most common causes. Spinal stenosis, epidural abscess, epidural tumor, and primary spinal cord tumors are much less common causes. Severity (increasing irritation and pressure over the cervical root) is determined by the degree of functional impairment, as follows: sensory symptoms only (80% to 85%); sensorimotor symptoms with loss of spinal reflex, motor strength, or muscle atrophy (15%); and spinal cord compression with long tract signs (<1%).

SYMPTOMS Most patients have numbness or tingling in particular fingers. A few patients describe an electrical-type pain over the scapula or radiating from the base of the neck down the arm. Advanced cases may be associated with loss of grip strength (C8) or pushing (C7) or lifting (C6) capacity.

"My fingers feel like they are coming out of Novocain."

"My hand feels numb."

"I think I have a pinched nerve."

"I have shooting pains down my arm that feel like someone is driving nails into the muscles of my arm."

"It's like your foot goes to sleep—like the nerve is coming out of it."

"I was working on a ladder, and when I looked straight up, I felt this electric shock in the base of my neck."

"I've been dropping things."

EXAM Muscle irritability in the upper back and neck, the range of motion of the neck (particularly in rotation), and the neurologic function of the upper extremities are examined in each patient.

EXAM SUMMARY

1. Abnormal upper extremity neurologic exam
2. Loss of full rotation of the neck and limited extension
3. Positive Spurling's sign
4. Relief with manually applied vertical traction
5. Paracervical tenderness

(1) Findings in the upper extremity neurologic exam are abnormal. Two-point discrimination, light touch, or pinprick sensation may be lost in selected fingers. Deep

tendon reflexes may be asymmetric. Grip, triceps, or biceps strength may be impaired in advanced cases. It is important to test strength two or three times to assess the power reserve of the specific muscle groups. (2) The range of motion of the neck is impaired, especially in rotation and extension. (Normal rotation of the neck is 90 degrees.) The loss of rotation correlates directly with the degree of underlying arthritis or the degree of secondary muscular irritation. (3) Nerve root irritation can be produced by 10 seconds of pressure or by tapping or downward pressure over the top of the cranium (Spurling's maneuver). (4) Nerve root irritation is improved by neck traction applied manually by the examiner. (5) Signs of cervical strain may be present (p. 3).

X-RAYS   A cervical spine series (including postero-anterior, lateral, odontoid, and oblique views) always is recommended. Plain films of the neck may show a loss of the normal cervical lordosis or foraminal encroachment (nearly 90% of cervical radiculopathy is caused by hypertrophic spurs compressing the nerve root at the foraminal level). Because spur formation can occur at multiple levels, the neurologic findings must be correlated with the radiographic abnormalities. Symptoms and signs involving the sixth root should correlate with the radiographic changes of foraminal encroachment at vertebral level C5-C6.

SPECIAL TESTING   MRI should be performed when neurologic findings are severe at presentation, when symptoms and signs persist despite reasonable treatment, and when the cervical spine series fails to show significant (at least 50% narrowing) foraminal encroachment in the oblique views.

DIAGNOSIS   The diagnosis of cervical radiculopathy is based on a history of radicular pain and paresthesia, neurologic impairment on exam, and correlating abnormalities on x-rays.

TREATMENT   The goals of treatment are to reduce pressure over the nerve, improve neurologic function, and improve neck flexibility. Ice, a muscle relaxant at night for 7 to 10 days, and rest and protection of the neck are the initial treatments of choice for sensory radiculopathy. Cervical traction, neurosurgical consultation, or both are the treatment recommendations for acute sensorimotor radiculopathy.

■ **STEP 1**   Perform a complete upper extremity neurologic examination, order neck x-rays or MRI (depending on the severity), and measure the baseline range of motion of the neck.
  Apply ice to the base of the neck and to the upper back to relieve muscle spasm.
  Offer a nighttime muscle relaxant (daytime use of a muscle relaxant may aggravate the condition).

Advise on the proper posture.
Advise on proper nighttime sleeping posture: The patient should sleep with the head and neck aligned with the body (using a small pillow under the neck when lying on the back or several pillows when lying on the side).
Offer a soft cervical collar (p. 245) or a Philadelphia collar for severe muscle irritability (p. 245).
Underscore the importance of stress reduction.
Recommend seat belts and an air bag.
Apply massage and heat to the upper neck and back (p. 267).
Prescribe an NSAID (e.g., ibuprofen) for pain control.
Restrict neck rotation, bending, and flexion.

■ **STEP 2 (2 TO 3 WEEKS FOR PERSISTENT CASES)**   Re-evaluate neurologic function.
  Begin gentle stretching exercises in rotation and lateral bending in sets of 20, performed after heat is applied (p. 268).
  Apply vertical cervical traction. A physical therapist can initiate this type of therapy; however, daily traction has to be performed by the patient at home. A water bag traction unit should be prescribed. Traction is begun at 5 lb for 5 minutes. At intervals of 7 days, the weight and timing are increased gradually to a maximum of 12 to 15 lb for 10 minutes twice a day (p. 269).
  Prescribe a stronger muscle relaxant.

■ **STEP 3 (4 TO 6 WEEKS FOR CHRONIC CASES)**   Re-evaluate neurologic function.
  Maximize vertical cervical traction.
  Consider consultation with an anesthesiologist or pain management specialist for epidural steroid injection.
  Consult with a neurosurgeon if symptoms persist.

PHYSICAL THERAPY   Physical therapy plays an integral part in the treatment of cervical radiculopathy and in the prevention of recurrent nerve impingement.

PHYSICAL THERAPY SUMMARY
1. Cautious muscle-stretching exercises, passively performed
2. Cautious stretching plus heat and massage
3. Avoid ultrasound
4. Gradually increase the weight and length of vertical cervical traction

Acute Period   Ice applications, massage, and gentle muscle-stretching exercises are used to reduce secondary muscular irritation. (All the treatments used for cervical strain can be applied cautiously to cervical radiculopathy.)
Heat and massage to the upper back and the base of the neck provide temporary relief of pain and muscle

spasm. These modalities can be combined with a nighttime muscle relaxant for additional effects.

Stretching exercises to reduce reactive muscular irritation and spasm must be used carefully (p. 268). The extremes of rotation and lateral bending may irritate the nerve roots (especially in foraminal encroachment disease). The tolerance of neck stretching must be assessed in the office before home exercise. *Ultrasound* probably should be avoided; it may aggravate nerve impingement.

Recovery and Rehabilitation After the acute irritation has subsided, stretching exercises are combined with vertical cervical traction. *Stretching exercises* are continued to maintain neck flexibility and to counteract muscular spasm. *Vertical cervical traction* performed daily decreases the direct pressure on the cervical roots and nerves. Radiculopathy secondary to foraminal encroachment uniformly responds to traction (gradually over 4 to 6 weeks). Radiculopathy secondary to a herniated disk responds less predictably. A poor response to vertical traction suggests severe muscle spasm or herniated disk.

INJECTION TECHNIQUE Local injection is not performed routinely. If cervical strain is present, local injection of the trapezius muscle can be performed (p. 5). Facet joint injections should be performed by a neurosurgeon or by an interventional radiologist.

SURGICAL PROCEDURE Depending on the cause, foraminotomy and diskectomy are the two most common procedures.

PROGNOSIS All patients with radiculopathy need plain films of the cervical spine to assess alignment, the degree of age-related disk disease, and the role of foraminal encroachment. Patients with advanced or progressive neurologic impairment (sensorimotor or sensorimotor with lower extremity long tract signs) must undergo MRI. Medical therapy is successful in nearly 90% of patients with sensory or early sensorimotor cervical radiculopathy. Response to traction may be slow, however. It is not unusual to require 4 to 6 weeks to resolve. Patients with reflex loss or dramatic motor weakness have a poorer response to medical treatment and should have an early workup with MRI and an electromyogram to define the extent of neurologic impairment. Patients failing to respond to conservative therapy over 3 to 4 weeks and patients with advanced neurologic symptoms and signs should be evaluated by MRI and should be referred to a neurosurgeon.

GREATER OCCIPITAL NEURITIS

Enter 1 inch lateral to the midline and 1 inch caudal to the superior nuchal line of the skull (the base of the skull).

Needle: $1^1/2$-inch, 22-gauge
Depth: $^1/2$ to $^3/4$ inch down to the fascia, then an additional $^1/4$ inch into the muscle
Volume: 3 to 4 mL of anesthesia, 1 mL of D80, or both

NOTE: Lightly advance the needle to feel the outer fascia, then enter the body of the muscle. Triamcinolone should not be used because of the greater chance of atrophy of muscle or overlying subcutaneous tissue.

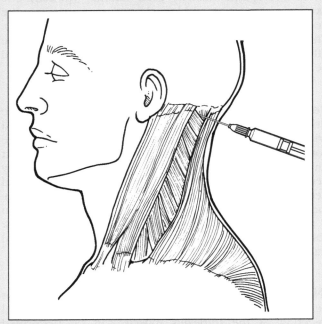

FIGURE 1–3. Injection of the greater occipital nerve as it exits the semispinalis capitis muscle.

DESCRIPTION Greater occipital neuritis is an isolated compression neuropathy of the greater occipital nerve as it courses from the upper cervical roots through the paracervical muscles to enter the subcutaneous tissue over the scalp. The nerve is composed solely of sensory fibers that provide pain, light touch, temperature, and vibration sensation to half of the scalp. Irritation and inflammation of the nerve occur as it penetrates the paracervical muscles.

SYMPTOMS The patient complains of a unilateral headache, variable degrees of paresthesias or hypesthesias, and symptoms reflecting the underlying cervical strain.

"I have a migraine on the left side of my head."

"My scalp is tingling, like the skin is crawling."

"My head is pounding, my neck is tight, and my skull is extremely tender."

"I have these shooting pains over the top of my head."

EXAM The patient is examined for signs of cervical strain, local tenderness at the base of the skull, and abnormal sensation over the scalp.

EXAM SUMMARY

1. Signs of cervical strain (spasm and tenderness of the trapezius and paraspinal muscles)
2. Local tenderness at the base of the skull
3. Sensory abnormalities over the scalp
4. Neurologic exam of the upper extremities is normal

(1) Spasm and tenderness of the trapezius and paraspinal muscles reflect the underlying cervical strain. Depending on the degree of muscle irritation, the range of motion of the neck may be limited. (2) Focal tenderness the size of a quarter is located 1 inch off the midline and $^1/2$ to 1 inch below the base of the skull. This tenderness corresponds to the site of penetration of the greater occipital through the trapezial fascia. (3) Variable degrees of sensory abnormality can be shown over the scalp on the ipsilateral side of the skull. (4) In an uncomplicated case, the neurologic exam of the upper extremities is normal. (5) Bony structures of the neck, shoulder, and upper back usually are not tender.

X-RAYS A cervical spine series (including postero-anterior, lateral, odontoid, and oblique views) is recommended. No specific radiographic changes are seen in most cases. Patients with moderate to severe muscular spasm may show a loss of the normal cervical lordosis alignment, however. Patients with dramatic loss of range of motion may show significant degenerative arthritic change, including foraminal encroachment at the C2 and C3 levels.

SPECIAL TESTING Special testing is rarely necessary. Patients who present with dramatic loss of range of motion or additional neurologic symptoms should have MRI to evaluate the integrity of the spinal cord and vertebral bodies.

DIAGNOSIS The diagnosis is based on a history of a unilateral headache that is associated with sensory abnormalities over the ipsilateral scalp and on physical findings of cervical strain and focal tenderness over the site of penetration of the greater occipital nerve through the upper trapezial fascia. Plain x-rays of the cervical spine are used to assess the severity of the underlying cervical strain, to assess the degree of upper cervical degenerative arthritis, and to exclude underlying bony pathology. Regional anesthetic block over the site of penetration of the greater occipital nerve is used to confirm the diagnosis and to differentiate this local cause of a unilateral headache from simple tension headache or common migraine.

TREATMENT The goals of treatment are to decrease the muscular irritation associated with the underlying cervical strain; to reduce the inflammation of the greater occipital nerve; and to perform passive stretching of the neck, cervical traction, or both to prevent future recurrences of neuritis.

STEP 1 Assess the quality and distribution of the headache and perform an upper extremity neurologic exam if there is any sign of radiculopathy.

Suggest simple changes in lifestyle, including sitting straight with the shoulders held back, sleeping with the head and neck aligned with the body (a small pillow under the neck), driving with the arms slightly shrugged (arm rests), and avoiding straps over the shoulders.

Restrict movement of the head, limiting rotation, bending, and flexion.

Recommend ice applications to control acute muscular spasms.

Perform neck massage after heating (e.g., manual, shower massager).

STEP 2 (3 TO 4 WEEKS FOR PERSISTENT CASES) Order x-rays of the neck to assess the alignment of the cervical spine.

Prescribe a muscle relaxant for nighttime use only at a dosage strong enough to cause mild sedation.

Perform local anesthesia with or without corticosteroid injection with D80 for refractory symptoms.

STEP 3 (6 TO 8 WEEKS FOR CHRONIC CASES) Repeat injection with D80.

Combine the injection with a soft Philadelphia collar to maintain good posture and assist in reducing the reactive muscle spasms.

Perform gentle passive stretching exercises in rotation and lateral bending to complete the recovery.

PHYSICAL THERAPY Physical therapy plays a major role in the initial treatment and prevention of greater occipital neuritis. Emphasis is placed on reducing the cervical muscle spasm.

PHYSICAL THERAPY SUMMARY

1. Ice
2. Heat before stretching of the neck and upper back muscles
3. Deep-muscle massage
4. Therapeutic ultrasound
5. Gentle vertical cervical traction, performed manually or with a traction unit

Acute Period Ice applications several times a day reduce the intensity of the cervical muscle spasm. The cold application must be left in place for 20 to 25 minutes to reach the affected muscles effectively. Subsequently, heat, massage, and gentle stretching exercises are used to reduce muscular irritation. These exercises should be performed daily at home. *Heat and massage* to the upper back and to the base of the neck provide temporary relief of pain and spasm. These modalities can be combined with a nighttime muscle relaxant for greater effects. *Stretching exercises* always are recommended to regain flexibility and to counteract muscular spasm (p. 268). Heat and a muscle relaxant may enhance the effects of stretching. More advanced or protracted cases may need deep-pressure massage or *ultrasound treatment* from a licensed therapist.

Recovery and Rehabilitation Muscular stretching exercises and cervical traction are used to treat persistent or chronic cases. *Stretching exercises* must be continued three times a week to maintain neck flexibility. Occasionally, chronic cases benefit from gentle *cervical traction,* beginning with a low weight of 5 to 10 lb for 5 minutes once or twice a day (p. 269). Severely irritated cervical muscles must be stretched cautiously. Traction can be irritating if applied too long, too frequently, or with too heavy a weight. The patient's tolerance to traction is assessed by applying vertical traction in the office, using either manual traction or a cervical traction unit.

INJECTION Local injection of anesthetic, corticosteroid, or both is used to treat an acute headache that has failed to respond to ice, a muscle relaxant or analgesic, and gentle stretching exercises.

Positioning The patient is placed prone, with the head aligned with the torso.

Surface Anatomy and Point of Entry The midline over the cervical spinous processes and the base of the skull are palpated and marked as appropriate (hairline). The greater occipital nerve penetrates through the paracervical muscles approximately 1 inch lateral to the spinous processes.

Angle of Entry and Depth The needle is inserted into the skin at a perpendicular angle. The depth is ³/₄ to 1 inch down to the trapezial muscle fascia.

Anesthesia Ethyl chloride is sprayed on the skin. The patient is asked to take several deep breaths before spraying the volatile liquid. Local anesthetic is placed at the outer fascial plane (1 mL) and just inside the belly of the muscle (1 mL).

Technique The success of injection depends on the accurate placement of the anesthetic and corticosteroid above and below the fascial plane of the trapezial muscle. While holding the syringe as lightly as possible, the needle is passed through the subcutaneous layer until the moderate tissue resistance of the outer fascia is met, approximately ³/₄ to 1 inch in depth. (*Note:* The needle will not enter the muscle unless pressure is applied.) Holding the syringe lightly allows identification of the outer fascial layer. Local anesthetic (1 to 2 mL) is injected just outside the muscle. With firmer pressure, the needle is passed into the muscle belly an additional ¹/₄ to ³/₈ inch

beyond the outer fascia. Often a "giving way" or "popping" is felt as the fascia is penetrated. Alternatively, if the fascia is not readily identified as the needle is advanced, the proper depth can be confirmed by applying vertical traction to the overlying skin. If the needle is above the fascia, it should move freely in the dermis when applying skin traction. Similarly, the needle sticks in place if the tip has penetrated the fascia. For optimal results, 0.5 to 1 mL of anesthetic, 0.5 mL of corticosteroid, or both are injected above and below the fascia.

INJECTION AFTERCARE

1. *Rest* the neck for the first 3 days by avoiding direct pressure, neck rotation, and lateral bending.
2. Recommend a soft Philadelphia *collar* for 3 to 7 days for severe cases.
3. Use *ice* (15 minutes every 4 to 6 hours), *acetaminophen* (1000 mg twice a day), or both for postinjection soreness.
4. *Protect* the neck for 30 days by limiting neck rotation and lateral bending and by maintaining good posture.
5. Begin passively performed *rotation stretching exercises* of the neck at 2 to 3 weeks.
6. Repeat the *injection* at 6 weeks if overall improvement is less than 50%.
7. Re-evaluate the patient for abnormal cervical lordosis, osteoarthritis, or disk disease with repeat *plain x-rays or MRI* of the cervical spine.
8. Consider referral to a *neurologist* for a standard workup for headaches if symptoms fail to respond to two consecutive injections and physical therapy.

GREATER OCCIPITAL NERVE INJECTION

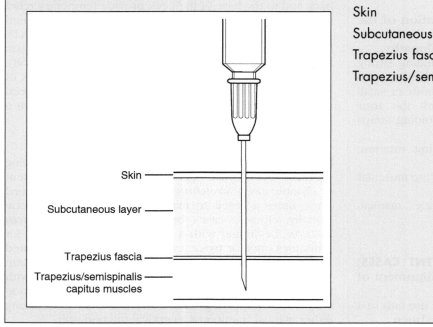

Skin
Subcutaneous layer
Trapezius fascia
Trapezius/semispinalis capitus muscles

Skin
Subcutaneous layer
Trapezius fascia
Trapezius/semispinalis capitus muscles

SURGICAL PROCEDURE No surgical procedure is available.

PROGNOSIS Greater occipital neuritis is a self-limited condition. Local anesthetic block with or without corticosteroid injection is uniformly successful in the short-term (relief lasting weeks or a few months). Long-term results demand attention to stress, posture, and physical therapy stretching exercises, however, to prevent recurrent episodes. Patients who fail to respond to treatment warrant a more extensive evaluation of the cervical spine and a standard workup for chronic headaches.

TEMPOROMANDIBULAR JOINT ARTHRITIS

With the jaw fully opened, enter the joint $^1/_4$ to $^3/_8$ inch directly anterior to the tragus in the depression formed over the joint; angle perpendicular to the skin.

Needle: $^5/_8$-inch, 25-gauge
Depth: $^1/_4$ to $^1/_2$ inch into the joint
Volume: 0.5 to 1 mL of anesthesia, 0.5 mL of K40, or both

NOTE: Identify and mark the course of the temporal artery and enter on either side of it. If arterial blood enters the syringe, exit the skin, hold pressure for 5 minutes, and re-enter either slightly anterior or posterior to the artery.

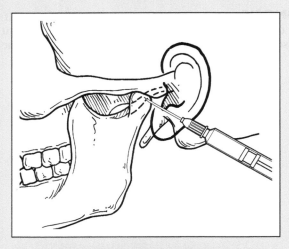

FIGURE 1-4. Injection of the TMJ.

DESCRIPTION   The temporomandibular joint (TMJ) is a hinge joint located between the zygoma of the temporal bone and the mandible. It is supported by two strong hinge ligaments (lateral temporomandibular and medial sphenomandibular ligaments), the muscles of mastication (medial and lateral pterygoid and the masseter muscles), and a thick joint capsule. In between the mandible and the temporal bone is a meniscal-like cartilage—the articular disk—located in the center of the joint.

Arthritis of the joint is relatively uncommon. Post-traumatic osteoarthritis and rheumatoid arthritis are the most common causes of acute joint inflammation. TMJ syndrome is a recurring or chronic irritation of the TMJ secondary to malocclusion, nighttime grinding of teeth, and stress. Patients complain of pain when chewing, clicking, inability to open the mouth (pterygoid muscle spasm), or rarely a locked position of the jaw.

SYMPTOMS   The patient complains of jaw pain, popping, or difficulties with chewing.

"While I'm still in bed, I just have to see if I can open my mouth.... My jaw is sore when I get up in the morning."

"I'll be in the middle of a sentence when my jaw jumps off track and I can't talk."

"My jaw pops every time I chew gum or eat a steak."

"My dentist says my teeth are wearing down too fast"

"My jaw gets stuck when I yawn. I have to jiggle it back and forth before I can open and close it again."

"I can't open my mouth wide enough to eat. My jaw hurts, and I have this awful pain in the back of my throat."

EXAM   The patient with acute TMJ symptoms is examined for local tenderness over the joint, degree of muscle spasm, and maximum mouth opening (MMO). Patients with chronic TMJ symptoms also are examined for general function of speech and chewing, the movement of the mandible, the condition of the teeth, and the integrity of the articular disk.

EXAM SUMMARY

1. The mechanical function of chewing, speech, and movement of the jaw
2. MMO
3. Local TMJ tenderness
4. Clicking or popping of the joint
5. Pterygoid and masseter muscle spasm

(1) The mechanical function of the TMJ can be assessed initially by noting the pattern of speech, by noting the ability to chew a stick of sugarless gum, and by asking the patient to move the mandible back and forth. *(2)* Physical measurement of the distance between the upper and lower teeth—the MMO—provides an objective measurement of the severity of arthritis and the degree of accompanying muscle spasm. *(3)* TMJ tenderness is located just anterior to the tragus of the ear or just inside the auditory canals. *(4)* Clicking and popping may be audible in recurrent or chronic cases. More subtle clicking may be felt by placing the tips of the index fingers in the auditory canals. *(5)* Pterygoid muscle spasm and tenderness is best assessed by running the gloved finger down the inner aspect of the lower alveolar ridge to the anterior tonsillar

pillar. Muscle spasm of the masseter muscle is rarely as tender as that in the pterygoid muscles.

X-RAYS Plain films of the skull provide little more than an assessment of the integrity of the mandible, maxilla, and temporal bones. Skull films do not provide adequate detail of the joint. Panorex films of the entire mouth and TMJ provide the detail necessary to evaluate the condition.

SPECIAL TESTING MRI assesses the position and integrity of the articular disk, determines the degree of arthritic change, and estimates the presence of intra-articular fluid. Displacement of the articular disk is characterized as *reducing displaced disk* or *nonreducing displaced disk*.

DIAGNOSIS The diagnosis is based on a history of painful chewing, loss of joint flexibility, and lateral facial pain over the TMJ combined with the physical findings of joint tenderness, impaired MMO, and spasm of the muscles of mastication. Intra-articular placement of local anesthesia can be used to confirm the diagnosis and distinguish TMJ from conditions affecting the ear, parotid gland, and temporal artery.

TREATMENT The goals of treatment are to reduce the inflammation of the joint, relieve the secondary spasm of the muscles of mastication, and prevent further accelerated wear of the joint or teeth.

STEP 1 Thoroughly examine the joint, the adjacent bones, and teeth; measure the MMO; order panorex x-rays of the mouth and jaw for long-standing symptoms; and perform an intra-articular injection of local anesthesia if the diagnosis is in question.

Apply ice to the joint.

Recommend a full liquid diet until acute pain is controlled.

Protect the joint and muscles of mastication by restricting chewing, avoiding meat, nuts, hard candy, and gum.

Prescribe a nighttime muscle relaxant, especially if stress plays a major role in the condition, or there is a history of grinding of the teeth.

Educate the patient regarding the role of stress, *"Personal and physical stress often manifests itself just at night by clenching of the jaw and grinding of the teeth."*

STEP 2 (3 TO 4 WEEKS FOR PERSISTENT CASES)
Order Panorex x-rays of the jaw.

Perform an intra-articular injection of K40.

Continue the liquid diet and advance to a soft diet as the condition improves.

Review the issue of stress, and determine its impact on the joint.

STEP 3 (6 TO 8 WEEKS FOR CHRONIC CASES)
Repeat the corticosteroid injection with K40.

Recommend the use of a bite-block if there is a history of grinding or signs of significant teeth wear and tear.

Consider a consultation with a dentist experienced in treating TMJ disorders.

PHYSICAL THERAPY Physical therapy plays a minor role in the treatment of TMJ syndrome.

PHYSICAL THERAPY SUMMARY

1. Ice
2. Heat before stretching

Acute Period Ice applications over the joint are not well tolerated because of the sensitivity of the face and ear and possible effects on the balance center of the inner ear.

Recovery and Rehabilitation Muscular stretching exercises of the muscles of mastication may need to be performed if the MMO has been reduced dramatically, or the joint has undergone dislocation or surgical intervention.

INJECTION TECHNIQUE Local injection of anesthetic is necessary to distinguish involvement of the TMJ from conditions affecting the ear, parotid gland, or intra-oral structures. Corticosteroid injection or hyaluronic acid is used when a restricted diet and muscle relaxant fail to reduce the pain and inflammation of the joint.

Positioning The patient is placed in the lateral decubitus position with a pillow supporting the head.

Surface Anatomy and Point of Entry The tragus, temporal artery, and articular tubercle of the zygomatic arch are palpated and marked. The patient is asked to open and close the mouth while the clinician feels the concavity of the joint. The point of entry is directly over the center of the joint, halfway between the articular tubercle of the zygoma and the head of the mandible (the condylar process).

Angle of Entry and Depth The needle is inserted into the skin at a perpendicular angle. The depth is $3/8$ to $1/2$ inch.

Anesthesia The patient is asked to take several deep breaths and then hold his or her breath. Ethyl chloride is sprayed on the skin. Local anesthetic is placed under the skin, just over the firm resistance of the joint capsule (0.5 mL) and intra-articularly (0.5 mL).

Technique The success of injection depends on an accurate intra-articular injection. The patient is asked to

TEMPOROMANDIBULAR JOINT INJECTION

Skin

Subcutaneous layer

Parotid fascia/parotid lateral temporomandibular ligament

Synovial membrane

Joint

Skin

Subcutaneous layer

Parotid fascia/parotid lateral TM ligament
Synovial membrane
Joint

open the jaw to its maximum point. While holding the syringe as lightly as possible, the needle is passed slowly and carefully through the subcutaneous layer until the tissue resistance of the joint capsule is met, approximately $3/8$ to $1/2$ inch in depth. If arterial blood enters the syringe, the needle is withdrawn, pressure is held for 5 minutes, and a point of entry either anterior or posterior to the artery is chosen. Local anesthetic (0.5 mL) is injected just outside the joint capsule. With firmer pressure, the needle is passed into the joint, an additional $1/4$ to $3/8$ inch beyond the joint capsule. Often a "giving way" or "popping" is felt as the fascia is penetrated. An intra-articular injection of 0.5 mL of anesthetic, corticosteroid, or both is performed. A successful injection reduces joint pain, allows freer opening and closing of the jaw, and decreases the acute pterygoid muscle spasm.

INJECTION AFTERCARE
1. *Rest* the joint for the first 3 days by avoiding direct pressure, chewing, and grinding of the teeth at night.
2. Use *ice* (15 minutes every 4 to 6 hours), *acetaminophen* (1000 mg twice a day), or both for postinjection soreness.
3. *Protect* the joint for 30 days by limiting chewing and grinding of the teeth at night.

4. Prescribe a *muscle relaxant* to be taken at bedtime in a dosage sufficient to cause mild sedation; reduce the acute pterygoid and masseter muscle spasm, and help curb the degree of grinding.
5. *Repeat* the injection at 6 weeks if overall improvement is less than 50%.
6. Obtain *Panorex x-rays* of the teeth and mandible to assess for intrinsic pathology of the teeth, mandible, and TMJ.
7. Obtain a *consultation* with an oral surgeon who specializes in TMJ disorders if treatment fails to provide long-term benefits.

SURGERY   Patients refractory to conservative care, patients with documented disorders of the articular disk, and patients with radiographic signs of arthritis should be evaluated by an oral surgeon specializing in TMJ disorders.

PROGNOSIS   Greater than 90% of patients with acute TMJ symptoms respond to a comprehensive program of restricted diet, jaw rest, a muscle relaxant, and counseling. Less than 10% of patients fail to response to these measures and require injection. Patients with persistent subacute or chronic TMJ symptoms should undergo special testing and consultation with an oral surgeon.

DIFFERENTIAL DIAGNOSIS OF SHOULDER PAIN

Diagnoses	Confirmations
Rotator cuff syndromes (most common)	
Impingement syndrome	Passive painful arc
Rotator cuff tendinitis	Lidocaine injection test
Rotator cuff tendon thinning	X-ray—shoulder series showing a narrow subacromial space
Rotator cuff tendon tear	Diagnostic arthrogram
Frozen shoulder	Loss of range of motion (ROM); normal x-ray
Acromioclavicular (AC) joint	
Osteoarthritis	X-ray—shoulder series
AC separation	X-ray—weighted views of the shoulder
Osteolysis of the clavicle	X-ray—shoulder series
Subscapular bursitis	Local anesthetic block
Sternoclavicular joint	
Strain or inflammatory arthritis	Local anesthetic block
Septic arthritis (intravenous drug abuse)	Aspiration and culture
Glenohumeral joint	
Osteoarthritis	X-ray—shoulder series (axillary view)
Inflammatory arthritis	Synovial fluid analysis
Septic arthritis	Synovial fluid culture
Multidirectional instability of the shoulder	
Dislocation	X-ray—shoulder series
Subluxation	Abnormal sulcus sign
Glenoid labral tear	Double-contrast arthrography
Referred pain	
Cervical spine	Neck rotation; x-ray; MRI
Lung	Chest x-ray
Diaphragm	Chest x-ray; CT scan
Upper abdomen	Chemistries; ultrasound

IMPINGEMENT SYNDROME

Enter 1 to 1½ inches below the midpoint of the acromial process; follow the angle of the acromion to the subacromial bursa.

Needle: 1½-inch, 22-gauge
Depth: 1 to 1½ inches to 3½ inches (obese patients)
Volume: 2 to 3 mL of anesthesia, 1 mL of D80

NOTE: Never inject under pressure or if the patient experiences dramatic pain (intratendinous or periosteal); if pain develops or resistance to injection is encountered, withdraw ½ inch and redirect.

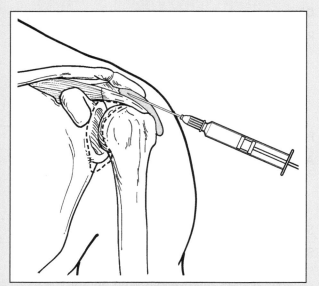

FIGURE 2–1. Subacromial bursal injection from the lateral approach.

DESCRIPTION *Impingement syndrome* is the term used to describe the symptoms that result from the compression of the rotator cuff tendons and the subacromial bursa between the greater tubercle of the humeral head and the undersurface of the acromial process. It is the mechanical component and principal cause of subacromial bursitis, rotator cuff tendinitis, rotator cuff tendon tear, and Milwaukee shoulder. In most patients, impingement syndrome precedes active rotator cuff tendinitis and subacromial bursitis. Injection of the subacromial bursa provides rapid control of the inflammation caused by the pressure and friction of repeated impingement.

SYMPTOMS The patient complains of shoulder pain aggravated by overhead motions or of inability to move the shoulder because of pain. The patient grabs the flesh over the lateral shoulder or rubs the hand up and down the deltoid muscle when describing the pain.

"It's too painful to raise my arm up."

"It feels like a leather strap is holding my shoulder down."

"My shoulder gets so sore after casing mail for an hour."

"If I sleep with my arm above my head, I hurt all the next day."

"It feels like my bones are rubbing together."

"I've had to stop reaching up to the high shelves in the kitchen. I have to stand on the footstool to put my dishes away."

EXAM Signs of subacromial impingement and the anatomic position (acromial angle) of the acromial process are assessed in each patient.

EXAM SUMMARY

1. Pain with the painful arc maneuver—subacromial impingement
2. Focal subacromial tenderness, just below the middle of the acromion
3. *Painless* testing of resisted abduction (supraspinatus), external rotation (infraspinatus), adduction (subscapularis), and elbow flexion (biceps), isometrically performed
4. Normal ROM of the glenohumeral joint
5. Preserved strength in all directions

(1) The hallmark physical finding of impingement syndrome is pain reproduced by the painful arc maneuver. Passive abduction of the arm at a predictable and reproducible angle causes shoulder pain. This maneuver brings the greater tubercle of the humeral head into contact with the lateral edge of the acromion. When impingement is severe, it is often accompanied by muscle spasm and muscle guarding and involuntary contraction of the trapezius muscle. *(2)* Focal subacromial tenderness is invariably present, although firm to hard pressure with the thumb between the greater tubercle of the humerus and just under the anterior third of the acromial process

may be necessary to show subacromial tenderness. This tenderness is identical to the local tenderness that occurs with rotator cuff tendinitis. *(3)* Tendon inflammation signs are not present with pure impingement syndrome. Isometric testing of midarc abduction, adduction, and internal and external rotation is painless. *(4)* ROM of the glenohumeral joint should be normal, unless frozen shoulder has developed or underlying glenohumeral arthritis is present. *(5)* Abduction and external rotation strength should be normal.

X-RAYS Routine x-rays of the shoulder (including posteroanterior, external rotation, Y-outlet, and axillary views) are optional in patients presenting with a first episode of impingement. Patients with recurrent or persistent cases should undergo radiographic testing. Calcification may be present in the rotator cuff tendons (30%) and always underscores the chronicity of the condition. More useful information focuses on the anatomic relationships of the acromion and humeral head. A high-riding humeral head—loss of the normal 1-cm space between the undersurface of the acromion and the top of the humeral head—indicates degenerative thinning of the rotator cuff tendons or a large rotator cuff tendon tear (1%). Long-standing cases of impingement may show erosive changes at the greater tubercle or bony sclerosis (severe and chronic impingement). Patients with the abnormal down-sloping acromial angle (rounded shoulder appearance) are at higher risk for recurrent or chronic impingement.

SPECIAL TESTING Diagnostic ultrasound, arthrography, and MRI often are ordered in persistent or chronic cases to exclude the possibility of rotator cuff tendon tear.

DIAGNOSIS The diagnosis of impingement syndrome is based on the history of lateral shoulder pain, the abnormal signs of local subacromial tenderness and a painful arc maneuver on exam, and the absence of signs of active tendinitis.

TREATMENT The goals of treatment are to increase the subacromial space, reducing the degree of impingement, and to prevent the development of tendinitis and tendon rupture. The pendulum-stretching exercise combined with restrictions on overhead reaching and positioning are the treatments of choice.

STEP 1 Assess the patient's overall shoulder function (reaching overhead, the Apley scratch sign, overall muscularity), estimate the patient's external rotation strength, and order plain x-rays of the shoulder (optional).

> Strongly suggest rest and restriction of overhead positioning and reaching.
> Recommend ice applications over the deltoid muscle to control pain.

> Demonstrate weighted pendulum-stretching exercises using 5 to 10 lb, recommending 5 minutes once or twice a day (p. 271); emphasize the importance of relaxing the shoulder muscles (passive stretching).
> Restrict overhead positioning, overhead reaching, and lifting until the pain is substantially improved.

STEP 2 (2 TO 4 WEEKS FOR PERSISTENT CASES) Prescribe a nonsteroidal anti-inflammatory drug (NSAID) (e.g., ibuprofen [Advil, Motrin]) given in full dose for 3 to 4 weeks if subtle signs of rotator cuff tendinitis are present.

> Discourage the use of a simple arm sling (p. 246). Immobilization in a susceptible patient (e.g., patients with a low pain threshold, high stress, or both) may hasten the development of frozen shoulder.

STEP 3 (6 TO 8 WEEKS FOR PERSISTENT CASES) Reemphasize the pendulum-stretching exercise.

> If symptoms persist, perform an empirical subacromial injection. Impingement syndrome is a mechanical problem with little accompanying inflammation. Local injection with corticosteroids has little therapeutic effect, unless tendon inflammation is present.
> Recommend general toning exercises in external rotation and internal rotation to enhance muscular support of the glenohumeral joint and to reduce impingement (p. 272).
> Suggest a long-term restriction of any repetitious overhead work or positioning for patients with recurrent or persistent impingement.

STEP 4 (3 TO 6 MONTHS FOR CHRONIC CASES) Consider orthopedic consultation for patients with symptoms refractory to rest, restricted use, physical therapy, NSAIDs, and an empirical corticosteroid injection (3% to 5%).

PHYSICAL THERAPY Physical therapy exercises are the treatments of choice for impingement syndrome.

PHYSICAL THERAPY SUMMARY

1. Ice
2. Weighted pendulum-stretching exercises, performed passively with relaxed shoulder muscles
3. Toning exercises for the infraspinatus, performed isometrically
4. Avoidance of simple slings or other shoulder immobilizers

Acute Period Ice and the weighted pendulum-stretching exercises are used to reduce impingement.

Ice, in the form of a bag of frozen corn, blue ice, or a plastic ice bag, is used for temporary relief of pain. The *weighted pendulum-stretching exercise* is fundamental to stretching the subacromial space. Initially the exercise is performed with the weight of the arm. With improvement, a hand-held 5- to 10-lb weight is added to increase the stretch (patients with hand and wrist arthritis should use Velcro weights placed just above the wrists). It is crucial to keep the arm vertical and relaxed when performing this exercise. Excessive bending at the waist may aggravate subacromial impingement.

Recovery and Rehabilitation

The weighted pendulum-stretching exercises are continued through the recovery period, and the isometric toning exercises are begun 4 to 6 weeks after the acute irritation has resolved. The *weighted pendulum-stretching exercise* performed three times a week is effective in preventing the symptoms of recurrent impingement.

Isometric toning exercises of the infraspinatus muscle are used to enhance the stability of the glenohumeral joint and to open the subacromial space (p. 272). Preferential toning of the infraspinatus muscle has the theoretical advantage of increasing the distance between the humeral head and the acromion (vector analysis suggests that preferential toning of the infraspinatus, located between the greater tubercle and the inferior angle of the scapula, leads to a resultant vector in the downward direction and a downward force on the humeral head).

INJECTION Local injection of anesthetic is used to confirm the diagnosis of impingement, and corticosteroid injection is used to treat impingement accompanied by active rotator cuff tendinitis (p. 21). Pure impingement syndrome is a mechanical problem and as such does not respond predictably to corticosteroid injection. Corticosteroid is definitely indicated, however, when signs of impingement accompany active rotator cuff tendinitis. Injection may be indicated in patients presenting with impingement and minor or subclinical degrees of rotator cuff tendinitis. If a subacromial bursal injection of anesthetic (lidocaine injection test) substantially reduces the patient's pain, improves the overall function of the shoulder, and reduces signs of impingement as noted during physical exam, an empirical injection of corticosteroid may be beneficial.

SURGICAL PROCEDURE Acromioplasty, performed arthroscopically or by open shoulder exposure, is the surgical procedure of choice for refractory impingement. Exact indications for this procedure have not been defined clearly, however. The most common indications for this surgery are (1) subacromial impingement, with or without rotator cuff tendinitis, in patients who fail to improve after several months of physical therapy (pendulum-stretching exercises and external and internal rotation isometric toning exercises) and one or two subacromial corticosteroid injections; (2) symptoms of refractory impingement with high-grade acromial angle (type III acromion, according to Neer's classification); and (3) radiographic changes at the greater tubercle—bony erosions or sclerosis.

PROGNOSIS Shoulder impingement is a potential problem for everyone. Who hasn't experienced soreness and pain in the shoulder after unaccustomed work overhead, such as painting a ceiling or trying to unscrew a stubborn ceiling light fixture? The diagnosis of impingement syndrome is made when these same symptoms become persistent and begin to interfere with activities of daily living. Repeated impingement eventually leads to subacromial bursal inflammation, rotator cuff tendinitis, greater tubercle degenerative change, and, if left untreated, degenerative thinning or rupture of the rotator cuff tendons.

The overall prognosis for impingement is excellent. Codman's weighted pendulum exercises combined with isometrically performed toning exercises effectively treat most patients. Only a small percentage of patients experiences refractory impingement that requires surgical consultation. Patients with an extreme down-sloping acromial process (approaching 45 degrees) and patients who have had a humeral neck fracture with angulation are at higher risk for chronic impingement.

ROTATOR CUFF TENDINITIS

Enter 1 to 1¹/₂ inches below the midpoint of the acromial process; follow the angle of the acromion to the subacromial bursa.

Needle: 1¹/₂-inch, 22-gauge
Depth: 1 to 1¹/₂ inches to 3¹/₂ inches (obese patients)
Volume: 2 to 3 mL of anesthesia, 1 mL of D80

NOTE: *Never* inject under pressure; if hard resistance of bone or the rubbery firm resistance of tendon is encountered, withdraw ¹/₂ inch and redirect. Restrict use for 3 days, and protect the shoulder for 30 days.

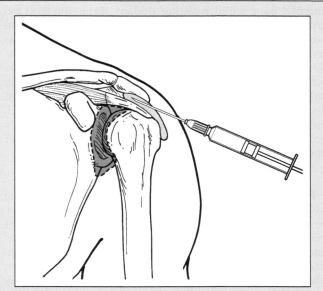

FIGURE 2–2. Subacromial bursal injection from the lateral approach.

DESCRIPTION Rotator cuff tendinitis is an inflammation of the supraspinatus (abduction) and infraspinatus tendons (external rotation) lying between the humeral head and the acromial process. Repetitive overhead reaching, pushing, pulling, and lifting with the arms outstretched—repeated abduction, elevation, and torque to the shoulder—lead to compression and irritation of the tendons (subacromial impingement). The subacromial bursa, located just under the inferior surface of the acromion, functions to protect the rotator tendons from compressive forces of the two bones. If the bursa fails to provide an appropriate amount of lubrication, the rotator cuff tendons become inflamed. Common shoulder tendinitis must be distinguished from frozen shoulder (loss of ROM), rotator cuff tendon tear (persistent weakness), and biceps tendinitis (painful arm flexion).

SYMPTOMS The patient complains of shoulder pain aggravated by overhead reaching and positioning or inability to move the shoulder because of pain. The patient typically places the hand over the outer deltoid, rubbing the muscle in an up-and-down direction when describing the pain.

"Every time I reach over my head, I get this achy pain in my outer shoulder."

"I can't lift my arm over my head because it hurts so bad."

"I can't sleep on my shoulder. Every time I roll over in bed, my shoulder wakes me up."

"I can't reach up or back anymore."

"Whenever I move suddenly or reach back, I get this sharp, deep pain in my shoulder."

"The only way I can stop the pain is to hang my arm over the side of the bed."

EXAM Signs of subacromial impingement, tendon inflammation, and weakness of the supraspinatus and infraspinatus muscles are looked for in each patient.

EXAM SUMMARY
1. Focal subacromial tenderness
2. Subacromial impingement, a positive painful arc maneuver
3. Pain with resisted midarc abduction and external rotation, isometrically performed
4. Normal ROM of the glenohumeral joint
5. Preserved strength of midarc abduction and external rotation (lidocaine injection test)

(1) Subacromial tenderness is located between the greater tubercle of the humerus and the acromial process. Typically, this tenderness is a dime-sized area just under the anterior third of the acromion. Diffuse subacromial tenderness usually indicates subacromial bursal inflammation. *(2)* The impingement sign is always present. Passive abduction of the arm with simultaneous downward pressure on the acromion (the painful arc) reproduces the

patient's pain as the swollen tendons and the subacromial bursa are mechanically compressed. *(3)* The degree of tendon inflammation is assessed by reproducing the patient's pain when resisting midarc abduction and external rotation isometrically. *(4)* ROM of the glenohumeral joint should be normal unless frozen shoulder has developed or underlying glenohumeral arthritis is present. *(5)* Abduction and external rotation strength should be normal in an uncomplicated case of tendinitis. If the patient's pain interferes with an accurate measurement of strength, a lidocaine injection test should be performed. The strength of the affected arm should be at least 75% of the strength of the unaffected side, unless a rotator cuff tendon tear is present.

X-RAYS Routine x-rays of the shoulder (including posteroanterior, external rotation, Y-outlet, and axillary views) are optional in patients presenting with a first episode of tendinitis. Patients with recurrent or chronic tendinitis should be tested, however, to evaluate for high-grade impingement or degenerative change. Tendon calcification—the body's attempt at tendon repair—may be seen in approximately 30% of cases. A high-riding humeral head (loss of the normal 1-cm space between the undersurface of the acromion and the top of the humeral head) indicates either degenerative tendon thinning or rotator cuff tendon tear (1%). Long-standing cases may have arthritic changes at the glenohumeral joint (<1%).

None of these radiographic changes provides conclusive evidence of active tendinitis. The specific diagnosis and the specific treatment recommendations must be based on the clinical exam.

SPECIAL TESTING Cases accompanied by greater than 50% loss of midarc abduction or external rotation strength and cases with equivocal lidocaine injection tests should be evaluated for rotator cuff tear. Contrast arthrography shows subtendinous tears, small tendon splits, and large transverse tears. MRI shows moderate to large tears and assesses the degree of muscle atrophy and contracture.

Patients older than 62 years who have experienced a fall onto the outstretched arm or a direct blow to the shoulder are at increased risk for rotator cuff tendon rupture, especially if they have experienced previous episodes of tendinitis. One third of 70-year-old patients with persistent symptoms have either a partial rotator cuff tendon rupture or a full-thickness rupture.

DIAGNOSIS The diagnosis of rotator cuff tendinitis is based on the history of shoulder pain aggravated by reaching; evidence of subacromial impingement; and pain with isometric testing of the supraspinatus, infraspinatus, or subscapularis. The diagnosis is confirmed by regional anesthetic block in the subacromial bursa. Rotator cuff tendon ruptures can accompany rotator cuff tendinitis in 1% to 3% of cases. It is important to perform a lidocaine injection test to exclude an underlying rotator cuff tendon rupture before giving a local corticosteroid injection.

TREATMENT The goals of treatment are to reduce tendon swelling and inflammation; to increase the subacromial space, reducing the degree of impingement; and to prevent progressive damage to the tendons (calcification, thinning, and rupture). The pendulum-stretching exercise combined with an effective anti-inflammatory treatment is the treatment of choice.

STEP 1 Assess the patient's overall shoulder function, order plain x-rays of the shoulder (if the patient is >60 years old or has a history of recurrent tendinitis), and estimate the patient's external rotation strength.

Suggest shoulder rest and restriction of overhead positioning, overhead reaching, and lifting until the pain is substantially improved.

Recommend ice applied over the deltoid muscle to reduce inflammation and acute pain.

Demonstrate weighted pendulum-stretching exercises, emphasize the importance of relaxing the shoulder muscles (passive stretching), and begin using a 5- to 10-lb weight for 5 minutes once or twice a day (p. 271).

STEP 2 (2 TO 4 WEEKS FOR PERSISTENT CASES) Prescribe an NSAID (e.g., ibuprofen), which is given in full dose for 3 to 4 weeks.

Re-emphasize the importance and the proper way of performing the pendulum-stretching exercise.

Discourage the use of a simple arm sling (p. 246). Immobilization in a susceptible patient (e.g., a diabetic, a patient with a low pain threshold, or a patient with a high degree of stress) may hasten the development of frozen shoulder.

STEP 3 (6 TO 8 WEEKS FOR PERSISTENT CASES) Perform a lidocaine injection test to differentiate the degree of mechanical impingement, active tendinitis, tendon tear (true weakness), or frozen shoulder (true stiffness). When the patient's pain is controlled, the actual degree of loss of strength or loss of ROM can be determined more accurately.

Order an arthrogram or diagnostic ultrasound if the lidocaine injection test result is abnormal (<50% pain relief and <75% of normal strength in abduction or external rotation), or order an MRI if the patient has profound weakness and is a candidate for surgery.

Perform a local injection of D80 if the patient has a normal lidocaine injection test result (>50% pain relief and >75% of normal strength).

Repeat the injection in 4 to 6 weeks if symptoms and signs have improved, but linger at or below the 50% improvement level.

Recommend isometrically performed external and internal rotation exercises to recover any lost rotation strength, but these must be delayed until substantial improvement in pain has occurred (typically at 2 to 3 weeks).

Advise long-term use of the weighted pendulum exercises and isometric toning exercises to prevent recurrent tendinitis (pp. 271-272).

STEP 4 (≥3 MONTHS FOR CHRONIC CASES) Cautiously perform or limit overhead reaching.

Advise on a long-term restriction of any repetitive overhead work or positioning.

Consider orthopedic consultation if symptoms persist or if tendon rupture is present.

PHYSICAL THERAPY Physical therapy plays an active role through the treatment of rotator cuff tendinitis and plays an important role in the prevention of recurrent tendinitis.

PHYSICAL THERAPY SUMMARY

1. Ice
2. Weighted pendulum-stretching exercises, performed passively with relaxed shoulder muscles
3. Toning exercises for the infraspinatus and supraspinatus tendons, isometrically performed
4. Avoidance of simple slings or other shoulder immobilizers

Acute Period Ice and the weighted pendulum-stretching exercises are used to reduce swelling and impingement. *Ice*, in the form of a bag of frozen corn or an ice bag, is used for temporary relief of pain and as an initial treatment for inflammation. The *weighted pendulum-stretching* exercise is fundamental to stretching the subacromial space, allowing the rotator cuff tendons room to contract and helping to prevent frozen shoulder (p. 271). Initially the subacromial space is stretched by the weight of the arm. With improvement, a 5- to 10-lb weight is used as tolerated. It is crucial to keep the arm vertical and relaxed when performing this exercise. Excessive bending at the waist may aggravate subacromial impingement. Active use of the shoulder muscles (as opposed to relaxing them and allowing them to stretch) may aggravate the underlying tendon inflammation.

Recovery and Rehabilitation The *weighted pendulum-stretching exercise* is continued through the recovery period. Continuing this exercise should be strongly encouraged in patients with high-grade impingement and in patients who have had more than one episode of tendinitis. Maintenance exercises three times a week reduce the chance of recurrent tendon compression.

Isometric toning exercises of the infraspinatus and supraspinatus muscles are used to strengthen the weakened tendons, to stabilize the glenohumeral joint, and to open the subacromial space (p. 272). These exercises are begun 4 to 6 weeks after the acute pain and swelling have

resolved. (Toning exercises begun too soon can re-ignite tendon inflammation.) Preferential toning of the infraspinatus muscle has the theoretical advantage of increasing the distance between the humeral head and the acromion.

INJECTION Local injection of anesthetic and corticosteroid is used (1) to confirm the diagnosis of an uncomplicated rotator cuff tendinitis, (2) to treat active rotator cuff tendinitis that has persisted for 6 to 8 weeks or that has failed to improve with treatment steps 1 through 4, (3) to treat rotator cuff tendinitis that accompanies frozen shoulder, and (4) to palliate the symptoms that accompany rotator cuff tendon tear in patients who are unable to undergo surgery (Tables 2-1 and 2-2).

Positioning The patient is placed in the sitting position, with the hands placed in the lap. The patient is asked to relax the shoulder and neck muscles. If the patient is unable to relax, traction applied to the flexed elbow may be necessary to open the subacromial space.

2-1 CLINICAL OUTCOMES OF ROTATOR CUFF TENDINITIS AFTER SUBACROMIAL INJECTION OF METHYLPREDNISOLONE (DEPO-MEDROL) 80 mg/mL

Complete resolution	
One injection	48
Two injections 6 weeks apart	8
Total	56 (62%)
Recurrence (averaged 5-6 mo)	
Reinjected once	14
Reinjected twice	7
Multiple injections	3
Total	24 (27%)
Failed to respond; chronic tendinitis	7 (8%)
Rotator cuff tendon rupture (developed in follow-up period)	3 (3%)
Lost to follow-up	9
Total	*99*

Note: Diagnosis confirmed with local anesthetic block; 1 mL of D80; home physical therapy; pendulum stretching exercises plus isometric toning exercises; 18-month prospective follow-up of 91% of patients enrolled.
Data collected at the Medical Orthopedic Clinic, Sunnyside Medical Center, Portland, Oregon.

2-2 ADVERSE REACTIONS TO A SUBACROMIAL INJECTION OF METHYLPREDNISOLONE (DEPO-MEDROL) 80 mg/mL

None	48 (49%)
Pain	32 (33%)
Inflammatory flare reaction (pain, heat, swelling)	7 (7%)
Vasovagal reaction	4 (4%)
Bruise	4
Stiffness	2
Swelling; itching; nausea; flushing	1 each
Postinjection infection	0
Postinjection tendon rupture (within 6 wk of injection)	1

Data collected at the Medical Orthopedic Clinic, Sunnyside Medical Center, Portland, Oregon.

SUBACROMIAL BURSAL INJECTION

Skin
Subcutaneous layer
Deltoid fascia
Deltoid muscle
Subacromial wall
Subacromial bursa

Skin
Subcutaneous layer
Deltoid fascia
Deltoid muscle
Subacromial wall
Subacromial bursa

Surface Anatomy and Point of Entry The lateral edge of the acromion is located, and its midpoint is marked. The point of entry is 1 to 1¹/₂ inches below the midpoint.

Angle of Entry and Depth The angle of entry should *parallel* the patient's own acromial angle (averaging 50 to 65 degrees). The depth varies according to the patient's weight and muscle development (1¹/₂ inches in an asthenic patient and 3¹/₂ inches in an obese patient >30% ideal body weight). The depth and angle of injection can be measured directly off a posteroanterior shoulder x-ray using a metal marker placed at the point of entry. This marker is particularly helpful in an obese patient or a patient with a well-developed deltoid muscle.

Anesthesia Ethyl chloride is sprayed on the skin. Local anesthetic is placed in the deltoid muscle (1 mL), the deep deltoid fascia (0.5 mL), and the subacromial bursa (1 to 2 mL). The subacromial bursa accepts only 2 to 3 mL of total volume. If this volume is exceeded, the medication flows out of the bursa and down to the deltoid insertion at the midhumerus or along the superior border of the supraspinatus.

Technique Successful treatment depends on the accurate injection of the subacromial bursa using no more than 3 mL of total volume. The lateral approach is the most accessible and safest method. The intratendinous injection is nearly impossible when paralleling the angle of the acromion because the position of the needle is tangential to the tendon. The needle is advanced through the subcutaneous tissue and the deltoid muscle until the subtle resistance of the deep deltoid fascia is encountered. If firm or hard tissue resistance is encountered (deltoid tendon

or periosteum, often painful), the needle is withdrawn ¹/₂ inch, and the angle is redirected 5 to 10 degrees up or down. A "giving way" or "popping" sensation often is appreciated when the subacromial bursa is entered. After administering 1 to 2 mL of anesthesia (the needle can be left in place), the patient's strength is retested. If pain is reduced by 50%, and the strength of abduction and external rotation is 75% to 80% of the unaffected side, 1 mL of D80 is injected. *Note:* Never inject under moderate to high pressure. If high injection pressure is encountered, first try rotating the syringe 180 degrees. If tension is still high and the patient is obviously anxious, ask the patient to take a deep breath and try to relax the shoulder muscles. If tension remains high, reposition the needle by ¹/₄-inch increments or by altering the angle of entry by 5 to 10 degrees.

INJECTION AFTERCARE

1. *Rest* for 3 days, avoiding direct pressure, reaching, overhead positioning, lifting, pushing, and pulling.
2. Use *ice* (15 minutes every 4 to 6 hours and *acetaminophen (Tylenol ES)* (1000 mg twice a day) for postinjection soreness.
3. *Protect* the shoulder for 30 days by limiting reaching, overhead positioning, lifting, pushing, and pulling.
4. Resume passively performed *pendulum-stretching exercises* on day 4.
5. Begin *isometric toning exercises* of abduction and external rotation at 3 to 4 weeks, after the acute pain and inflammation have resolved.

6. Repeat *injection* at 6 weeks if overall improvement is less than 50%.
7. Delay *regular activities, work, and sports* until most of lost muscular tone has been recovered.
8. Obtain *plain x-rays* in all patients who fail to experience at least 2 months of relief. Plain films of the shoulder are used to measure the subacromial space distance (normal 10 to 11 mm), assess the AC joint for inferior-directed osteophytes, or to identify signs of high-grade impingement (roughening or erosive changes at the greater tubercle). Obtain a shoulder MRI arthrogram for patients at risk for rotator cuff tendon tear.

SURGICAL PROCEDURE Surgery is indicated for chronic or persistent rotator cuff tendinitis complicated by high degrees of subacromial impingement or tendon tear. The various procedures attempt (1) to reduce impingement (subacromial decompression and acromioplasty devised by Neer), (2) to remove devitalized tissue (excision of calcific deposits or necrotic tendons), and (3) to repair torn tissue (primary tendon repair). Surgical treatment is successful only about 70% to 75% of the time.

The procedure often reduces pain, but fails to return the patient to his or her original level of function. The patient must be advised that the success of surgery as a rule depends on the degree of irreparable tendon damage and degeneration.

PROGNOSIS Uncomplicated rotator cuff tendinitis treated with one or two injections 6 weeks apart does extremely well; 85% to 90% of patients respond completely, with approximately one in three requiring repeat treatment in the next few years. The prognosis is governed by the accuracy of injection; the use of a concentrated, long-acting corticosteroid; the degree of subacromial impingement; the degree of chronic tendon degeneration (the number of recurrences and the width of the subacromial space); and the compliance of the patient (exercises and restrictions). Patients with persistent or progressive loss of flexibility (frozen shoulder) require ROM measurements and plain films of the shoulder to evaluate for frozen shoulder. Patients who fail to restore external rotation or abduction strength need plain films of the shoulder and MRI arthrography to evaluate for rotator cuff tendon tear.

FROZEN SHOULDER (ADHESIVE CAPSULITIS)

Frozen shoulder can be injected at the subacromial bursa or intra-articularly. The intra-articular injection enters just below the coracoid and is directed outward (fluoroscopy is strongly recommended when performing dilation).

Needle: 1¹/₂-inch versus 3¹/₂-inch spinal needle, 22-gauge
Depth: 1¹/₂ to 2¹/₂ inches
Volume: 4 mL of anesthetic, 10 to 12 mL of saline for dilation, 1 mL of K40

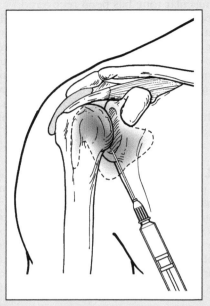

FIGURE 2–3. Intra-articular injection for frozen shoulder.

DESCRIPTION *Frozen shoulder* is a descriptive term that refers to a stiff shoulder joint—a glenohumeral joint that has lost significant ROM (abduction and rotation being most affected). Pathologically the glenohumeral joint capsule has lost its normal distensibility. In long-standing cases, adhesions may form between the joint capsule and the humeral head (adhesive capsulitis). Rotator cuff tendinitis, acute subacromial bursitis, fractures about the humeral head and neck, and paralytic stroke are common causes. Protracted cases with severe restriction of motion may be complicated by hand swelling, finger discoloration, Sudeck atrophy of bone, and an unusual pattern of pain that radiates up and down the arm (reflex sympathetic dystrophy).

SYMPTOMS The patient complains of a gradual loss of shoulder function and motion. The patient often rubs the outer shoulder and shows the inability to move it in certain directions when describing the condition.

"My shoulder is stiffening up."

"I can't reach up over my head."

"I can't reach back to fasten my bra. I have to fasten it in front and rotate it around."

"It's getting harder and harder to put on my coat."

"I can't shave under my armpit anymore."

"My shoulder used to be quite sore and tender. The pain has gotten a lot better, but I can't move it now."

EXAM The ROM of the glenohumeral joint is measured, and a specific cause of local pain or inflammation (e.g., rotator cuff tendinitis, fracture, dislocation) is identified in each patient.

EXAM SUMMARY

1. An abnormal Apley scratch test (inability to scratch the lower back)
2. Restricted abduction and external rotation, measured passively
3. No radiographic evidence of glenohumeral arthritis
4. Hand swelling, finger discoloration, synovitis (complicating reflex sympathetic dystrophy)

(1) General function of the shoulder is assessed by asking patients to raise their arms overhead and to scratch the lower back (the Apley scratch test). These simple maneuvers are used to assess glenohumeral motion rapidly. Patients with normal glenohumeral motion should be able to raise their arms straight overhead and scratch the midback at the T8-T10 vertebral level. Patients with frozen shoulder lack full overhead reaching and are unable to scratch even the lower back at the L4-L5 level. *(2)* Next, individual motions are measured. In many patients, abduction and external rotation are reduced and should be estimated or measured with a goniometer (measurements are made passively). The glenohumeral

joint normally rotates externally to 90 degrees and abducts to 90 to 110 degrees. To measure abduction accurately, shrugging must be prevented by placing downward pressure over the acromion. *(3)* Frozen shoulder must be distinguished from advanced glenohumeral arthritis; on examination, glenohumeral arthritis seems similar to frozen shoulder. Arthritis often shows loss of motion in all directions, however, and has characteristic changes on plain x-rays of the shoulder. *(4)* Severe frozen shoulder (months in duration) may be associated with diffuse hand pain and swelling, finger discoloration, abnormal patterns of sweating, or unilateral joint synovitis (reflex sympathetic dystrophy).

X-RAYS   X-rays are not required to diagnose or stage frozen shoulder. Routine views (including posteroanterior, external rotation, Y-outlet, and axillary views) often are obtained, however, because of the protracted nature of the condition and to satisfy the patient's expectations. Most plain films are nondiagnostic, although rotator cuff tendon calcification is found in 30% of cases.

SPECIAL TESTING   No special studies are required or used routinely. Shoulder arthrography, often ordered to rule out subtle glenohumeral arthritic change or rotator cuff tendon tear, may show the characteristic changes of a contracted glenohumeral capsule. Normally the glenohumeral joint easily fills with 8 to 10 mL of radiopaque contrast material. An advanced case of frozen shoulder may accept only 4 to 5 mL of contrast.

DIAGNOSIS   The diagnosis of frozen shoulder requires showing a loss of ROM of the glenohumeral joint, a loss that is not attributable to glenohumeral arthritis or to a painful periarticular process, such as tendinitis or fracture. X-rays of the shoulder are required to rule out arthritis of the glenohumeral joint. A lidocaine injection test is used to reduce the dramatic levels of pain and muscle spasm that can interfere with an accurate measurement of the ROM of the joint.

TREATMENT   The goals of treatment are to treat any underlying periarticular or bony process, to stretch out the glenohumeral joint lining gradually, and to restore normal ROM to the shoulder. Weighted pendulum-stretching exercise combined with passively performed glenohumeral stretches in abduction and external rotation is the treatment of choice.

■ **STEP 1**   Determine the general function of the shoulder, rule out glenohumeral osteoarthritis with plain x-rays, and perform a lidocaine injection test to obtain accurate measurements of abduction and external rotation.

Restrict active overhead positioning, overhead reaching, and lifting to avoid aggravating any underlying tendinitis or arthritis.

Educate the patient about the slow recovery time, especially in diabetic and stroke patients: "It may take 6 to 18 months to recover."

Begin twice-a-day pendulum-stretching exercises (p. 271).

Recommend an individualized program of passively performed stretching exercises in the directions of motion with the greatest loss, commonly abduction and external rotation (p. 273).

Advise on the application of heat to the anterior shoulder before stretching.

Prescribe an NSAID (e.g., ibuprofen) for pain control, noting that inflammation is not prominent in pure frozen shoulder.

■ **STEP 2 (6 TO 8 WEEKS FOR ROUTINE FOLLOW-UP) Re-evaluate the ROM.**

Reinforce the specific passive stretching exercises.

Consider a subacromial or intra-articular injection of corticosteroid, especially if an underlying tendinitis is present or if the ROM of the glenohumeral joint fails to improve over 6 to 8 weeks of physical therapy (p. 21).

■ **STEP 3 (3 MONTHS WITH PERSISTENT LOSS OF ROM) Re-evaluate the ROM.**

Encourage the patient.

Consider intra-articular dilation with lidocaine and saline in patients who have lost greater than 50% of external rotation, abduction, or both.

■ **STEP 4 (6 TO 12 MONTHS FOR CHRONIC CASES)**   Resume normal activities gradually as motion improves.

Suggest pendulum-stretching exercises to prevent a recurrence.

Begin external and internal rotation isometric exercises to recover the lost rotation strength; begin these when 75% of normal ROM has been restored.

Consider referral to an orthopedic surgeon for patients who fail to recover ROM over 12 to 18 months, including patients who are refractory to stretching, subacromial and intra-articular injection, and saline dilation (1% to 2%).

Resort to shoulder manipulation under general anesthesia if symptoms fail to improve.

PHYSICAL THERAPY   The principal treatment for frozen shoulder involves an individualized program of shoulder-stretching exercises.

PHYSICAL THERAPY SUMMARY
1. Heating of the shoulder
2. Weighted pendulum-stretching exercise twice a day, performed passively with relaxed shoulder muscles

Continued

3. Daily stretching exercises in the directions most affected, performed passively
4. Rotator cuff muscle toning after motion has been significantly restored, performed isometrically

Acute Period and Recovery Heat, weighted pendulum-stretching exercises, and passive stretching exercises are used to restore glenohumeral flexibility. The shoulder is *heated* for 10 to 15 minutes with moist heat or in a bathtub or shower.

Weighted pendulum-stretching exercises are performed for 5 minutes (p. 271). The arm is kept vertical while the patient bends slightly at the waist. The patient should be instructed on relaxing the shoulder muscles when performing this exercise: "This is a pure stretching exercise; don't swing the weight more than 1 foot in distance or diameter; let the weight do the work." *Passive stretching exercises* are performed after the pendulum-stretching exercises. Recommendations should be individualized. Emphasis should be on stretching exercises that focus on the directions in which the patient has had the greatest loss, usually abduction and external rotation (p. 273). The abduction stretching should be limited to no higher than shoulder level, especially if the frozen shoulder resulted from rotator cuff tendinitis. The need to stretch to the point of tension, but not pain, should be emphasized. Multiple repetitions performed twice a day gradually stretch the glenohumeral capsule. General

rotator cuff tendon toning exercises may play a minor role in recovery, especially if rotator cuff tendinitis preceded the frozen shoulder (p. 272).

INJECTION A subacromial injection of corticosteroid is indicated when concurrent rotator cuff or bicipital tendinitis is present (p. 21). A glenohumeral intra-articular injection combined with saline dilation is indicated when greater than 50% of ROM has been lost despite an adequate trial of physical therapy, subacromial injection, or both.

Positioning The patient should be recumbent with the head raised to 30 degrees.

Surface Anatomy and Point of Entry The coracoid process is located and marked. The point of entry is $^{1}/_{2}$ to $^{3}/_{4}$ inch caudal to the coracoid.

Angle of Entry and Depth The angle of entry is perpendicular to the skin and angled slightly outward. The depth is $1^{1}/_{2}$ to $2^{1}/_{2}$ inches. Fluoroscopy is strongly advised if dilation is performed.

Anesthesia Ethyl chloride is sprayed on the skin. Local anesthetic is placed at the pectoralis major fascia (1 mL), at the subscapularis fascia (1 mL), and at the periosteum of the glenoid or humeral head (approximately 1 to 2 mL).

Technique Successful treatment combines an intra-articular injection of corticosteroid with saline dilation of the joint. Fluoroscopy is recommended to ensure an accurate intra-articular injection. Ethyl chloride is sprayed on the skin. The needle is advanced to the firm resistance of the pectoralis major fascia, to the firm resistance of the subscapular fascia, and finally to the hard resistance

---

GLENOHUMERAL JOINT INJECTION

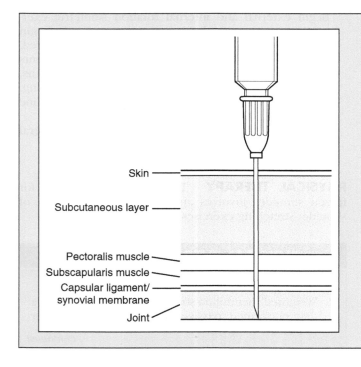

Skin
Subcutaneous layer
Pectoralis muscle
Subscapularis muscle
Capsular ligament/synovial membrane
Joint

of the periosteum of the glenoid or the humeral head. Anesthesia is placed at each tissue plane followed by 2 to 3 mL of radiopaque contrast material to confirm the intra-articular position. Subsequently, 10 to 15 mL of normal saline is injected slowly but gradually. The volume is determined by the increasing pressure to injection and the patient's awareness of a sense of tightening. At the completion of dilation, 1 mL of K40 is injected.

INJECTION AFTERCARE

1. *Rest* for 3 days, avoiding direct pressure, reaching, overhead positioning, lifting, pushing, and pulling.
2. Use *ice* (15 minutes every 4 to 6 hours) and *acetaminophen* (1000 mg twice a day) for postinjection soreness.
3. *Protect* the shoulder for 30 days by limiting reaching, overhead positioning, lifting, pushing, and pulling.
4. Resume passively performed *pendulum-stretching exercises* and passively performed *stretching exercises* of abduction and external rotation on day 4.
5. Begin *isometric toning exercises* of abduction and external rotation after 75% of normal ROM has been restored.
6. Repeat *injection* at 2 to 3 months if overall improvement is less than 50%.
7. Delay *regular activities, work, and sports* until most of the shoulder's ROM has been recovered and at least 75% of muscular tone has been restored.
8. Request a *consultation* with an orthopedic surgeon if the ROM fails to increase by an average of 10% to 15% per month. Steady improvement in the ROM can be assessed by the ability to rotate the shoulder and place the thumb on the spinous processes of the back. On average, the patient should be able to place the thumb 1 to 2 inches higher each month.

SURGICAL PROCEDURE Arthroscopic dilation of the glenohumeral joint and manipulation under general anesthesia are the most common procedures performed for refractory frozen shoulder (<2%).

PROGNOSIS Frozen shoulder is a reversible condition. Given enough time and a rigorous daily physical therapy stretching program, shoulder flexibility gradually returns in most patients. Most patients recover 95% to 100% of their lost ROM. Patients with insulin-dependent diabetes, patients who have had difficulty performing physical therapy, and patients with loss of ROM approaching 50% of normal should be considered for glenohumeral joint dilation and corticosteroid injection; these patients are at greater risk for incomplete recovery and permanent stiffness. The British method of intra-articular dilation (*Br Med J* 1991; 302:1498-1501) is extremely successful and should be considered when physical therapy stretching fails to improve ROM over 2 months or when the patient presents with a dramatic loss of motion. This procedure reduces pain, allows more active participation in physical therapy, and hastens the return to normal function. Arthroscopic dilation—a replacement for the archaic manipulation under general anesthesia—is indicated for refractory cases of adhesive capsulitis.

ROTATOR CUFF TENDON TEAR

Transverse or longitudinal tendon tears occur at the "musculoskeletal" juncture—the anatomic area at risk for the greatest degree of impingement and the watershed area of poorest tendon blood flow.

"Milwaukee shoulder" is a combination of a large tendon tear, a large joint effusion, and radiographic changes of glenohumeral joint osteoarthritis.

Diagnostic testing includes plain x-rays, shoulder arthrography, diagnostic ultrasound, and MRI.

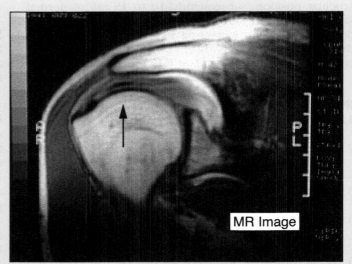

MR Image

FIGURE 2–4. Rotator cuff tendon tear. (*Arrow* shows irregularity of the supraspinatus under the acromion.)

DESCRIPTION Rotator cuff tendon tears—loss of the normal integrity of the infraspinatus tendon or supraspinatus tendon or both—occur as the end result of chronic subacromial impingement and progressive tendon degeneration, as a result of traumatic injury, or as a result of a combination of these conditions. Risk factors for tendon disruption include (1) mucinoid degenerative tendon thinning; (2) injury from a fall or a direct blow to the shoulder; (3) age older than 62 years; (4) history of recurrent tendinitis; (5) a narrow "subacromial space" (normal width 1/2 inch); and (6) weakness of external rotation, abduction, or both that is not attributable to the pain of active rotator cuff tendinitis, disuse atrophy, or suprascapular nerve irritation.

Repeated subacromial impingement over many years causes chronic tendon inflammation, which leads to progressive mucinoid degeneration, tendon thinning, and ultimately tendon rupture. Injuries that most commonly are associated with rotator cuff tendon tears include falls onto the outstretched arm, falls directly onto the outer shoulder, vigorous pulling on a lawn mower cable, and unusual heavy pushing and pulling. Tears are classified anatomically as tendon splits or transverse ruptures and functionally as partial or complete. Rotator cuff tendon tears are common, although many elude clinical detection. Cadaver studies show an incidence of 15% of tendon disruption.

SYMPTOMS The patient complains of weakness of the shoulder, localized pain over the upper back, or a popping sensation whenever the shoulder is moved. The patient often tries to reach over the shoulder attempting to touch the affected area of the upper back when describing the condition or asks the examiner to listen to the popping sound.

"Every time I roll my shoulder, it pops."

"I can't sleep on my back anymore. There's this spot of pain over my shoulder blade."

"I can't sit against a hard-backed chair."

"Doc, what makes my shoulder pop all the time?"

"I work at an assembly table. I have to reach back and forth. The back of my shoulder began to hurt when I took this new job."

"That cortisone shot for my bursitis really took the pain away. I could finally get back to my gardening; however, when I was rototilling, my arm was jerked forward. It felt like a .22 shell went off in my shoulder. Now the pain is worse than ever and I can't lift my arm."

EXAM General function of the shoulder, specific weakness of glenohumeral external rotation and abduction, and signs of active rotator cuff tendinitis are examined in each patient.

EXAM SUMMARY

1. Loss of smooth overhead motion
2. *Weakness* and pain with isometric testing of midarc abduction, external rotation, or both
3. The painful arc maneuver is usually positive (p. 18)
4. Subacromial tenderness
5. Atrophy of the infraspinatus or supraspinatus muscles or both noted over the scapula

(1) The general function of the shoulder is assessed first. Large tears dramatically affect shoulder mobility and strength, interfering with the ability to reach overhead (large tear), to lift a 2- to 5-lb weight overhead (moderate tear), to lift an object with an outstretched arm (moderate tear), or to raise the arm smoothly overhead (small tear). *(2)* The integrity of the specific tendons is assessed by strength testing. Weakness of external rotation (the function of the infraspinatus tendon) or midarc abduction (the function of the supraspinatus tendon) is the hallmark sign of rotator cuff tendon tear. Because pain often accompanies weakness (concurrent rotator cuff tendinitis), a lidocaine injection test is often necessary to isolate true weakness from weakness resulting from pain or poor effort. *(3)* As with active rotator cuff tendinitis, the painful arc maneuver is positive. *(4)* Tenderness is present in the subacromial area. *(5)* Moderate to large tears that have been present for several weeks to months are associated with atrophy of the infraspinatus and supraspinatus muscles in their respective scapular fossae. Lastly, some cases show crepitation or popping with passive circumduction of the shoulder.

X-RAYS   Plain x-rays of the shoulder (including posteroanterior, external rotation, Y-outlet, and axillary views) always are recommended if a rotator cuff tendon tear is suspected. A subacromial space measurement less than 1 cm—the distance between the undersurface of the acromion and the head of the humerus—suggests degenerative thinning, tear, or both. Calcification is present in 30% of cases, but does not correlate directly with the presence of tendon disruption.

SPECIAL TESTING   Cases accompanied by greater than 50% loss of midarc abduction or external rotation strength after a lidocaine injection test (and cases with an equivocal lidocaine injection test) warrant either arthrography or MRI of the shoulder to evaluate for rotator cuff tear. All patients who have three of the major risk factors for tear should undergo further testing with shoulder arthrography, diagnostic ultrasound if available, or MRI.

Patients older than 62 years who have had a fall onto the outstretched arm or a direct blow to the shoulder are at increased risk for rotator cuff tendon rupture. One third of 70-year-olds with persistent symptoms have either a partial rotator cuff tendon rupture or a full-thickness rupture.

DIAGNOSIS   A presumptive diagnosis of tendon tear can be made in the setting of rotator cuff tendinitis with persistent weakness after a lidocaine injection test. If the patient is elderly, has serious medical comorbidities, or elects to avoid an operation, further testing is unnecessary. A definitive diagnosis of tendon tear requires special testing, however. Shoulder arthrography shows subtendinous tears, small splits, and large tendon tears. MRI shows large tears. MRI cannot distinguish a small tear from active tendinitis.

TREATMENT   The treatment of rotator cuff tears varies according to age, the overall general health of the patient, if the dominant side is affected, and if concurrent rotator cuff tendinitis is present. The goals of treatment are to recover and improve lost strength in external rotation and abduction, to improve the global function of the shoulder, and to treat any concurrent rotator cuff tendinitis. The treatment of choice is immediate surgical consultation in a 50- to 62-year-old patient with a large, dominant shoulder tear. For an elderly patient with major medical problems, for patients with medium-sized tears (especially on the nondominant side), and for patients with small tears, physical therapy toning exercises of external rotation and abduction are the nonsurgical treatments of choice. Medical treatment can be considered for "partial" or small tears with modest loss of abduction and external rotation strength.

STEP 1   Assess the patient's overall shoulder function, order plain x-rays of the shoulder, and evaluate the patient's strength of external rotation.

> Order a diagnostic arthrogram or MRI immediately for a 50- to 62-year-old man who shows clinical findings of a large tear of the dominant shoulder (e.g., profound weakness, inability to raise the arm above shoulder level) and refer to an orthopedic surgeon with experience in shoulder surgery.
>
> If the clinical exam suggests a "partial" or small tear with modest loss of abduction and external rotation strength, advise on the following medical treatments:
>
> Suggest a restriction of overhead positioning and reaching.
>
> Apply ice over the deltoid muscle to reduce pain and inflammation acutely.
>
> Perform weighted pendulum-stretching exercises passively, using a 5- to 10-lb weight for 5 minutes once or twice a day (p. 271).
>
> Begin isometric toning exercises at a level that does not cause pain or soreness during the exercise, hours later, or the next day.

STEP 2 (2 TO 4 WEEKS FOR PERSISTENT CASES) Prescribe an NSAID (e.g., ibuprofen) in full dose for 3 to 4 weeks.

> Perform a local corticosteroid injection if the signs of tendinitis predominate, the patient has mild to moderate weakness, and the subacromial space is greater than 6 to 7 mm in diameter (mild degenerative change only).
>
> Re-emphasize the pendulum-stretching exercises, passively performed.
>
> Continue isometric toning exercises at a level that does not cause pain or soreness during the exercise, hours later, or the next day.
>
> Discourage the use of a simple arm sling (p. 246). Immobilization in a susceptible patient (often with a low pain threshold or with stress) may hasten the development of frozen shoulder.

STEP 3 (6 TO 8 WEEKS FOR PERSISTENT CASES)
Order an arthrogram or diagnostic ultrasound if symptoms and signs fail to improve with steps 1 and 2 and if surgery is contemplated.

Consider referral to an orthopedic surgeon for primary repair of small to medium-sized tears if symptoms persist.

STEP 4 (≥3 MONTHS FOR CHRONIC CASES) Prescribe weighted pendulum-stretching exercises and toning exercises in abduction and external rotation to prevent a recurrence (p. 271).

Restrict or avoid any repetitive overhead work or positioning, pushing, and pulling in a patient with chronic symptoms arising from medium-sized to large tears.

Consider consultation with an orthopedic surgeon who specializes in shoulder repair and replacement if symptoms persist, function is dramatically interfered with, and the patient is willing to undergo the risks of surgery.

PHYSICAL THERAPY Physical therapy plays an essential role in the active treatment and rehabilitation of small to medium-sized rotator cuff tendon tears and a significant role in the postoperative recovery of surgically repaired medium-sized to large tears.

PHYSICAL THERAPY SUMMARY

1. Ice to control acute pain or swelling
2. Weighted pendulum-stretching exercises, performed passively with relaxed shoulder muscles
3. Isometrically performed toning exercises in external rotation and abduction
4. Active exercises as tolerated

Acute Period and Recovery Exercises to stretch the glenohumeral space are combined with toning exercises and restricted use. Daily *isometric toning exercises* of glenohumeral abduction and external rotation are essential to the rehabilitation of small to medium-sized rotator cuff tendon tears (p. 272). These exercises are performed with low tension and high repetition, using a TheraBand, large rubber bands, a spring tension chest expander, or similar aid. Enough tension is used to stress the rotator cuff tendon muscles, but not enough to aggravate an underlying tendinitis. The toning is enhanced if it is preceded by heating of the shoulder for 10 to 15 minutes and by stretching of the subacromial space with *weighted pendulum-stretching exercises* (p. 271). These exercises also are crucial to the overall success of the surgical repair of complete rotator cuff tendon tears.

Rehabilitation General care of the shoulder coupled with a long-term restriction of overhead work is necessary to prevent further tendon degeneration. Emphasis is placed on prevention, using the *weighted pendulum-stretching exercises* and *isometric toning exercises.*

INJECTION A subacromial injection of anesthetic is used to confirm the diagnosis of rotator cuff tendinitis complicated by tear (the lidocaine injection test showing persistent weakness despite adequate control of pain). Patients with medium-sized to large tears, persistent pain, and persistent loss of shoulder function should undergo diagnostic MRI arthrography and be evaluated by an orthopedic surgeon. Patients with small to medium-sized tears can be treated cautiously with physical therapy and medication. Corticosteroid injection is used to treat concomitant tendinitis and to palliate symptoms in non-surgical candidates (p. 21). In a few patients, the control of the inflammatory component enables the patient to participate fully in the physical therapy recovery exercises. Corticosteroid injection also can be used to palliate the pain and swelling in an elderly patient who is unable to undergo surgical repair (p. 21). In these cases, injection must be combined with immobilization to counter any adverse effect the corticosteroid may have on the healing process. An abduction pillow immobilizer or a simple shoulder immobilizer should be used concurrently for 30 days—the duration of action of the long-acting injectable corticosteroid.

SURGICAL PROCEDURE Primary tendon repair can be combined with a procedure to reduce impingement, such as acromioplasty.

PROGNOSIS Fifteen percent of patients with rotator cuff tendinitis have tendon tears of various degrees (arthrographic data and the results of autopsy study). Most of these tears heal as the active inflammation is relieved and the recovery exercises are completed. Less than 1% of these patients have profound weakness and dramatic loss of shoulder function suggesting large transverse tears. These patients require plain x-rays and MRI to define the pathology and prepare for possible surgical repair. In addition, if the patient has two or three of the five major risk factors, special studies should be obtained.

Small to medium-sized tears with loss of 25% to 50% of strength and function can be treated medically. At least half of these smaller tears respond to treatment that includes restrictions in use, physical therapy exercises, and, in selected cases, a subacromial injection of corticosteroid. The duration of treatment often exceeds 6 months. Patients who do not respond to 4 weeks of conservative care should be referred promptly to an orthopedic surgeon.

Medium-sized to large tears, especially in a working man 50 to 62 years old, should be referred to an orthopedic surgeon immediately. Unnecessary delays in referral may lead to muscle atrophy, making surgical recovery more difficult and prolonged.

ACROMIOCLAVICULAR SPRAIN AND OSTEOARTHRITIS

Enter just over the end of the clavicle (1 1/2 inches medially to the lateral edge of the acromion).

Needle: 5/8-inch, 25-gauge
Depth: 3/8 to 5/8 inch, down to the periosteum of the clavicle
Volume: 1 mL of anesthetic, 0.5 mL of K40

NOTE: The needle does not enter the joint directly. The injection is placed under the synovial membrane.

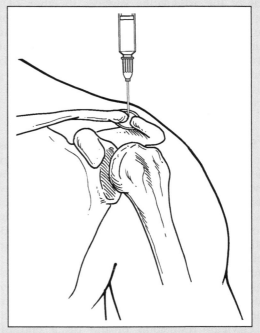

FIGURE 2–5. Injection of the acromioclavicular (AC) joint at the distal clavicle just under the synovial membrane.

DESCRIPTION   The AC, coracoclavicular, and coracoacromial ligaments are attached tightly to the periosteum and hold the acromion, clavicle, and coracoid together. Falls on an outstretched arm, a dramatic blow to the anterior shoulder (tackling in football), or a fall landing directly on the anterior portion of the shoulder can cause the ligaments to be sprained, partially torn, or completely disrupted (first-degree, second-degree, and third-degree AC separations or sprains). Later in life, degenerative arthritis dominates the diagnoses at the AC joint. Over a lifetime of use, the articular cartilage wears down (normal width 3 to 5 mm), the bones become sclerotic, and bony osteophytes form on the ends of the clavicle and the acromion. These nearly universal osteoarthritic changes cause symptoms in a very small percentage of the population (<5%).

SYMPTOMS   The patient complains of shoulder pain or swelling at the AC joint. The symptoms often are so localized that when describing the condition, the patient points to the end of the collarbone with the index finger.

"Whenever I reach up or across my shoulder, I get a pain right here [pointing to the AC joint]."

"I fell off my mountain bike and landed right on my shoulder. Ever since then I have had achy pain and swelling right here [pointing to the AC joint]."

"If I reach up, I feel a grinding in my shoulder."

"The bones seem to be rubbing against one another."

"I can't lie on my shoulder. Sharp pain wakes me up."

EXAM   Each patient is examined for joint inflammation, arthritic change, and disruption of the ligaments that support the joint.

EXAM SUMMARY

1. AC joint enlargement or deformity
2. AC joint tenderness (with or without swelling)
3. Pain aggravated by forced adduction of the shoulder, performed passively
4. Pain and deformity aggravated by downward traction on the arm
5. AC joint widening with downward traction on the arm

(1) Simple inspection may reveal that the AC joint is distorted by tissue swelling, bony osteophytes, or elevation of the clavicle (third-degree separation). *(2)* Local tenderness (most common sign) is located at the top of

the joint, approximately $1^1/_2$ inches medial to the lateral edge of the acromion. *(3)* Pain is consistently aggravated by passively adducting the arm across the chest, forcing the ends of the articulating surfaces together. *(4)* Pain may be aggravated by placing downward traction on the arm. In second-degree and third-degree separations, this pain may be accompanied by a widening of the gap between the clavicle and the acromion (palpable or visible in asthenic patients and in patients with high-grade separations). *(5)* The diagnosis is supported by a local anesthetic block placed just over the joint.

X-RAYS X-rays of the shoulder (including postero-anterior, external rotation, Y-outlet, and weighted views of the AC joint) are recommended. Plain films of the shoulder may show degenerative change, such as narrowing, sclerosis, "squaring-off" of the bones of the clavicle or proximal acromion, or osteophytic spurring. Weighted views of the shoulder (with and without hand-held weights) may show excessive widening between the end of the clavicle and the acromial process (>5 mm).

Severe osteophytic enlargement of the AC joints can contribute to subacromial impingement. Large, inferiorly directed osteophytes (4 to 5 mm in length) can irritate the subacromial bursa or the rotator cuff tendons. Osteolysis of the clavicle—resorption of the distal end of the clavicle—is a rare complication of injury to the joint.

SPECIAL TESTING Weighted views of the AC joint are used to determine the severity of AC separation.

DIAGNOSIS The diagnosis of AC joint disease is made easily by physical examination. The degree of osteo-arthritis or the extent of AC separation is determined by x-rays.

TREATMENT The goal of treatment is to reduce direct pressure and traction at the AC joint to allow the ligaments to reattach to their respective bony insertions. The treatments of choice are restriction of reaching and direct pressure over the outer shoulder, combined with immobilization.

STEP 1 **Examine the joint, order weighted views of the AC joints, and determine the stage of the injury (first, second, or third degree) and the degree of osteoarthritic change.**

Recommend applications of ice to control swelling and pain.

Advise the patient to avoid sleeping on either side.

Recommend restriction of reaching over the head and across the chest.

Limit lifting to 10 to 20 lb held close to the body.

Prescribe a Velcro shoulder immobilizer (p. 247) for 3 to 4 weeks for shoulder separation (less so for osteoarthritic flares).

Educate the patient: "If the ligaments aren't allowed to reattach to the bone, symptoms may recur over and over."

STEP 2 (2 TO 4 WEEKS FOR PERSISTENT CASES) **Re-emphasize the restrictions.**

Perform a local injection with anesthetic to confirm the diagnosis and differentiate it from bicipital or subscapularis tendinitis or with corticosteroid injection (K40) to treat osteoarthritis and first-degree sprains with prominent swelling.

Perform a second injection 4 to 6 weeks after the first injection, and combine it with a Velcro shoulder immobilizer to protect the injection and the joint.

STEP 3 (8 TO 10 WEEKS FOR CHRONIC CASES) **Recommend general conditioning of the major shoulder muscles to minimize the stresses and strains of the joint (no single muscle supports the joint directly).**

Advise on long-term restrictions of reaching, pushing, pulling, and lifting (military press, bench press, and pull-downs must be discontinued) for refractory cases.

Consider an orthopedic referral for persistent symptoms or severe functional impairment.

PHYSICAL THERAPY Physical therapy plays a minor role in the treatment of AC strain and degenerative arthritis of the AC joint. Ice over the AC joint can provide temporary symptomatic relief. There are no effective isometric toning exercises or stretching exercises that provide direct support to the joint. General shoulder conditioning is recommended for athletes.

PHYSICAL THERAPY SUMMARY

1. Ice
2. General shoulder conditioning

INJECTION Local injection of anesthetic is used to confirm the diagnosis (to differentiate it from concurrent rotator cuff disease and bicipital tendinitis). Corticosteroid injection is used to control the symptoms of an acute arthritic flare or shoulder separation unresponsive to immobilization.

Positioning The patient is placed in the sitting position with the shoulders held back and the hands in the lap.

Surface Anatomy and Point of Entry The acromion and clavicle are identified. The AC joint is located as a $^1/_4$-inch depression at the distal end of the clavicle or $1^1/_2$ inches medial to the lateral edge of the acromion. The point of entry is over the anterosuperior portion of the distal clavicle.

ACROMIOCLAVICULAR JOINT INJECTION

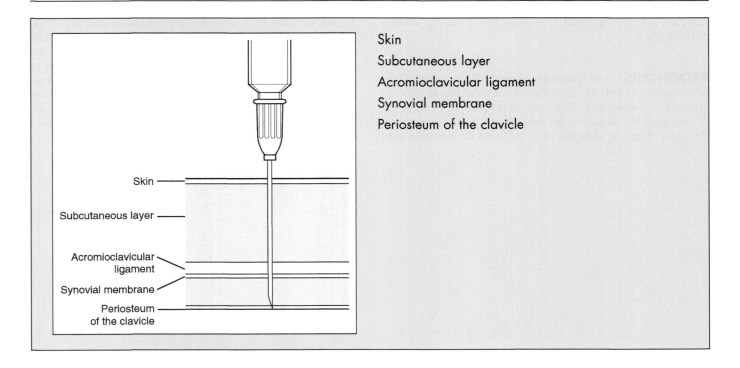

Skin
Subcutaneous layer
Acromioclavicular ligament
Synovial membrane
Periosteum of the clavicle

Skin
Subcutaneous layer
Acromioclavicular ligament
Synovial membrane
Periosteum of the clavicle

Angle of Entry and Depth A 25-gauge needle is inserted at a perpendicular angle. The depth is $^3/_8$ to $^5/_8$ inch.

Anesthesia Ethyl chloride is sprayed on the skin. Local anesthetic is placed in the subcutaneous tissue (0.5 mL) and $^1/_4$ inch above the periosteum of the distal clavicle (0.5 mL). All anesthesia is injected $^1/_4$ inch above the joint, providing the highest concentration of corticosteroid to the joint.

Technique The success of treatment depends on an undiluted intra-articular injection of corticosteroid either layered atop the joint or placed just under the synovial lining that attaches to the adjacent bone. This technique uses an *indirect method* of injecting cortisone into the joint, taking advantage of the anatomic attachment of the synovial membrane to the adjacent bone. The synovial membrane is approximately 1 cm in length (see Figure 2-5). Instead of attempting to perform the injection into the center of the joint directly, which is difficult, painful, and potentially dangerous (cartilage damage), the 25-gauge needle is advanced through the synovial membrane and down to the bone adjacent to the joint line. The center of the joint is *not* entered directly. After achieving anesthesia placed just above and outside the synovium, the 25-gauge needle is advanced gently down to the firm resistance of the periosteum of the clavicle. Using a separate syringe, 0.5 mL of K40 is injected flush against the bone. The joint does not accommodate much medication. If the patient experiences increasing pressure, the needle should be withdrawn $^1/_8$ inch and

the remaining steroid layered atop the joint, just outside of the synovial membrane.

INJECTION AFTERCARE

1. *Rest* for 3 days, avoiding overhead reaching, reaching across the chest, lifting, leaning on the elbows, and sleeping directly on the shoulder.
2. Use a *shoulder immobilizer* with the injection to maximize protection of the joint (optional).
3. Use *ice* (15 minutes every 4 to 6 hours) and *acetaminophen* (1000 mg twice a day) for postinjection soreness.
4. *Protect* the shoulder for 30 days by limiting overhead reaching, reaching across the chest, lifting, leaning on the elbows, and sleeping directly on the shoulder.
5. Begin *general shoulder conditioning* 3 to 4 weeks after most of the pain and inflammation have resolved.
6. Repeat the *injection* and combine it with 3 to 4 weeks of immobilization at 6 weeks if overall improvement is less than 50%.
7. Delay *regular activities, work, and sports* until the pain has resolved.
8. Request *consultation* with an orthopedic surgeon if two injections are unsuccessful.

SURGICAL PROCEDURE Second-degree and third-degree separations are most likely to remain symptomatic. A variety of stabilization procedures are available to eliminate the movement of the clavicle against the acromion. Distal clavicle resection remains the definitive procedure for arthritis, second-degree and third-degree separations, osteolysis, and arthritis with inferiorly directed osteophytes that are encroaching on the rotator cuff tendons.

PROGNOSIS All patients should have plain films performed of both AC joints to determine the degree of arthritis or weighted views to determine the stage of AC separation. Patients with first-degree AC separation or the early stage of arthritis respond well to injection and immobilization. Patients with second-degree and third-degree separations and advanced arthritic changes respond much less predictably.

The success of medical treatment for higher stage AC separations is determined by adequate and anatomic healing of the injured ligaments. The emphasis of treatment must be on immobilization rather than on the anti-inflammatory action of injection. Because proper reattachment of the ligaments does not always occur, recurrent injury is seen frequently. Surgical consultation can be considered in recurrent cases, although distal clavicle resection or internal fixation is performed infrequently.

BICEPS TENDINITIS

Enter 1 to $1^1/_4$ inch below the anterolateral corner of the acromion, directly over the bicipital groove.

Needle: $1^1/_2$-inch, 25-gauge
Depth: $^1/_2$ to $^3/_4$ inch to either tubercle and $^3/_4$ to 1 inch to the bottom of the bicipital groove
Volume: 1 to 2 mL of anesthetic, 1 mL of D80

NOTE: Gently locate the periosteum of the tubercle, anesthetize the bone, and carefully "walk down" the bone to the bottom of the groove.
CAUTION: Maintain the bevel of the needle parallel to the fibers of the tendon.

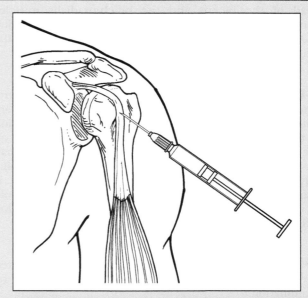

FIGURE 2–6. Bicipital groove injection for bicipital tendinitis.

DESCRIPTION Biceps tendinitis is an inflammation of the long head that results from the mechanical friction and irritation as it passes through the bicipital groove of the anterior humerus. Repetitive lifting and overhead reaching lead to a spectrum of pathologic changes that include simple inflammation, microtearing, chronic inflammation, mucinoid degenerative change, and tendon rupture. Vigorous or unusual lifting can lead to the spontaneous rupture of a chronically inflamed tendon. The risk of rupture approaches 10% to 12%, which is the highest spontaneous rupture rate of any tendon in the body. Risk factors for tendon rupture include (1) mucinoid degenerative change, (2) unusual or vigorous lifting injury, (3) age older than 62 years, and (4) a history of recurrent tendinitis.

SYMPTOMS The patient has shoulder pain aggravated by lifting or overhead reaching. The patient often takes one finger and points directly to the bicipital groove when describing the condition.

"The front of my shoulder hurts every time I lift my mail tray."

"I get this pain right here [pointing to a vertical line of pain running up the upper arm] whenever I move my shoulder."

"My shoulder has been sore for a long time. Yesterday, I tried to place my trailer on the trailer hitch when I felt and heard this loud pop."

"My shoulder used to hurt a lot every day. Two days ago, it stopped hurting. Now I have this big bruise near my elbow, and the muscle seems bigger."

EXAM The patient is examined for swelling and inflammation of the long head of the biceps in the bicipital groove for signs of tendon rupture and for associated subacromial impingement.

EXAM SUMMARY

1. Local tenderness in the bicipital groove
2. Pain aggravated by flexion of the elbow, isometrically performed
3. A positive painful arc maneuver if impingement is present (p. 18)
4. A bulge in the antecubital fossa, signifying long head tendon rupture

(1) Local tenderness is present in the bicipital groove approximately 1 inch below the anterolateral tip of the acromion. The bicipital groove can be identified by identifying the lesser and greater tubercles of the anterior humeral head. The groove is identified by palpating the anterior humerus, passively internally and externally rotating the arm, and feeling the groove move back and forth. *(2)* Pain is aggravated by resisting elbow flexion isometrically. The patient describes a line of pain along the anterior humerus. *(3)* Pain may be aggravated by passively abducting the arm (the painful arc maneuver), as the long head tendon traverses between the humeral head and the undersurface of the acromion on its way to attach to the glenoid process. *(4)* Rupture of the tendon usually is manifested by a bulge several inches above the antecubital

fossa and a large ecchymosis present along the inner aspect of the distal arm. The strength of elbow flexion usually is preserved, however. The strength of the short head of the biceps and the brachioradialis muscles combine to make up 80% of the strength of elbow flexion and compensate easily for the loss of strength from the long head.

X-RAYS X-rays of the shoulder (including postero-anterior, external rotation, Y-outlet, and axillary views) are not always necessary. Plain films may show calcification in the bicipital groove. Treatment decisions are based on the clinical findings of the exam, however, rather than on the presence or absence of calcification. If bicipital rupture is present, and the painful arc maneuver is dramatically positive, plain x-rays of the shoulder should be obtained to evaluate for concurrent rotator cuff tendon inflammation or rotator cuff tendon tear.

SPECIAL TESTING Arthrography or MRI is indicated if concurrent rotator cuff tendon tear is suggested by examination.

DIAGNOSIS The diagnosis is suggested by a history of anterior humeral pain and by an exam showing local tenderness in the bicipital groove that is aggravated by resisted elbow flexion. A regional anesthetic block in the bicipital groove may be necessary to differentiate biceps tendinitis from referred pain from the rotator cuff tendons or pain arising from the glenohumeral joint.

TREATMENT The goals of treatment are to reduce the inflammation and swelling in the tendon, to strengthen the biceps muscle and tendon, and to prevent rupture. Restriction of lifting and reaching combined with an effective anti-inflammatory regimen is the treatment of choice.

STEP 1 Assess the patient's overall shoulder function, estimate the patient's strength of elbow flexion, evaluate the risk factors for tendon rupture, and examine the antecubital area for evidence of tendon rupture.
Eliminate lifting.
Restrict over-the-shoulder positions and reaching.
Apply ice over the anterolateral shoulder.
Begin the weighted pendulum-stretching exercise to reduce the pressure over the tendon (the long head tendon courses through the subacromial space to attach to the superior glenoid labrum).
Suggest an NSAID (e.g., ibuprofen) for 3 to 4 weeks.
Educate the patient: "If restrictions aren't followed, there is a 5% to 10% risk of rupture."

STEP 2 (2 TO 4 WEEKS FOR PERSISTENT CASES) Perform a local injection of D80 in the bicipital groove

for patients younger than 50 years old or in the subacromial bursa for patients older than 50.
Repeat the injection in 4 to 6 weeks if symptoms have not decreased by at least 50%.
Combine the injection with a simple sling or shoulder immobilizer to provide maximum protection against rupture (pp. 246-247).
Begin isometric strengthening of elbow flexion, and follow this by active biceps curls to recover and enhance the strength of the short and long heads of the biceps and the brachioradialis muscles. These are begun after 50% of the pain and inflammation have subsided.

STEP 3 (2 TO 3 MONTHS FOR CHRONIC CASES) Consider an orthopedic consultation for persistent symptoms or if rupture has occurred. Surgery is rarely indicated.

PHYSICAL THERAPY Physical therapy plays a minor role in the treatment of bicipital tendinitis and bicipital tendon rupture.

PHYSICAL THERAPY SUMMARY

1. Ice
2. Phonophoresis
3. Weighted pendulum-stretching exercises, performed passively with relaxed shoulder muscles
4. Toning exercises for the short head of the biceps and brachioradialis tendons (with rupture)

Acute Period Ice, phonophoresis, and the weighted pendulum-stretching exercises are used in the early treatment of bicipital tendinitis. *Ice* placed over the anterior humeral head provides temporary relief of pain. *Phonophoresis* over the anterior humeral head may provide relief of pain and swelling in thin patients. For an uncomplicated case of bicipital tendinitis, *weighted pendulum-stretching exercises* are performed daily (p. 271). Increasing the subacromial space can provide the long head tendon more freedom of motion.

Recovery and Rehabilitation Weighted pendulum-stretching exercises are combined with isometric toning of the elbow flexors. *Weighted pendulum-stretching exercises* are continued through the recovery period. When these exercises are performed three times a week, the chance of recurrent tendinitis is reduced.
Isometric toning exercises of elbow flexion are begun 3 to 4 weeks after the acute pain has resolved. These exercises should be performed at 45 degrees of passive abduction of the shoulder to minimize the amount of friction in the bicipital groove. Daily toning exercises are particularly important when bicipital tendon rupture

has occurred. Strengthening the short head of the biceps and brachioradialis just 15% to 20% counteracts the loss of strength from the rupture of the long head of the biceps.

INJECTION   Several methods of injection can be used based on age and the risk of tendon rupture. Local injection of anesthetic placed directly into the bicipital groove is used to confirm the diagnosis of active tendinitis, and corticosteroid injection is used to treat the active inflammation. Because tendon rupture is rare in individuals younger than age 50, bicipital groove injection—the most precise anatomic injection—is the preferred injection in this age group. With advancing age (>50 years old) and especially in patients with recurrent tendinitis, a subacromial bursal injection (p. 21) or a glenohumeral intra-articular injection (p. 26) is preferred. These latter two injections avoid the hazard of direct needle penetration of the tendon associated with the bicipital groove injection.

Positioning   The patient is placed in the sitting position with the hands placed in the lap. The patient is asked to relax the shoulder and neck muscles.

Surface Anatomy and Point of Entry   The humeral head and the lateral edge of the acromion are located and marked. The point of entry is directly over the bicipital groove. It is located 1 to $1^{1}/_{4}$ inches caudal to the antero-lateral edge of the acromion. When the examiner's fingers are over the anterolateral humeral head, the groove is

palpable when the arm is passively rotated internally and externally.

Angle of Entry and Depth   The angle of entry is perpendicular to the skin. The depth is $^{1}/_{2}$ to $^{3}/_{4}$ inch to either bony prominence and $^{3}/_{4}$ to 1 inch to the bottom of the groove.

Anesthesia   Ethyl chloride is sprayed on the skin. Local anesthetic is placed at the firm tissue resistance of the lesser or greater tubercle (0.25 to 0.5 mL) and at the bottom of the bicipital groove (1.0 mL).

Technique   The success of treatment depends on the effective control of the inflammation of the bicipital tendon. If a *bicipital groove injection* is employed, it is imperative to maintain the bevel of the needle parallel to the fibers of the tendon during the entire procedure. The needle is advanced gently down to the hard tissue resistance of the periosteum of either the lesser or the greater tubercle, anesthetizing one or both. Having identified the adjacent bone, the needle is withdrawn $^{1}/_{4}$ to $^{3}/_{8}$ inch and redirected into the groove ($^{1}/_{4}$ inch deeper) until the rubbery, firm resistance of the tendon or the hard resistance of the humerus is felt. Injection should be done only under light pressure. Resistance when injecting suggests either an intratendinous or a periosteal injection. If re-examination shows less local tenderness and less pain from isometric testing of arm flexion (>50%), 1 mL of D80 is injected. Alternatively a subacromial injection should be used in patients older than 50 years or in patients with significant risk factors for tendon rupture.

BICIPITAL TENDINITIS INJECTION

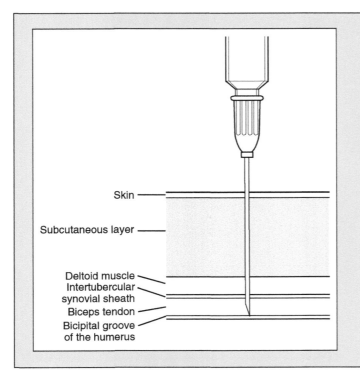

Skin

Subcutaneous layer

Deltoid muscle

Intertubercular synovial sheath

Biceps tendon

Bicipital groove of the humerus

INJECTION AFTERCARE

1. *Rest* for 3 days, avoiding all lifting.
2. Use *ice* (15 minutes every 4 to 6 hours) and *acetaminophen* (1000 mg twice a day) for postinjection soreness.
3. *Protect* the tendon for 30 days by avoiding or at least limiting lifting (held close to the body, with low weight) and overhead reaching and positioning (the biceps tendon is located under the acromion).
4. Resume passively performed *pendulum-stretching exercises* on day 4.
5. Begin isometric *elbow flexion exercises* after the pain has resolved (several weeks).
6. Repeat *injection* at 6 weeks if overall improvement is less than 50% (accompanied by a discussion of the risk factors for tendon rupture: age >50, recurrent tendinitis, previous tendon rupture, poor general shoulder conditioning, and rheumatoid arthritis).
7. Delay *regular activities, work, and sports* until the lost tone has been recovered fully.

SURGICAL PROCEDURE   Surgery for bicipital tendinitis or bicipital tendon rupture is rarely indicated. Repair of the long head of the biceps is rarely necessary because the short head of the biceps and the brachioradialis provide 80% of the strength of flexion, and their combined strength can be enhanced by flexion exercises.

PROGNOSIS   Bicipital tendinitis responds well to restricted use, the pendulum-stretching exercises, and corticosteroid injection. A significant number of patients develop mucinoid degenerative changes in the tendon. Spontaneous rupture occurs in 10% of cases. Special x-rays or scans are not needed to distinguish tendinitis from tendon rupture. Little functional disability results because the short head of the biceps and the brachioradialis provide 80% of the strength of elbow flexion. Rupture often cures the problem, but leads to a minor deformity. For these reasons, surgical repair is performed infrequently. Heavy laborers, violinists, and other patients who demand the utmost from their upper extremities should be referred for surgical consultation.

SUBSCAPULAR BURSITIS

Enter directly over the second or third rib, whichever is closest to the superomedial angle of the scapula.

Needle: 1¹/₂-inch, 22-gauge
Depth: ³/₄ to 1¹/₄ inches down to the periosteum of the rib
Volume: 1 to 2 mL of anesthetic, 1 mL of K40

NOTE: Place one finger above and one finger below the rib in the intercostal spaces and enter between these two; never advance more than 1¹/₄ inches (too deep—pleura).

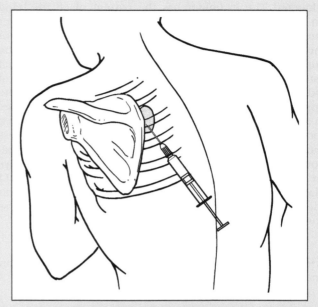

FIGURE 2–7. Subscapular bursa injection.

DESCRIPTION Subscapular bursitis or scapulothoracic syndrome is a focal inflammation caused by friction between the superomedial angle of the scapula and the second and third ribs (the difference in terminology reflects the confusion over the exact nature of the structure; it is neither a true bursa nor a true articulation, simply a friction point of the body). Inflammation of the bursa develops as a result of exaggerated movement of the scapula (mechanical pressure and friction develop between the superomedial angle of the scapula and the adjacent second and third ribs) or compression between the two bones from extrinsic pressure over the back. Conditions that are associated with excessive scapular movement include frozen shoulder, glenohumeral osteoarthritis, and chronic rotator cuff tendinitis (with the gradual loss of normal glenohumeral movement, disproportionate degrees of shrugging occur). Mechanical pressure and friction also can occur in thin patients with poor muscular development, patients with dorsokyphotic posture, workers who perform repetitive to-and-fro motion of the upper extremities (e.g., ironing, assembly work), and athletes who perform heavy bench press exercise. The condition must be distinguished from the more common rhomboid or levator scapular muscle irritation (posture, stress, whiplash) and the referred pain of the lower cervical roots.

SYMPTOMS The patient complains of localized pain over the upper back or a popping sound whenever the shoulder is shrugged. The patient often tries to reach over the shoulder in an attempt to touch the affected area of the upper back when describing the condition.

"Every time I roll my shoulder, it pops."

"I can't sit against a hard-backed chair."

"I work at an assembly table. I have to reach back and forth. The back of my shoulder began to hurt when I took this new job."

"I can't sleep on my back anymore. There's this spot of pain over my shoulder blade."

EXAM The patient is examined for localized tenderness under the superomedial angle of the scapula atop the second or third ribs.

EXAM SUMMARY

1. Local tenderness under the superomedial angle of the scapula, directly over the second and third ribs
2. Full ROM of the shoulder
3. No evidence of cervical root irritation or rhomboid or trapezius muscle strain
4. Confirmation with local anesthetic block

(1) Local tenderness is present in a half-dollar–sized area just under the superomedial angle of the scapula.

The tenderness is palpated along the second or the third rib, whichever is closer to the angle. Palpation of the exact site of irritation requires that the patient's arm be fully adducted. The examiner has the patient place the hand on the contralateral shoulder and then relax the shoulder muscles. *(2)* The condition does not affect the ROM of the glenohumeral joint directly. Shoulder ROM may be impaired, however, if frozen shoulder or glenohumeral osteoarthritis is an underlying cause. *(3)* Because cervical radiculopathy can refer pain in the identical area of the upper back, the neck must be examined in each case. In an uncomplicated case of bursitis, the ROM of the neck should be unaffected (a normal 90 degrees of painless rotation), and the upper extremity neurologic examination should be normal. *(4)* Local anesthetic block plays an integral role in the diagnosis. Lidocaine (1 to 2 mL) placed at the level of the periosteum of the closest rib should eliminate the patient's pain and local tenderness completely.

X-RAYS   X-rays of the shoulder are unnecessary in an uncomplicated case.

SPECIAL TESTING   No special testing is indicated.

DIAGNOSIS   Focal tenderness just under the supero-medial angle of the scapula suggests subscapular bursitis. To distinguish this local inflammatory condition from referred pain from the cervical roots or the muscular irritation of upper back strain, the diagnosis must be confirmed by local anesthetic block at the level of the adjacent rib.

TREATMENT   The goals of treatment are to reduce the acute inflammation, to discover any underlying cause, and to prevent further episodes by improvement in posture and in shoulder muscle tone. Local corticosteroid injection with K40 is the treatment of choice.

STEP 1   Perform a neck, shoulder, and upper back exam; define any underlying cause; and if symptoms are localized to the superomedial angle of the scapula, confirm the diagnosis with local anesthesia.

If the diagnosis is confirmed, perform an injection of 1 mL of K40.

Emphasize the importance of correct posture.

Advise on avoiding direct pressure over the scapula, especially reclining against hard surfaces.

Recommend limitations of reaching across the chest, to-and-fro motions, and overhead reaching of the affected arm.

STEP 2 (4 TO 6 WEEKS FOR PERSISTENT CASES)   Repeat the K40 injection if the symptoms and signs have not improved by at least 50%.

Re-emphasize correct posture.

Begin isometric internal and adduction toning exercises to enhance the tone and bulk of the subscapularis muscle, to be performed daily.

Perform therapeutic ultrasound for refractory cases.

PHYSICAL THERAPY   Physical therapy plays a minor role in the treatment of subscapular bursitis. General shoulder conditioning can be combined with enhancement of the subscapularis muscle tone. Increases in the tone and bulk of the shoulder's principal internal rotator have the theoretical advantage of providing a natural padding between the ribs and the undersurface of the scapula. This exercise must be combined with improvements in sitting posture to be effective.

INJECTIONS   Local injection of anesthetic is used to confirm the diagnosis, and corticosteroid injection is used to treat the active inflammation. NSAIDs are not effective for this condition because of poor tissue penetration.

Positioning   The patient is placed in the sitting position. To expose the bursa fully, the shoulder on the affected side is fully adducted. The patient is asked to place his or her hand on the contralateral shoulder.

Surface Anatomy and Point of Entry   The supero-medial angle of the scapula is identified. With the shoulder fully adducted, the second and third ribs are identified and marked. With one finger in the intercostal space above and one finger in the intercostal space below, the needle is inserted directly over the rib.

Angle of Entry and Depth   The angle of entry is perpendicular to the skin. The depth is $3/4$ inch in thin patients and $1 1/4$ inches in heavier patients. *Caution*: Never advance deeper than $1 1/4$ inches (pleura). If periosteum has not been encountered at $1 1/4$ inches, withdraw the needle and redirect.

Anesthesia   Ethyl chloride is sprayed on the skin. Local anesthetic is placed at the firm tissue resistance of the periosteum of the rib (1 to 2 mL). Putting anesthesia into the muscular layer above the rib is avoided so as to differentiate the degree of bursitis from any associated involvement of the overlying rhomboid muscles.

Technique   The successful injection of the bursa depends on the proper positioning of the patient and the accurate placement of medication at the level of the periosteum of the rib. The needle is advanced through the trapezius and the levator scapulae muscle to the hard resistance of the periosteum of the rib. Alternatively the needle is advanced no more than $3/4$ inch beyond the outer fascia of the trapezius if the hard resistance of the periosteum of the rib cannot be identified positively (the trapezius and the rhomboid muscles are approximately $3/8$ inch thick each, total $3/4$ inch). Anesthetic and corticosteroid are injected at the level of the periosteum.

INJECTION AFTERCARE

1. *Rest* for 3 days, avoiding all direct pressure and to-and-fro shoulder motions.
2. Use *ice* (15 minutes every 4 to 6 hours) and *acetaminophen* (1000 mg twice a day) for postinjection soreness.

SUBSCAPULAR BURSA INJECTION

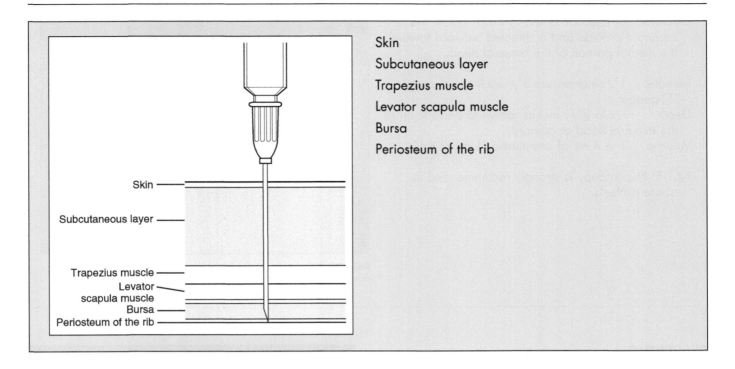

Skin
Subcutaneous layer
Trapezius muscle
Levator scapula muscle
Bursa
Periosteum of the rib

Skin
Subcutaneous layer
Trapezius muscle
Levator scapula muscle
Bursa
Periosteum of the rib

3. *Protect* the shoulder for 30 days by limiting direct pressure and the extremes of shoulder motion.
4. Re-emphasize the need for good *posture*.
5. Begin *isometric toning exercises* of internal rotation and adduction at 3 weeks. If the bulk and tone of the subscapularis muscle can be increased, the scapula would be less likely to rub against the underlying ribs.
6. Repeat the *injection* at 6 weeks if overall improvement is less than 50%.
7. Delay *regular activities, work, and sports* until the pain and inflammation have resolved, and improvement in adduction and internal rotation strength is substantial.

SURGICAL PROCEDURE No surgical procedure is available.

PROGNOSIS Local injection of anesthesia followed by corticosteroid is highly effective in treating the acute inflammation of subscapular bursitis. To avoid recurrences and to ensure a long-term benefit, a full exam of the glenohumeral joint and neck are performed to identify any underlying cause. Shoulder and cervical plain films are used to identify underlying glenohumeral joint arthritis, chronic rotator cuff tendinitis with thinning, and degenerative cervical disk disease. Prevention of recurrent bursitis depends on correcting posture, reducing muscular stress, and enhancing the tone and bulk of the subscapularis muscle. Long-term complications do not occur.

GLENOHUMERAL OSTEOARTHRITIS

Intra-articular injection enters $1/2$ inch below the coracoid process and is directed outward toward the medial portion of the humeral head.

Needle: $1^1/_2$-inch versus $3^1/_2$-inch spinal needle, 22-gauge
Depth: $1^1/_2$ to $2^1/_2$ inches, down to periosteum of the humeral head or glenoid
Volume: 3 to 4 mL of anesthesia, 1 mL of K40

NOTE: Fluoroscopy is strongly recommended in obese patients.

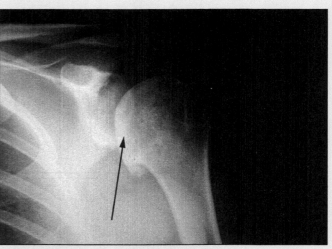

FIGURE 2–8. Intra-articular injection of the shoulder. (*Arrow* indicates direction of injection.)

DESCRIPTION Osteoarthritis of the glenohumeral joint—wear-and-tear of the articular cartilage of the glenoid labrum and humeral head—is an uncommon problem. In most cases, it is the long-term consequence of trauma to the shoulder, the injury having occurred years or decades earlier. Injuries that are associated with the development of osteoarthritis include previous dislocation, humeral head or neck fracture, large rotator cuff tendon tears, and rheumatoid arthritis. X-rays are diagnostic and show osteophyte formation at the inferior humeral head, flattening and sclerosis of the humeral head, and narrowing of the inferior portion of the articular cartilage, which has a normal width of 3 to 4 mm.

SYMPTOMS The patient complains of the gradual development of shoulder pain and stiffness over months to years. The patient often rubs the front of the shoulder when describing the symptoms.

"My shoulder is stiff."

"I can't reach back to put my coat on."

"I dislocated my shoulder in football. The coach said I would get arthritis in my shoulder. Now I'm 58 years old and my shoulder is gradually losing its motion ... it's getting stiffer and stiffer."

"My shoulder makes this terrible clunking noise, like the front of my car when the steering went out."

EXAM The patient is examined for local glenohumeral joint line tenderness and swelling, loss of ROM of external rotation and abduction, and crepitation.

EXAM SUMMARY

1. Local tenderness located anteriorly, just under the coracoid process
2. Restricted abduction and external rotation, measured passively
3. Crepitation with circumduction or clunking on release of isometric tension
4. Swelling of the infraclavicular fossa or general fullness to the shoulder

(1) Tenderness is located anteriorly, just under the thumb-shaped projection of the coracoid process. Firm outward and slightly upward pressure is necessary to assess the irritation along the anterior glenohumeral joint line. *(2)* End-point stiffness and restricted ROM are the hallmark physical signs of arthritis of the shoulder. The global function of the shoulder is reduced. Overhead reaching and reaching to the lower lumbosacral spine (Apley scratch test) are impaired. Loss of glenohumeral abduction and external rotation predominate and are used to gauge the severity of the condition. *(3)* Noise arising from the joint is common. Crepitation or a clunking sound is palpable anteriorly over the shoulder and can be reproduced best by resisting abduction in midarc and feeling for the crepitation as the tension placed across the shoulder is released (the humeral head rapidly moves across the irregular glenoid cartilage, causing the noise). These sounds may be audible in patients with moderate to severe arthritis. *(4)* Dramatic involvement of the glenohumeral joint is associated with a joint effusion. Small effusions are usually too subtle to detect. Patients with moderate to large effusions present with infraclavicular swelling or

general fullness to the shoulder. General fullness is best assessed by looking down on the joint from above and comparing the posteroanterior dimension with the unaffected side.

X-RAYS Plain x-rays of the shoulder (including posteroanterior, external rotation, Y-outlet, and axillary views) are strongly recommended. The earliest changes include narrowing of the articular cartilage and irregularities at the inferior glenoid fossa. As the disease progresses, the distance between the inferior glenoid and the humeral head gradually decreases, and spurring off the inferior portion of the humeral head gradually increases. Advanced arthritis presents with a large humeral head spur, a flattening of the humeral head, and obliteration of the articular cartilage at the inferior glenoid.

SPECIAL TESTING Special testing is unnecessary in moderate to advanced cases with well-established changes on plain x-rays. To detect early disease, CT arthrography can be ordered. Iodine contrast arthrography with CT is indicated to detect subtle irregularities of the inferior glenoid labral cartilage or early thinning of the articular cartilage in a young, active patient who has had trauma to the shoulder. These patients tend to complain of deep anterior shoulder pain, loss of smooth motion, and crepitation with movement, and they show hypermobility on examination.

DIAGNOSIS A diagnosis of osteoarthritis is suggested by a history of progressive loss of ROM, crepitation or crunching with circumduction, and documentation of a loss of external rotation and abduction. Because the findings on physical examination of frozen shoulder are nearly identical to the findings of glenohumeral osteoarthritis, plain x-rays are needed to confirm the diagnosis. Early presentations of osteoarthritis may require CT arthrography to show clearly the early thinning of the inferior glenoid articular cartilage.

TREATMENT The goals of treatment combine exercises to improve ROM and muscular support with ice applications and medication to reduce the inflammation. Weighted pendulum-stretching exercises performed daily and isometric toning exercises of external rotation and abduction are the initial treatments of choice.

STEP 1 **Determine the severity of the condition by assessing the patient's reaching overhead and reaching to the lower back (Apley scratch test), by measuring the loss of abduction and external rotation, and by estimating the strength of external rotation.**

Obtain baseline x-rays of the shoulder.

Educate the patient about the slowly progressive nature of the condition: "This is a wear-and-tear type of arthritis that progresses very slowly."

Suggest an elimination of heavy work, overhead reaching, and forceful pushing and pulling.

Recommend ice applications to the anterior shoulder to control pain and swelling.

Heat the anterior shoulder and perform daily weighted pendulum-stretching exercises with the shoulder muscles relaxed (p. 271).

Follow the pendulum-stretching exercises with passive stretching exercises in the directions of motion with the greatest loss, commonly abduction and external rotation (p. 273).

Prescribe an NSAID (e.g., ibuprofen) in full dose for 3 to 4 weeks, then substitute it with *acetaminophen*, 1000 mg twice a day.

Consider a Velcro shoulder immobilizer for severe arthritic flare, but strongly advise concurrent daily stretching exercises to prevent further stiffening of the shoulder (i.e., development of frozen shoulder).

Prescribe glucosamine sulfate, 1500 mg/day.

STEP 2 (6 TO 8 WEEKS FOR ROUTINE FOLLOW-UP) **Re-evaluate the ROM.**

Reinforce the specific passive stretching exercises.

Perform an intra-articular injection of corticosteroid or refer patient to a radiologist to perform this under fluoroscopic control.

Evaluate and treat any concurrent rotator cuff tendinitis.

After the pain and inflammation of the acute flare subside, begin isometric toning exercises of external and internal rotation to improve the stability of the joint.

STEP 3 (3 MONTHS FOR FOLLOW-UP) **Re-evaluate the ROM.**

Encourage the patient.

Perform repeat x-rays if the patient has lost significant ROM, and symptoms have been relentlessly progressive.

STEP 4 (6 TO 12 MONTHS FOR CHRONIC CASES) **Gradually increase activities of daily living, as tolerated.**

Consider consultation with an orthopedic surgeon specializing in shoulder replacement when treatment fails to control pain and improve overall shoulder function.

PHYSICAL THERAPY Physical therapy plays a significant role in the rehabilitation of acute osteoarthritic flare and a vital role in the prevention of future episodes.

PHYSICAL THERAPY SUMMARY
1. Ice placed over the anterior shoulder
2. ROM exercises to restore or enhance lost external rotation and abduction *Continued*

3. Gentle pendulum-stretching exercises, as tolerated
4. Isometrically performed toning exercises in rotation and abduction, followed by more active exercises

Acute Period and Recovery Heat, the weighted pendulum-stretching exercises, and passive stretching exercises are used to improve glenohumeral flexibility. The shoulder is *heated* for 10 to 15 minutes with moist heat or in a bathtub or shower. *Weighted pendulum-stretching exercises* are performed for 5 minutes (p. 271). The arm is kept vertical, and the patient bends slightly at the waist. The patient should be instructed on relaxing the shoulder muscles when performing this exercise: "This is a pure stretching exercise; don't swing the weight in a diameter greater than 1 foot; let the weight do the work." *Passive stretching exercises* are performed after the pendulum-stretching exercises. Recommendations should be individualized. Emphasis is on stretching exercises that address the directions in which the patient has suffered the greatest loss, usually abduction and external rotation (p. 273). The abduction stretch is limited to no higher than shoulder level, especially if rotator cuff tendinitis accompanies arthritis. The need to stretch to the point of tension, but not pain, is emphasized. Multiple repetitions performed daily gradually stretch the glenohumeral capsule.

General *rotator cuff tendon toning exercises* may play a major role in recovery, especially if arthritis is complicated by rotator cuff tendinitis (p. 272). Gradually increasing the tone of the infraspinatus tendon (external rotation) and the subscapularis tendon (internal rotation) enhances stability, provides greater support, and reduces arthritic flare-ups. Activities of daily living should be postponed until muscle tone in external and internal rotation is restored.

INJECTION Local injection of anesthetic is used to confirm the diagnosis (e.g., to separate it from concurrent rotator cuff disease). Corticosteroid injection is used to control the symptoms of the acute arthritic flare.

SURGICAL PROCEDURE Shoulder replacement (arthroplasty) for intractable symptoms or loss of 50% ROM is the procedure of choice.

PROGNOSIS Osteoarthritis of the glenohumeral joint is a slowly progressive process. Radiographs are needed to confirm the diagnosis and to assist in determining the severity of the problem. Physical therapy exercises combined with intra-articular injection are effective in controlling the acute inflammatory flare. Maintenance toning exercises in external and internal rotation are necessary to enhance stability, improve motion, and reduce the frequency of arthritic flares. Total shoulder replacement is indicated when overall function is impaired, activities of daily living are significantly affected, and pain is intractable.

MULTIDIRECTIONAL INSTABILITY OF THE SHOULDER

The treatment of choice is isometric toning exercises involving internal and external rotation. These exercises are performed with the shoulder kept in neutral position; resistance is accomplished using a TheraBand, bungee cord, an inner tube, or a similar aid.

Isometric internal rotation

Isometric external rotation

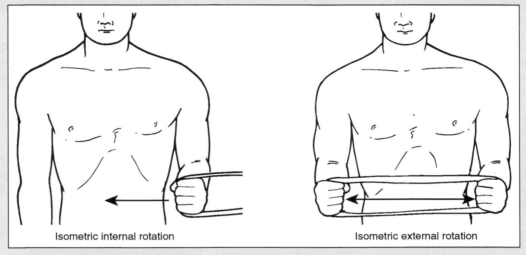

Isometric internal rotation   Isometric external rotation

FIGURE 2–9. Multidirectional instability of the shoulder.

DESCRIPTION   Multidirectional instability of the shoulder is synonymous with *subluxation, loose shoulder,* or *partial dislocation.* It is more common in young women with poor muscular support of the shoulder, in patients with large rotator cuff tendon tears (loss of support as exemplified in a patient with Milwaukee shoulder), and in athletic patients younger than age 40 (especially swimmers and throwers). The shoulder exam includes the following abnormal signs: (1) the "sulcus sign," when downward traction is applied to the upper arm; (2) translocation of the humeral head in the glenoid fossa, when force is applied in the anteroposterior direction; (3) variable degrees of crepitation or popping; and (4) apprehension when performing the extremes of ROM (especially rotation). This abnormal movement places the shoulder at risk for rotator cuff tendinitis. Nonsurgical treatment involves (1) maximizing the tone and strength of the infraspinatus and subscapular tendons (internal and external rotation isometric toning exercises) to enhance the support to the glenohumeral joint, (2) restricting reaching and lifting, and (3) treating any concurrent rotator cuff tendinitis. It is an uncommon problem after age 40 because of the natural stiffening of the tissues around the shoulder.

SYMPTOMS   The patient complains of looseness of the shoulder, a noisy shoulder, or anterolateral shoulder

pain typical of rotator cuff tendinitis. The patient often grabs hold of the deltoid muscle, securing it in place, or rubs over it when describing the condition.

"It feels like my shoulder is going to pop out."

"Every time I try to lift something heavy, my shoulder seems to slip."

"My shoulder seems weak."

"My shoulder makes this crunching sound."

"I'm afraid to rock-climb because I can't trust my shoulder."

EXAM   The patient is examined for the degree of instability (subluxation), for the presence of subacromial impingement and tendon inflammation, and for early signs of glenohumeral osteoarthritis.

EXAM SUMMARY
1. Downward traction on the arm causing the sulcus sign
2. Increased anteroposterior mobility of the humeral head (relative to the glenoid fossa)

Continued

3. Painful arc maneuver may be positive
4. Positive apprehension sign when the arm is placed at 70 to 80 degrees of abduction and passively rotated externally

(1) The hallmark sign of hypermobility is the sulcus sign, an objective measurement of the looseness of the glenohumeral joint. By placing downward traction on the arm (pressure applied to the antecubital fossa when the elbow is flexed to 90 degrees), the humerus can be observed to pull away from the acromion. A gap of $^1/_2$ to $^3/_4$ inch that forms between the humeral head and the undersurface of the acromion indicates severe hypermobility. By contrast, it is impossible to create a subacromial gap in patients with fibromyalgia, stress, or highly toned muscles. *(2)* Hypermobility can be confirmed by applying pressure to the humeral head in the anteroposterior direction, while simultaneously holding the acromion in a fixed position. The humeral head can be felt to move in the glenoid with moderate to severe hypermobility. Sharp pain or a grinding crunch may indicate osteoarthritic change or a tear of the glenoid labrum. *(3)* Rotator cuff tendinitis can accompany hypermobility. The painful arc may be positive, and anterolateral shoulder pain may be reproduced by isometric testing of midarc abduction (supraspinatus) and external rotation (infraspinatus). *(4)* An apprehension sign can be shown in patients with true dislocation. With the arm passively abducted to 70 to 80 degrees, tolerance of forced passive external rotation is assessed.

X-RAYS   Plain x-rays of the shoulder (including posteroanterior, external rotation, Y-outlet, and axillary views) are highly recommended for patients with persistent pain, loss of ROM, or persistent signs of rotator cuff tendinitis.

SPECIAL TESTING   CT arthrography is the test of choice to assess the integrity of the glenoid labral cartilage (thinning or tears) and to determine the degree of early osteoarthritis of the glenohumeral joint (early inferior glenoid osteophyte formation or loss of glenoid articular cartilage). The most common indication for this test is poor response to isometric toning exercises, persistent lack of full ROM, or persistent clicking or crepitation with circumduction of the shoulder.

DIAGNOSIS   The diagnosis of hypermobility is made by clinical exam.

TREATMENT

The goals of treatment are similar to the recommendations for rotator cuff tendinitis. Emphasis is placed on performing isometric toning exercises to improve the stability of the glenohumeral joint and reduce the risk of osteoarthritis. Isometric toning exercises in external and internal rotation are the treatment of choice.

■ **STEP 1   Assess the patient's degree of hypermobility, estimate the ROM, and order x-rays of the shoulder.**
Advise rest and restriction of overhead positioning, reaching, pushing, pulling, and lifting.
Recommend ice for concurrent rotator cuff tendinitis.
Prescribe isometric toning exercises in external and internal rotation, beginning at low tension.

■ **STEP 2 (2 TO 4 WEEKS FOR PERSISTENT CASES)   Prescribe an NSAID (e.g., ibuprofen) in full dose for 3 to 4 weeks or perform a subacromial injection of D80.**
Re-emphasize the isometric toning exercises in external and internal rotation.

■ **STEP 3 (6 TO 8 WEEKS FOR PERSISTENT CASES)   Order CT arthrography to exclude a glenoid labral tear if symptoms fail to respond to exercises and an empirical injection of D80.**
Repeat the injection in 4 to 6 weeks if symptoms and signs have improved but linger at or below the 50% improvement level.

■ **STEP 4 (≥3 MONTHS FOR CHRONIC CASES)   Emphasize the need to continue the toning exercises to maintain stability.**
Recommend cautious performance of or limitations of overhead reaching.
Tell a patient with recurrent or persistent symptoms to avoid all repetitive overhead work or positioning.
Refer the patient to an orthopedic surgeon with experience in shoulder surgery for a stabilization procedure.

PHYSICAL THERAPY   Isometric toning exercises in external and internal rotation combined with general shoulder conditioning are the mainstays of treatment for hypermobility of the shoulder.

PHYSICAL THERAPY SUMMARY

1. Ice if concurrent rotator cuff tendinitis is present
2. Isometrically performed toning exercises in external and internal rotation
3. General shoulder conditioning with emphasis on rotation and deltoid muscle toning

Acute Period   *Ice* can provide temporary relief of pain and swelling if rotator cuff tendinitis is present.

Recovery and Rehabilitation *Isometric toning exercises* of the external rotation (infraspinatus muscle) and internal rotation (subscapularis muscle) are combined to enhance the stability of the glenohumeral joint and to counteract the hypermobility (p. 272). Ideally the strength of external rotation should equal the strength of internal rotation, which should be close to the strength of the biceps muscle. When rotation is enhanced, *general shoulder conditioning* can be started. These exercises should be performed daily until tone is enhanced, then three times a week indefinitely.

INJECTION   Local anesthetic injection can be used to identify the presence or degree of subclinical or overt rotator cuff or bicipital tendinitis (p. 21). If subacromial or bicipital groove anesthetic block improves pain and function significantly, empirical corticosteroid injection can be performed.

SURGICAL PROCEDURE   Variations of the Putti-Platt procedure to remove redundant capsule and to reinforce the anterior joint capsule with the subscapularis tendon is the procedure of choice. Each of the procedures strives to achieve greater stability of the joint while attempting to avoid excessive tightening of the joint (loss of ROM or impairment of muscular strength).

PROGNOSIS   Physical therapy strengthening exercises in internal and external rotation are the principal means of reducing the frequency of dislocation and degree of subluxation. Unless the patient has a complicating rotator cuff tendinitis, anti-inflammatory medication and corticosteroid injection are not indicated. Patients experiencing anterior shoulder pain, limited ROM, and clicking arising from the glenohumeral joint should have shoulder x-rays and MRI performed. Radiographic studies are necessary to define fully secondary glenoid labral tears, anterior glenoid rim fractures, rotator cuff tendon tears, and degree of glenohumeral osteoarthritis.

The need for surgical consultation depends on the overall impairment of shoulder function and the number of episodes and frequency of dislocation or complicating shoulder tendinitis. Many milder cases can be managed medically because the natural history of the condition is to improve slowly as the body gradually stiffens during the 40- to 50-year age range. Patients with frequent dislocation and recurrent tendinitis should be evaluated, however, by an orthopedic surgeon for consideration of a stabilization procedure. Recurrent dislocation must be managed properly to avoid glenohumeral osteoarthritis later in life.

DIFFERENTIAL DIAGNOSIS OF ELBOW PAIN

Diagnoses	Confirmations
Lateral epicondylitis (most common)	Local anesthetic block
Brachioradialis muscle strain	Exam
Medial epicondylitis	Local anesthetic block
Olecranon bursitis	
Draftsman's elbow	Aspiration; hematocrit
Septic bursitis	Aspiration; Gram stain/culture
Bursitis secondary to gout	Aspiration; crystal analysis
Hemorrhagic secondary to chronic renal failure	Aspiration; hematocrit; chemistries
Olecranon spur fracture	X-ray—elbow series
Triceps tendinitis	Exam
Radiohumeral arthritis	
Osteochondritis dissecans	X-rays; MRI; surgical exploration
Post-traumatic osteoarthritis	X-ray—elbow series
Inflammatory arthritis	Aspiration; cell count
Hemarthrosis	Aspiration; hematocrit
Cubital tunnel	Nerve conduction velocity testing
Bicipital tendinitis	
Biceps tendon rupture	Local anesthetic block
Referred pain	
Cervical spine	Neck rotation; x-ray; MRI
Carpal tunnel syndrome	Nerve conduction velocity testing
Rotator cuff tendinitis	Painful arc; subacromial tenderness; isometric testing of the tendons

LATERAL EPICONDYLITIS

Enter directly over the prominence of the lateral epicondyle; use *skin* traction to identify the interface of the subcutaneous fat and the extensor carpi radialis tendon.

Needle: 5/8-inch, 25-gauge
Depth: 1/4 to 1/2 inch, just above the tendon
Volume: 1 to 2 mL of anesthetic; 0.5 mL of D80

NOTE: *Never* inject under forced pressure or if the patient experiences sharp pain (too deep and likely intratendinous).

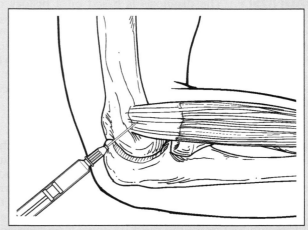

FIGURE 3–1. Injection for lateral epicondylitis at the interface of the dermis and the tendon

DESCRIPTION   Lateral epicondylitis (tennis elbow) is an injury of the common extensor tendons (most commonly extensor carpi radialis brevis) at the origin of the lateral epicondyle of the humerus. Unaccustomed or repetitive lifting, tooling, or hammering and sports activities involving tight gripping and repetitive impact cause microtearing, microsplitting, or microavulsion of the tendons. Secondary inflammation develops at the epicondyle after this mechanical injury. The condition tends to be resistant to treatment because of the constant traction that occurs with everyday use of the wrist and hand. The range of motion (ROM) and function of the radiohumeral joint are normal; lateral epicondylitis does not affect the joint because it is a classic example of a periarticular condition.

SYMPTOMS   The patient has elbow pain and weakness of the forearm. The patient points to the lateral epicondyle or rubs the outer aspect of the lower humerus with the fingertips when describing the condition.

"The pain in my elbow has gotten so bad that I can't even lift my coffee cup."

"After a couple of hours of using my screwdriver, my elbow starts to ache really badly."

"I was pounding nails over the weekend, and ever since then my elbow has been aching."

"Anytime I try to use my torque wrench, I get this sharp pain on the outside of my elbow."

"You've got to do something, doc. I can't spike the volleyball anymore."

EXAM   Each patient is examined for local irritation at the lateral epicondyle, for the strength and integrity of the

common extensor tendon mechanism, and for weakness of grip.

EXAM SUMMARY

1. Local epicondylar tenderness
2. Pain aggravated by resisting wrist extension and radial deviation, isometrically performed
3. Decreased grip strength
4. Full ROM of the elbow joint

(1) Local tenderness is the most common sign and is located over a dime-sized area at the lateral epicondyle. It is best identified with the elbow flexed to 90 degrees. A few patients have local tenderness between the radial head and the lateral epicondyle (the radial humeral bursa, an extension of the joint lining of the elbow). *(2)* This lateral elbow pain is aggravated by resisting wrist extension and radial deviation performed isometrically with the wrist held in neutral position. (The tendon most commonly involved in tennis elbow is the extensor carpi radialis brevis, whose function is to extend and radially deviate the wrist.) *(3)* Pain is aggravated by strong gripping. In severe cases, weakness of grip occurs not only from disuse, but also from the mechanical disruption of the injury. Objective measurement of grip strength and endurance with a dynamometer can be used to document severe involvement. *(4)* The ROM of the elbow is preserved. Loss of extension or flexion almost always indicates a primary elbow joint process.

X-RAYS   X-rays of the elbow are unnecessary. Routine films of the elbow are normal in nearly all cases.

SPECIAL TESTING   No special testing is indicated.

DIAGNOSIS   The diagnosis is based on a history of pain over the lateral epicondyle and on an examination showing local epicondylar tenderness and lateral elbow pain aggravated by isometric wrist extension or radial deviation. Regional anesthetic block at the epicondyle can be used to confirm the diagnosis and differentiate it from the referred pain of carpal tunnel syndrome, cervical radiculopathy, or rotator cuff tendinitis.

TREATMENT   The goals of treatment are to allow the microtorn common extensor tendon to reapproximate or reattach to the lateral epicondylar process, to reduce the secondary inflammation, and to restore forearm muscle strength. The treatment of choice comprises ice to reduce inflammation at the lateral epicondyle combined with immobilization of the wrist to prevent traction and tension.

STEP 1   Assess the integrity of the joint by evaluating flexion and extension, estimate the strength of gripping, and obtain baseline measurements of the patient's strength of wrist extension.

Recommend limitations on lifting, hammering, repetitious wrist motion, fine handwork, and supination and pronation of the forearm to reduce the tension and traction across the tendons.

Apply ice over the epicondyle to reduce pain and swelling.

Prescribe a Velcro wrist splint to protect the tendons against traction (p. 249).

Empirically prescribe a nonsteroidal anti-inflammatory drug (NSAID) (e.g., ibuprofen [Advil, Motrin]) for 3 to 4 weeks. Oral medication may not concentrate sufficiently in this relatively avascular tendon site.

Educate the patient: "You may feel the pain at the elbow, but it is the wrist and hand motions that aggravate the condition the most."

STEP 2 (3 TO 4 WEEKS FOR PERSISTENT CASES) Order a short-arm cast (p. 250).

Suggest a long-arm cast if supination and pronation during the forearm exam prominently affect the pain at the elbow.

Discontinue the NSAID at 4 weeks if symptoms have not responded dramatically.

Continue with applications of ice.

STEP 3 (6 TO 8 WEEKS FOR PERSISTENT CASES) Perform a local injection of D80, and strongly advise continued fixed immobilization with casting for an additional 3 weeks.

Repeat the injection in 4 to 6 weeks if symptoms have not been reduced by at least 50%.

STEP 4 (6 TO 10 WEEKS FOR CHRONIC CASES) Begin toning exercise (p. 275) after the pain has subsided.

Use a tennis elbow band (p. 248) to prevent a recurrence.

Advise the patient to delay regular activities, work, and sports until the forearm muscular tone and strength have been restored.

Demonstrate palms-up lifting and explain how this avoids putting direct tension on the elbow.

Consider an orthopedic referral for persistent symptoms, especially for laborers and carpenters.

PHYSICAL THERAPY   Physical therapy plays a minor role in the active treatment of lateral epicondylitis and a vital role in its rehabilitation and prevention.

PHYSICAL THERAPY SUMMARY

1. Ice
2. Phonophoresis with a hydrocortisone gel
3. Gripping exercises, isometrically performed
4. Toning exercises of wrist extension, isometrically performed

Acute Period   Ice and *phonophoresis* using a hydrocortisone gel provide temporary relief of pain and swelling. Ice routinely is recommended and is particularly helpful for inflammatory flare reactions after local corticosteroid injection. Phonophoresis is an alternative treatment that is used when inflammatory changes are prominent and have failed to respond to ice. Both must be combined with immobilization to be effective.

Recovery and Rehabilitation   Isometric exercises are used to restore the strength and tone of the extensor muscles. *Isometric toning exercises* are begun 3 to 4 weeks after the symptoms and signs have resolved (p. 276). Initially, *grip exercises* using grip putty, a small compressible rubber ball, or an old tennis ball are performed daily in sets of 20, with each hold lasting 5 seconds. The strength and endurance of the forearm flexor and extensor muscles are built up gradually. (When actively flexing the forearm muscles by gripping, the extensor muscles are activated as well.) These exercises are followed by *isometric toning exercises of wrist extension,* which are essential to restoring full strength to the forearm and to preventing future recurrences. Each episode of epicondylitis seems to weaken the common extensor mechanism. To overcome the loss of tensile strength, toning exercises must continue to be done three times a week and should be combined with an ongoing limitation on lifting, applying torque, and heavy gripping. For recurrent disease, these exercises should be continued for 6 to 12 months.

INJECTION Local injection with corticosteroid is indicated when initial management with immobilization fails to reduce symptoms sufficiently to allow participation in the physical therapy recovery exercises.

Positioning The patient is placed in the supine position, the elbow is flexed to 90 degrees, and the hand is placed under the ipsilateral buttock (for maximum exposure of the epicondyle).

Surface Anatomy and Point of Entry The lateral epicondyle is most prominent and readily palpated with the elbow flexed to 90 degrees. It is located $1/2$ inch proximal to the radial head (the radial head should rotate smoothly under the examiner's fingers when passively supinating and pronating the forearm). The point of entry is directly over the center of the epicondyle.

Angle of Entry and Depth Most patients have little subcutaneous tissue overlying the epicondyle. The depth down to the interface of the dermis and the extensor tendons averages $1/4$ to $3/8$ inch, but can be as superficial as $1/8$ inch. With so little overlying subcutaneous fat, it is necessary to create a space for the corticosteroid injection by pinching up the skin, entering the tented-up skin at an angle, and distending the area with 1 mL of anesthesia.

Anesthesia Ethyl chloride is sprayed on the skin. Local anesthetic is placed in the subcutaneous tissue only (0.5 mL).

Technique Successful injection requires the accurate placement of the medication at the interface of the subcutaneous fat and the tendon. The depth of injection can be determined accurately by gradually advancing the needle until the patient feels mild discomfort (the subcutaneous tissue is usually pain-free) or until the rubbery resistance of the tendon is felt. *Note:* A painful reaction to injection or firm resistance during injecting suggests that the needle is too deep, likely within the body of the tendon (withdraw $1/8$ inch). Alternatively the proper depth can be confirmed by applying traction to the overlying skin. If the needle is placed properly above the tendon, it should move freely in the dermis when applying skin traction. Conversely the needle sticks in place if the tip has penetrated the body of the tendon. In the latter case, the needle simply is withdrawn $1/8$ inch. The corticosteroid always should be injected at the interface between the subcutaneous fat and the tendon.

INJECTION AFTERCARE

1. *Rest* for 3 days, avoiding all lifting, typing, writing, turning of the forearms, tooling, hammering, and direct pressure over the epicondyle.
2. Use *ice* (15 minutes every 4 to 6 hours) and *acetaminophen (Tylenol ES)* (1000 mg twice a day) for postinjection soreness.
3. *Protect* the elbow for 3 to 4 weeks by the uninterrupted use of a Velcro wrist brace or a short-arm cast and by avoiding direct pressure. Because neither the Velcro wrist brace nor the short-arm cast device sufficiently restricts forearm supination or pronation, the examiner must emphasize the restriction of turning of door handles and keys.
4. Emphasize the need to perform *lifting palms up,* to use a wrist bar when typing, and to use thick, padded grips on tools.

LATERAL EPICONDYLITIS INJECTION

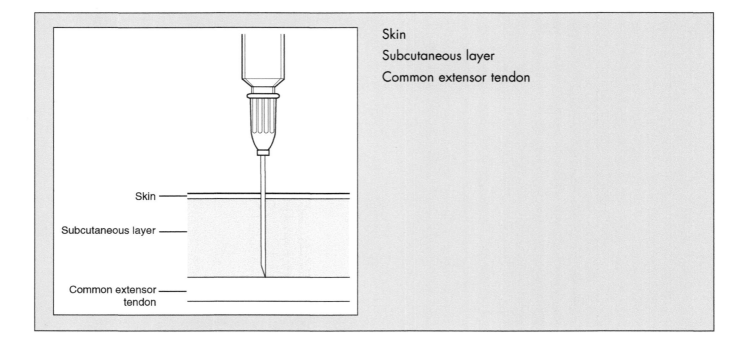

Skin

Subcutaneous layer

Common extensor tendon

5. Begin *gripping exercises* at half tension after the brace or cast is discontinued. Educate the patient: *"Begin with a half grip—just enough to firm the forearm muscles—and gradually build up over 1 to 2 weeks."*

6. With restoration of normal grip strength, *isometric toning exercises of wrist extension* are begun at low tension and increased slowly. The patient should exercise only to the edge of discomfort; patients experiencing forearm muscle soreness probably are exercising too aggressively. Exercises must be interrupted if the lateral epicondyle becomes progressively more irritated.

7. Repeat *injection* at 6 weeks if pain, tenderness, or forearm weakness persists, and especially if the aforementioned recovery exercises are poorly tolerated.

8. Delay *regular activities, work, and sports* until the pain and inflammation have resolved and grip and wrist extension strength has increased substantially (at least 80% of normal).

9. Obtain *plain x-rays* of the elbow and a *consultation* with an orthopedic surgeon for refractory or chronic symptoms.

SURGICAL PROCEDURE Tendon excision or débridement and tendon lengthening or tenotomy is performed infrequently (approximately 3% to 5% of cases). Surgery can be considered when two courses of immobilization combined with local ice applications and at least one local corticosteroid injection have failed to resolve the acute symptoms. *Note:* Surgery should be reserved for patients who have significant functional impairment of grip and forearm strength. Because surgery is capable of restoring only 90% of the tensile strength of the tendon, patients with grip-strength measurements less than 75% to 80% of normal have the best chance of realizing a functional benefit.

PROGNOSIS Of patients, 95% respond to a combination of rest and restricted use, wrist immobilization, and corticosteroid injection. The remaining 5% may respond to long-term physical therapy toning exercises with severe restrictions of forearm use. Patients failing to restore forearm and wrist function (chronic tendinitis—mucinoid degeneration of the tendon) can be considered for surgical exploration and tendon repair.

MEDIAL EPICONDYLITIS

Enter $^3/_8$ to $^1/_2$ inch distal to the prominence of the medial epicondyle; use skin traction to identify the interface between the subcutaneous fat and the tendon.

Needle: $^5/_8$-inch, 25-gauge
Depth: $^1/_4$ to $^1/_2$ inch, just above the tendon
Volume: 1 to 2 mL of anesthetic; 0.5 mL of D80

NOTE: *Never inject under forced pressure or if the patient experiences sharp pain (too deep—within the tendon).*

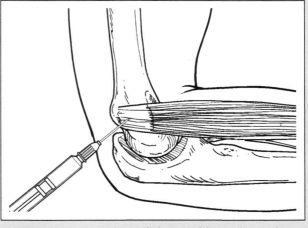

FIGURE 3–2. Injection for medial epicondylitis at the interface of the dermis and the tendon.

DESCRIPTION Medial epicondylitis (golfer's elbow) is an injury of the common flexor tendons at the medial epicondyle of the humerus. Unaccustomed or repetitive lifting, tooling, or hammering and sports activities involving tight gripping and repetitive impact cause microtearing, microsplitting, or microavulsion of the origin of the flexor carpi radialis tendon. Secondary inflammation develops at the epicondyle after this mechanical injury. Symptoms persist because of the constant tension and traction that occur during everyday use of the wrist and hand. The ROM and function of the radiohumeral joint are normal; lateral epicondylitis does not affect the joint because it is a classic example of a periarticular condition.

SYMPTOMS The patient has elbow pain and weakness of the forearm. The patient points to the medial epicondyle or rubs the inner aspect of the lower humerus when describing the condition.

"I have constant pain in my neck, shoulder, and arms because of my fibromyalgia. However, I have this very severe pain along the inside of my elbow."

"After a couple of hours of using my computer, my elbow starts to ache really badly."

"Every time I brush my elbow against my side, I get this sharp pain."

"I'm losing the strength of my grip … my elbow hurts so bad."

"I can't believe there's no swelling. My elbow (pointing to the inner aspect of the joint) hurts so badly I would think there would be something showing."

EXAM Each patient is examined for local irritation at the medial epicondyle, for the strength and integrity of the

common flexor tendon mechanism, and for weakness of grip.

EXAM SUMMARY

1. Local epicondylar tenderness
2. Pain aggravated by resisting wrist flexion and radial deviation, isometrically performed
3. Decreased grip strength
4. Full ROM of the elbow joint

(1) Local tenderness is the most common sign and is located over a dime-sized area just distal to the medial epicondyle. This tenderness is in contrast to the local tenderness of lateral epicondylitis, which occurs directly over the bone. *(2)* This medial elbow pain is aggravated by resisting wrist flexion and radial deviation performed isometrically (the flexor carpi radialis is the tendon most commonly involved, and its function is to flex and radially deviate the wrist). *(3)* Strong gripping aggravates pain. In severe cases, weakness of grip occurs not only from disuse, but also from the mechanical disruption of the tendon. Objective measurement of grip strength and endurance with a dynamometer can be used to document severe involvement. *(4)* The ROM of the elbow is preserved. Loss of flexion or extension almost always indicates a primary elbow joint process.

X-RAYS X-rays of the elbow are unnecessary. Routine films of the elbow are normal in most cases.

SPECIAL TESTING No special testing is indicated.

DIAGNOSIS   The diagnosis is based on a history of medial epicondylar pain and on an exam showing local tenderness and pain aggravated by isometric wrist flexion, radial deviation, or both. Regional anesthetic block at the epicondyle confirms the diagnosis and differentiates it from the pain of cubital tunnel syndrome or cervical radiculopathy or the referred pain of rotator cuff tendinitis.

TREATMENT   The goals of treatment are to allow the microtorn common flexor tendon to reapproximate or reattach to the medial epicondylar process, to reduce the inflammation at the epicondyle, and to restore forearm muscle strength by performing isometric toning exercises of gripping and wrist flexion. The treatment of choice comprises ice to reduce inflammation at the medial epicondyle combined with immobilization of the wrist to prevent traction and tension at the elbow.

STEP 1   **Assess the integrity of the joint by evaluating flexion and extension, obtain baseline measurements of patient's strength of wrist flexion, and estimate the strength of gripping.**

Recommend limitations on lifting, hammering, repetitious wrist motion, fine handwork, and supination and pronation of the forearm to reduce the tension and traction across the tendons.

Apply ice over the epicondyle.

Prescribe a Velcro wrist splint (p. 249).

Empirically prescribe an NSAID (e.g., ibuprofen [Advil, Motrin]) for 3 to 4 weeks; note that oral medication may not concentrate sufficiently in this relatively avascular tendon site.

Educate the patient: "You may feel the pain at the elbow, but it is the wrist and hand motions that aggravate the tendon."

STEP 2 (3 TO 4 WEEKS FOR PERSISTENT CASES)   **Prescribe a short-arm cast (p. 250) to replace the splint.**

Prescribe a long-arm cast if supination and pronation during the forearm exam prominently affect the pain at the elbow.

Discontinue the NSAID if the pain at the elbow has not responded at 3 to 4 weeks.

Continue with applications of ice.

STEP 3 (6 TO 8 WEEKS FOR PERSISTENT CASES)   **Perform a local injection of D80, and strongly advise continued fixed immobilization with casting for an additional 3 weeks.**

Repeat the injection in 4 to 6 weeks if symptoms have not been reduced by at least 50%.

STEP 4 (6 TO 10 WEEKS FOR CHRONIC CASES)   **Begin toning exercise (p. 276) after pain has subsided.**

Use a tennis elbow band (p. 248) to prevent a recurrence.

Advise the patient to delay regular activities, work, and sports until forearm muscular tone and strength have been restored.

Demonstrate palms-down lifting, and explain how this avoids putting direct tension on the elbow.

Consider an orthopedic referral for persistent symptoms, especially for laborers and carpenters.

PHYSICAL THERAPY   Physical therapy plays a minor role in the active treatment of tendinitis of common flexor origin, but a vital role in its rehabilitation and prevention.

PHYSICAL THERAPY SUMMARY

1. Ice
2. Phonophoresis with a hydrocortisone gel
3. Isometrically performed toning of gripping
4. Isometrically performed toning of wrist flexion

Acute Period   Ice and *phonophoresis* using a hydrocortisone gel provide temporary relief of pain and swelling. Ice routinely is recommended and is particularly helpful for inflammatory flare reactions after local corticosteroid injection. Phonophoresis is an alternative treatment used when inflammatory changes are prominent and have failed to respond to ice. Both must be combined with immobilization to be effective.

Recovery and Rehabilitation   Isometric exercises are used to restore the strength and tone of the flexor muscles. *Isometric toning exercises* are begun 3 to 4 weeks after the symptoms and signs have resolved (p. 276). Initially, *gripping exercises* using grip putty, a small compressible rubber ball, or an old tennis ball are performed daily in sets of 20, with each grip being held for 5 seconds. The strength and endurance of the forearm flexor muscles are built up gradually. These exercises are followed by *isometric toning exercises of wrist flexion*, which are essential to restore full strength to the forearm and to prevent recurrences. Each episode of epicondylitis seems to weaken the common flexor mechanism. To overcome the loss of tensile strength, toning exercises must continue to be performed three times a week and combined with an ongoing limitation on lifting, applying torque, and heavy gripping. For recurrent disease, these exercises should be continued for 6 to 12 months.

INJECTION   Local injection with corticosteroid is indicated when initial management with immobilization fails to reduce symptoms sufficiently to allow participation in the physical therapy recovery exercises.

Positioning   The patient is placed in the supine position, the elbow is flexed to 90 degrees, and the arm is rotated externally as far as comfortable.

Surface Anatomy and Point of Entry   The medial epicondyle is most prominent and readily palpated with

MEDIAL EPICONDYLITIS INJECTION

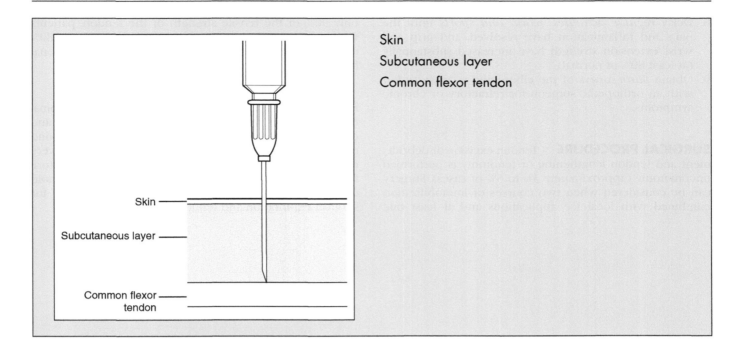

Skin
Subcutaneous layer
Common flexor tendon

Skin
Subcutaneous layer
Common flexor tendon

the elbow flexed to 90 degrees. The point of entry is $^1/_2$ inch distal to the center of the epicondyle.

Angle of Entry and Depth   Most patients have little subcutaneous tissue overlying the epicondyle. The depth down to the interface of the dermis and the flexor tendons averages $^1/_4$ to $^3/_8$ inch, but can be as superficial as $^1/_8$ inch. With so little overlying subcutaneous fat, it is necessary to create a space for the corticosteroid injection by pinching up the skin, entering the tented-up skin at an angle, and distending the area with 1 mL of anesthesia.

Anesthesia   Ethyl chloride is sprayed on the skin. Local anesthetic is placed in the subcutaneous tissue only (0.5 or 1 mL to create a greater space for the steroid).

Technique   Successful injection requires the accurate placement of the medication at the interface of the subcutaneous fat and the tendon. The depth of injection can be determined accurately by gradually advancing the needle until the patient feels mild discomfort (the subcutaneous tissue is usually pain-free) or until the rubbery tissue resistance of the tendon is felt. A painful reaction to injection or firm resistance during injection suggests the needle is too deep and within the body of the tendon (withdraw $^1/_8$ inch). Alternatively the proper depth can be confirmed by applying vertical traction to the overlying skin. If the needle is placed properly above the tendon, it should move freely in the dermis when applying skin traction. Similarly the needle sticks in place if the tip has penetrated the body of the tendon (withdraw $^1/_8$ inch). The corticosteroid always should be injected at the interface between the subcutaneous fat and the tendon.

INJECTION AFTERCARE

1. *Rest* for 3 days, avoiding all lifting, typing, writing, turning of the forearms, tooling, hammering, and direct pressure over the epicondyle.
2. Use *ice* (15 minutes every 4 to 6 hours) and *acetaminophen* (1000 mg twice a day) for postinjection soreness.
3. *Protect* the elbow for 3 to 4 weeks by the uninterrupted use of a Velcro wrist brace or a short-arm cast and by avoiding direct pressure. Because neither the Velcro wrist brace nor the short-arm cast device sufficiently restricts forearm supination or pronation, the examiner must emphasize the restriction of turning of door handles and keys.
4. Emphasize the need to perform *lifting palms down,* to use a wrist bar when typing, and to use thick, padded grips on tools.
5. Begin *gripping exercises* at half tension after the brace or cast is discontinued. Educate the patient: *"Begin with a half grip—just enough to firm the forearm muscles—and gradually build up over 1 to 2 weeks."*
6. With restoration of normal grip strength, *isometric toning exercises of wrist flexion* are begun at low tension and increased slowly. The patient should exercise only to the edge of discomfort; patients experiencing forearm muscle soreness probably are exercising too aggressively. Exercises must be interrupted if the lateral epicondyle becomes progressively more irritated.

7. Repeat *injection* at 6 weeks if improvement in pain, tenderness, or strength is less than 50%, and especially if the aforementioned recovery exercises are poorly tolerated.
8. Delay *regular activities, work, and sports* until the pain and inflammation have resolved, and grip and wrist extension strength have increased substantially (at least 80% of normal).
9. Obtain *plain x-rays* of the elbow and a *consultation* with an orthopedic surgeon for refractory or chronic symptoms.

SURGICAL PROCEDURE   Tendon excision or débridement and tendon lengthening or tenotomy is performed uncommonly (approximately 3% to 5% of cases). Surgery can be considered when two courses of immobilization combined with local ice applications and at least one local corticosteroid injection have failed to resolve the symptoms. *Note:* Surgery should be reserved for patients who have significant functional impairment of grip and forearm strength. Because surgery is capable of restoring only 90% of the tensile strength of the tendon, patients with grip-strength measurements less than 75% to 80% of normal have the best chance of realizing a functional benefit.

PROGNOSIS   Of patients, 95% respond to a combination of rest and restricted use, wrist immobilization, and corticosteroid injection. The remaining 5% may respond to long-term physical therapy toning exercises with severe restrictions of forearm use. Patients failing to restore forearm and wrist function (chronic tendinitis—mucinoid degeneration of the tendon) can be considered for surgical exploration and tendon repair.

OLECRANON BURSITIS

Enter at the base of the bursa paralleling the ulna; rotate the bevel so that it faces the bone; aspirate the entire contents either with the syringe or with manual pressure; send for fluid studies.

Needle: 1¹/₂-inch, 18-gauge
Depth: ¹/₄ to ³/₈ inch
Volume: 0.5 mL of anesthetic (only in the dermis) and 0.5 mL of K40

NOTE: Apply a compression dressing with gauze and Coban tape for 24 to 36 hours followed by a protective neoprene pull-on elbow sleeve for 3 weeks.

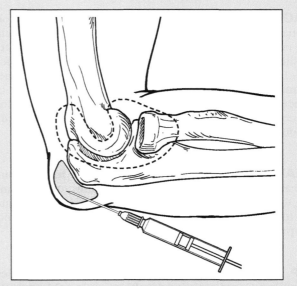

FIGURE 3-3. Olecranon bursa aspiration and injection.

DESCRIPTION   Olecranon bursitis is an inflammation of the bursal sac located between the olecranon process of the ulna and the overlying skin. It is a low-pressure bursa that is susceptible to external pressure. Most cases (90%) are caused by repetitive trauma in the form of pressure, commonly referred to as draftsman's elbow. It is one of two bursal sacs that are uniquely susceptible to infection (5% are caused by *Staphylococcus aureus* or *Streptococcus* infection). The remaining 5% of cases are caused by gout; gout is drug induced, as opposed to the classic inherited form that affects the feet primarily. Given the differential diagnosis, all bursal sacs should be aspirated at presentation to define the exact etiology. Septic bursitis should be treated with oral antibiotics plus repeated aspiration until clear. Intravenous antibiotics are indicated if the septic bursitis is accompanied by cellulitis. Nonseptic bursitis can be treated with the combination of treatments discussed subsequently.

SYMPTOMS   The patient complains of pain and swelling just behind the elbow. The patient rubs over the olecranon process or elevates the flexed elbow to show the swelling when describing the symptoms.

"Within 5 hours, I had this golf ball show up at the end of my elbow."

"I am a mapmaker. I slowly developed this swelling over my elbow."

"When I rub the skin over my elbow, I feel a bunch of little marbles."

"I've got this sack of fluid hanging off my elbow."

"All of a sudden I developed this red, hot, swollen area over my elbow."

EXAM   Bursal sac swelling, inflammation, and thickening are examined in each patient.

EXAM SUMMARY

1. Swelling, redness, and heat over the olecranon process
2. Full ROM of the elbow joint
3. A characteristic aspirate

(1) Cystic swelling, redness, heat, or all three are present over the proximal olecranon process, ranging from 1 to 2 inches in length. *(2)* The ROM of the elbow joint should be unaffected; the bursal swelling is extra-articular. *(3)* The diagnosis is confirmed by aspiration of fluid from the bursal sac. If redness extends beyond the immediate area of the bursa and is accompanied by induration, septic bursitis surrounded by cellulitis should be suspected.

X-RAYS   X-rays of the elbow are unnecessary. Routine films of the elbow show soft-tissue swelling over the olecranon. An olecranon spur may be present in approximately 20% of cases. Treatment rarely is influenced by radiographic studies.

SPECIAL TESTING   Special testing includes bursal fluid analysis.

DIAGNOSIS   The diagnosis is based on the laboratory evaluation of the bursal aspirate. Cell count, Gram stain, and crystal analysis help to differentiate acute traumatic bursitis from the inflammatory reaction of gout and infection. It is impossible to distinguish an acutely inflamed traumatic bursitis from septic bursitis based solely on clinical grounds. Every patient with acute bursitis must undergo aspiration and laboratory testing to determine the definitive cause accurately.

TREATMENT   The goals of treatment are to determine the cause of the swelling, to reduce swelling and inflammation, to encourage the walls of the bursa to reapproximate, and to prevent chronic bursitis. The treatment of choice comprises aspiration, drainage, and laboratory analysis.

STEP 1   Aspirate the bursa for diagnostic studies, including Gram stain and culture, uric acid crystals, and hematocrit.

Apply a simple compression dressing for 24 to 36 hours (gauze and Coban tape).

Ice applied over the olecranon process is effective in reducing pain and inflammation.

Avoid direct pressure.

Prescribe a solid, $1/4$-inch-thick neoprene pull-on elbow sleeve; apply immediately after the compression dressing (p. 248).

STEP 2 (1 TO 2 DAYS AFTER LABORATORY ANALYSIS) Prescribe an antibiotic for the infection (*S. aureus*), evaluate and treat for gout, or perform an intrabursal injection of K40 for traumatic bursitis.

Continue with the neoprene pull-on sleeve.

STEP 3 (4 TO 6 WEEKS FOR PERSISTENT CASES)   Repeat the aspiration and local injection with K40 if the bursa reaccumulates fluid in the first 3 to 4 weeks and if the tenderness persists.

Perform passive stretching of the elbow in flexion and extension in the uncommon event that the ROM of the elbow has been impaired.

Educate the patient: "In 10% to 20% of cases, there is persistence of swollen or thickened sacs."

STEP 4 (3 MONTHS FOR CHRONIC CASES)   Consider consultation with an orthopedist if thickening has developed and it is interfering with the patient's activities of daily living.

PHYSICAL THERAPY   Physical therapy does not play a significant role in the treatment or rehabilitation of olecranon bursitis.

INJECTION   Local injection with corticosteroid is indicated when initial management with simple aspiration and compression dressing fails to control swelling or thickening or both.

Positioning   The patient is placed in the supine position, the elbow is flexed to 90 degrees, and the arm is placed over the chest.

Surface Anatomy and Point of Entry   The bursal swelling is located directly over the olecranon process. The point of entry is at the base of the bursa along the ulna.

Angle of Entry and Depth   The angle of entry is parallel to the ulna. The depth is $1/4$ to $3/8$ inch from the surface.

Anesthesia   Ethyl chloride is sprayed on the skin. Local anesthetic is placed in the subcutaneous tissue only (0.5 mL), adjacent to the bursal wall. Intrabursal anesthesia is unnecessary because the bursal wall has little in the way of pain receptors.

Technique   Successful treatment—complete removal of the fluid, control of inflammation, and prevention of chronic thickening—requires thorough removal of fluid in a timely manner, appropriate anti-inflammatory medication, and postinjection compression of the bursal sac. After the subcutaneous tissue has been anesthetized, an 18-gauge needle is passed, bevel outward, into the center of the bursal sac. The bevel is rotated 180 degrees toward the ulna. Using a combination of aspiration suction and manual compression (milking the fluid with finger pressure on either side), complete decompression of the contents of the bursal sac is accomplished. If infection is suspected, the needle is withdrawn, immediate pressure is applied to avoid any postprocedure bleeding, a compression bandage is applied, and the fluid is sent for studies. For aseptic bursitis—sepsis excluded by lack of fever, few risk factors for infection, clear acellular serous fluid, and a negative Gram stain—the needle is left in place, and the bursa is injected with 0.5 mL of K40. Subsequently the needle is withdrawn, immediate pressure is applied to avoid any postprocedure bleeding, a compression bandage is applied, and the fluid is sent for studies.

INJECTION AFTERCARE

1. *Rest* for 3 days with the bulky compression dressing worn for the first 24 to 36 hours and avoidance of all direct pressure and extremes of ROM of the elbow.
2. Use *ice* (15 minutes every 4 to 6 hours) and *acetaminophen* (1000 mg twice a day) for postprocedure soreness.
3. *Protect* the elbow for 3 to 4 weeks with a pull-on neoprene elbow sleeve, worn continuously.
4. Prescribe daily passive flexion or extension *stretching exercises* over the next several weeks if ROM has been affected (the ROM of the elbow usually is preserved except in the case of septic bursitis accompanied by cellulitis).
5. *Repeat aspiration* of septic bursitis commonly is needed at 7 to 10 days because of the intense inflammatory response.
6. Repeat the *injection* at 6 weeks if swelling persists or chronic thickening develops ("*It feels like I have gravel under my skin.*").

OLECRANON BURSA ASPIRATION

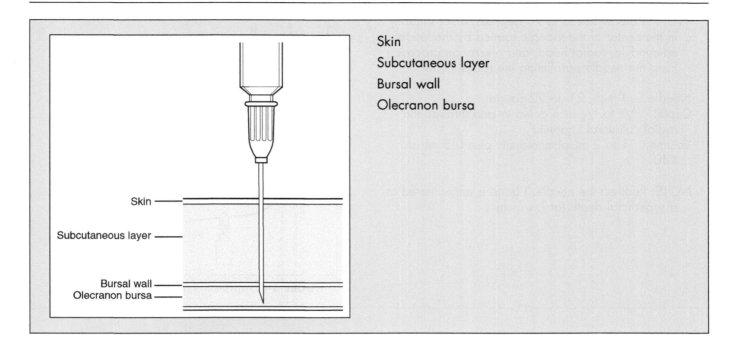

Skin
Subcutaneous layer
Bursal wall
Olecranon bursa

Skin ——

Subcutaneous layer ——

Bursal wall ——
Olecranon bursa ——

7. Avoid *direct pressure* for the next 6 to 12 months to decrease the chance of recurrence.
8. Obtain a *consultation* with an orthopedic surgeon if the bursal swelling, thickening, or both fail to dry up naturally over 6 months.

SURGICAL PROCEDURE   Bursectomy can be considered for persistent swelling or chronic bursal thickening that fails to improve with combined treatment modalities (aspiration, drainage, and injection of K40 on two successive attempts).

PROGNOSIS   Treatment success depends on an accurate diagnosis, appropriate therapy based on laboratory study, complete aspiration of the contents of the bursa, and protective padding to prevent recurrence. With these measures, 80% to 85% of cases resolve. Approximately 15% of cases develop some degree of chronic bursal thickening and require sequential treatment. Despite these measures, 5% of patients develop recurrent swelling and thickening of the bursal walls. These cases of chronic bursitis are considered for surgical bursectomy.

RADIOHUMERAL JOINT ARTHROCENTESIS

With the elbow flexed to 90 degrees, enter laterally in the center of the triangle formed by the lateral epicondyle, radial head, and olecranon process; keep the needle paralleling the radial head.

Needle: 1-inch, 21- to 22-gauge
Depth: $^5/_8$ to $^3/_4$ inch down to and through the radial collateral ligament
Volume: 1 to 2 mL of anesthetic plus 0.5 mL of K40

NOTE: Redirect the needle if bone is encountered at a superficial depth (at $^3/_8$ inch).

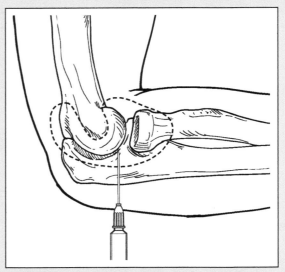

FIGURE 3–4. Aspiration and injection of the elbow.

DESCRIPTION Aspiration of the radiohumeral joint and synovial fluid analysis distinguish between hemarthrosis and inflammatory, noninflammatory, and septic elbow effusions. Rheumatoid arthritis, osteoarthritis secondary to trauma, and spondyloarthropathy with peripheral joint involvement are the rheumatic conditions most likely to cause elbow effusions. Septic arthritis is extremely rare.

SYMPTOMS The patient complains of an inability to move the elbow through a full ROM, of a pressure-like pain in the antecubital fossa, or both. When describing the condition, the patient actively flexes and extends the arm, demonstrates the lack of full extension or flexion of the joint, or, in the case of osteochondritis, tries to reproduce the recurrent popping sound.

"I can't straighten my arm."

"I feel a pressure buildup in my elbow."

"My elbow doesn't move smoothly anymore. It's like a ratchet that catches as I try to straighten it."

"I can't throw any more. My elbow hurts too much, and it's getting weaker."

EXAM Assessment of the ROM of the elbow in extension and flexion is the key to distinguishing involvement of the joint from involvement of the periarticular soft tissues. In addition, ROM measurements correlate directly with the severity of the arthritic process and the success of treatment. Combining these measurements with an assessment of crepitation, the smoothness of motion, end-

point stiffness, and the specific points of local tenderness allows the differentiation of an uncomplicated effusion of the elbow from osteoarthritis, osteochondritis dissecans, loose bodies, and radial head subluxation.

EXAM SUMMARY

1. Loss of full flexion, extension, supination, or pronation
2. Lack of smooth motion or catching (loose body or osteochondritis dissecans)
3. Lateral joint line tenderness and swelling (the bulge sign of elbow effusion)
4. End-point stiffness or pain with forced passive flexion or extension
5. Varus and valgus stress maneuvers show looseness (large chronic effusion)

(1) The hallmark finding of radiohumeral joint disease is a loss of full ROM. The earliest sign of an elbow effusion is a loss of full extension. As the condition advances, full flexion is restricted. If the radial head is involved with osteochondritis dissecans or osteoarthritis from previous injury, supination and pronation also are affected. In either case, there is end-point stiffness at the extremes of ROM. *(2)* Lack of smooth motion or locking with passive flexion and extension suggests an intra-articular loose body. Osteochondritis dissecans is the most common cause of this unique sign. *(3)* The characteristic swelling of the elbow joint is best observed laterally. With the elbow flexed to 90 degrees, a bulge sign should be

observable or palpable in the triangle formed by the radial head, lateral epicondyle, and olecranon process. *(4)* Endpoint stiffness or pain with passive flexion and extension is characteristic of osteoarthritis. *(5)* With ever-increasing amounts of elbow fluid over longer and longer intervals of time, the supporting ligaments begin gradually to loosen. Varus and valgus stress applied to the supporting ligaments of the joint show the looseness caused by this chronic distention.

X-RAYS X-rays of the elbow (including lateral and posteroanterior views) always are indicated when the elbow joint is involved. Osteoarthritic narrowing between the radius and the humerus or the olecranon and the humerus may be seen. Evidence of an old fracture may be present. Plain films may not show evidence of osteochrondritis dissecans with accompanying loose body, however.

SPECIAL TESTING If elbow signs persist, and true locking of the joint has been shown, MRI is advisable to evaluate for osteochondritis dissecans or intra-articular loose body.

DIAGNOSIS The diagnosis of radiohumeral joint disease is strongly suggested by the loss of full ROM of the joint. The diagnosis is confirmed by aspiration of joint fluid, improvement in pain and ROM after intra-articular injection of lidocaine, or both.

TREATMENT Because the treatment of choice depends solely on the etiology of the effusion, the first priority is to aspirate synovial fluid for laboratory analysis. Hemarthrosis simply requires drainage. Nonseptic effusions can be treated with corticosteroid injection. Septic arthritis requires immediate institution of parenteral antibiotics. Infection of the joint is rare. When the diagnosis is made, all patients require passive ROM exercises to restore the ROM of the joint.

STEP 1 Measure the ROM in extension and flexion; describe the size of the lateral joint line bulge sign; and aspirate the joint for diagnostic studies, including Gram stain and culture, uric acid crystal analysis, and cell count and differential.
  Apply ice over the entire anterior joint.
  Avoid repetitive bending and extension.
  Prescribe a long-arm posterior plaster splint to provide temporary support to the joint, taking into consideration the need to avoid excessive immobilization that could stiffen the joint.
  Prescribe a neoprene pull-on elbow brace (p. 248) to protect and support the joint.
  Prescribe an NSAID in full dose for 2 to 3 weeks, but only for nonseptic effusion (rheumatoid, osteoarthritic, or spondyloarthritic diagnoses).

STEP 2 (1 TO 3 DAYS AFTER LABORATORY ANALYSIS) After excluding infection, perform an intra-articular injection of K40 for the rheumatoid or osteoarthritic effusion.
  Continue use of the neoprene pull-on.
  Prescribe glucosamine sulfate, 1500 mg/day.
  Begin ROM exercises to restore full flexion and extension.

STEP 3 (3 TO 4 WEEKS FOR PERSISTENT CASES) Repeat the joint aspiration and local injection with K40 if there is persistent swelling and pain.
  Continue ROM exercises to restore full flexion and extension.

STEP 4 (3 MONTHS FOR CHRONIC CASES) If locking or effusion persists, consider an orthopedic consultation for joint débridement.

PHYSICAL THERAPY *Ice* placed over the outer elbow provides temporary control of pain and swelling. *Passive ROM exercises* are vital in restoring full ROM to the joint. These exercises are best performed after the acute symptoms of pain and swelling have subsided. After restoring the normal ROM of the joint, *isometric toning exercises* are performed to restore the strength of the biceps, brachioradialis, and triceps muscles.

PHYSICAL THERAPY SUMMARY

1. Ice placed over the outer elbow
2. ROM exercises in flexion and extension, passively performed
3. Isometrically performed toning of flexion and extension after the ROM has been restored

INJECTION Aspiration and drainage should be considered for tense, painful hemarthrosis. Corticosteroid injection is indicated for any inflammatory condition that is characterized by a persistent loss of 15 to 20 degrees of extension, flexion, or both or that has failed to respond to systemic therapy.
  Positioning The patient is placed in the supine position, the elbow is flexed to 90 degrees, and the arm is placed over the chest.
  Surface Anatomy and Point of Entry Joint swelling is seen most readily between the radial head, olecranon process, and lateral epicondyle when the elbow is flexed to 90 degrees (the bulge sign of an elbow effusion). The point of entry is at the center of the triangle formed by these three bony prominences.
  Angle of Entry and Depth The angle of entry is perpendicular to the skin, paralleling the radial head. The synovial cavity depth is $3/4$ inch.

RADIOHUMERAL JOINT ASPIRATION

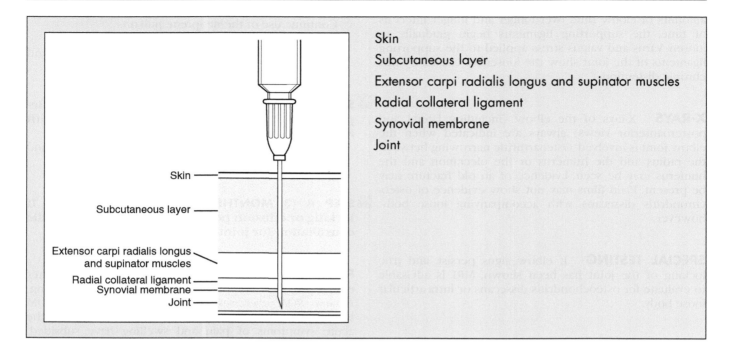

Skin
Subcutaneous layer
Extensor carpi radialis longus and supinator muscles
Radial collateral ligament
Synovial membrane
Joint

Skin
Subcutaneous layer
Extensor carpi radialis longus and supinator muscles
Radial collateral ligament
Synovial membrane
Joint

Anesthesia Ethyl chloride is sprayed on the skin. Local anesthetic is placed in the subcutaneous tissue (0.25 mL), at the hard resistance of any bony prominence encountered at a superficial depth (0.25 mL), and at the firm resistance of the deep ligaments (0.25 mL).

Technique Successful aspiration and drainage requires accurate localization of the point of entry and careful insertion of the needle into the synovial cavity located at the apex of the "inverted cone" formed by the olecranon, lateral epicondyle, and radial head. A *lateral approach* provides the best access. A 21- or 22-gauge needle is advanced gently down to the firm resistance of the radial collateral ligament, paralleling the radial head. If bone is encountered prematurely at a superficial level (³/₄ inch), local anesthesia is injected, and the needle is withdrawn ¹/₄ inch and redirected. After placing anesthesia just outside the radial collateral ligament, the needle is advanced ¹/₄ inch through the firm resistance of the ligament and joint capsule. Aspiration is attempted at this depth. If fluid is not obtained, the bevel of the needle is turned 180 degrees, and the aspiration is attempted again. For the aseptic effusion, the needle is left in place, and the joint is injected with 0.5 mL of K40.

INJECTION AFTERCARE

1. *Rest* for 3 days, avoiding all repetitious motion and tension at the elbow.

2. Use *ice* (15 minutes every 4 to 6 hours) and *acetaminophen* (1000 mg twice a day) for soreness.
3. *Protect* the elbow for 3 to 4 weeks with a pull-on neoprene elbow sleeve, worn continuously.
4. Begin daily passive flexion or extension *stretching exercises* as soon as the pain and swelling have abated.
5. Septic arthritis may need to be *reaspirated* at 7 to 10 days.
6. Repeat *injection* at 6 weeks for nonseptic, inflammatory effusions if swelling persists or chronic synovial thickening develops.
7. Obtain *MRI* and *consultation* with an orthopedic surgeon if full, smooth ROM is not restored (osteochondritis dissecans or loose body).

SURGICAL PROCEDURE   Arthroscopy is indicated to remove loose bodies, to evaluate and treat osteochondritis dissecans, or to débride the osteoarthritic joint.

PROGNOSIS   Local injection is effective in providing temporary improvement in the symptoms and signs of radiohumeral joint inflammatory effusions. Persistent elbow effusions that fail to respond to treatment are the most important indication of underlying osteoarthritis, osteochondritis dissecans, or loose body.

DIFFERENTIAL DIAGNOSIS OF WRIST PAIN

Diagnoses	Confirmations
Wrist sprain (most common)	
Simple wrist sprain (ligamentous)	Exam; normal x-rays
Sprain with chondral fracture	Persistent loss of grip, decreased range of motion (ROM), and persistent tenderness
Navicular fracture	Loss of 45% of ROM; sequential x-rays; bone scan
Kienböck's disease	Avascular necrosis of the lunate on serial x-rays of the wrist
Perilunate dislocation	Loss of normal bony alignment
Triangular cartilage fracture of the ulnocarpal joint	MRI or arthroscopy
Dorsal ganglion	
From the radiocarpal joint	Aspiration
From the tenosynovial sheath	Aspiration
Carpal tunnel syndrome (CTS)	Nerve conduction velocity (NCV) testing or local anesthetic block
De Quervain's tenosynovitis	Local anesthetic block
Radiocarpal arthritis	
Post-traumatic osteoarthritis	X-rays—wrist series
Rheumatoid arthritis	Synovial fluid analysis; erythrocyte sedimentation rate; rheumatoid factor
Gout or pseudogout	Crystal analysis
Referred pain to the wrist	
Carpometacarpal (CMC) osteoarthritis	X-rays—thumb series
Cervical spine	Neck rotation; x-rays; MRI
Pronator teres syndrome (mimicking CTS)	NCV testing

DE QUERVAIN'S TENOSYNOVITIS

Enter ³/₈ inch proximal to the tip of the radial styloid, angling at 45 degrees to the bone (approach the bone carefully owing to its sensitivity).

Needle: ⁵/₈-inch, 25-gauge
Depth: ³/₈ to ¹/₂ inch flush against the periosteum of the radial styloid
Volume: 2 to 3 mL of anesthetic and 0.5 mL of D80

NOTE: The injection should form a palpable "bubble," 1¹/₂ inches in length.

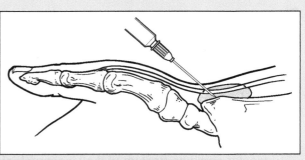

FIGURE 4–1. Injection and dilation of De Quervain's tenosynovitis.

DESCRIPTION De Quervain's tenosynovitis is an inflammation of the extensor and abductor tendons of the thumb. Repetitive or unaccustomed use of the thumb (gripping and grasping) leads to friction and irritation of the snuffbox tendons as they course over the distal radial styloid. Twenty percent of cases occur in young mothers within the first 6 months of their delivery (typically from repetitious and unaccustomed lifting of the newborn, but occasionally from inappropriate intravenous line placement). If left untreated, this friction-induced tenosynovitis can progress to fibrosis and to loss of flexibility of the thumb in flexion. The latter condition is called *stenosing tenosynovitis*.

SYMPTOMS The patient has wrist pain and difficulties with gripping. The patient often rubs over the distal styloid when describing the condition.

"I can't grip anymore."

"Every time I try to pick up my baby, I get this sharp pain in my wrist."

"I have had this sharp pain over my wrist [pointing to the end of the radius] ever since I had a needle stuck into my vein."

"It's very sore right here [pointing to the end of the radius], and it has begun to swell."

"My bone is getting bigger [pointing to the radial styloid]."

EXAM Each patient is examined for tenderness and swelling at the radial styloid process; for the degree of inflammation of the extensor pollicis longus, extensor pollicis brevis, and abductor pollicis longus tendons; and for the range of motion (ROM) of the thumb.

EXAM SUMMARY

1. Local tenderness at the tip of the radial styloid
2. Pain aggravated by resisting thumb extension or abduction, isometrically performed
3. A positive Finklestein test (pain aggravated by passive stretching the thumb in flexion)
4. A distensible tenosynovial sac

(1) Local tenderness is present over the distal portion of the radial styloid, adjacent to the abductor pollicis longus tendon. *(2)* Pain is aggravated by resisting thumb extension and abduction isometrically (thumb abduction moves the thumb perpendicular to the palm, and extension places the thumb in the "hitchhiker's position"). *(3)* Pain is aggravated by passively stretching the thumb tendons over the radial styloid in thumb flexion (Finklestein maneuver). This maneuver is so painful that the patient often responds by lifting the shoulder to prevent the examiner from stretching the tendons. *(4)* Tendon fibrosis is assessed by evaluating flexion and circumduction of the thumb and by assessing the distensibility of the tissues over the radial styloid. Normally the soft tissues over the radial styloid should distend readily with 2 to 3 mL of local anesthetic, forming a bubble 1¹/₂ inches long.

X-RAYS X-rays of the wrist and thumb are unnecessary. Plain films of the wrist and thumb are normal; calcification of these tendons does not occur.

SPECIAL TESTING No special testing is indicated.

DIAGNOSIS The diagnosis is suggested by a history of radial-side wrist pain and an exam showing local radial styloid tenderness and pain aggravated by resisting thumb extension. The diagnosis is confirmed by regional anesthetic block placed directly over the radial styloid. Effective relief of signs and symptoms excludes CMC arthritis and radiocarpal arthritis. A distensible tenosynovial sac essentially excludes stenosing tenosynovitis.

TREATMENT The goals of treatment are to reduce the inflammation in the tenosynovial sac, to prevent adhesions from forming, and to prevent recurrent tendinitis (by tendon-stretching exercises and by altering lifting and grasping). Corticosteroid injection placed at the radial styloid is the treatment of choice.

STEP 1 Confirm the diagnosis, and assess for stenosing tenosynovitis.

Suggest rest and restriction of thumb gripping and grasping.

Apply ice at the radial styloid.

Prescribe buddy taping of the thumb to the base of the first finger (p. 252), a dorsal hood splint (p. 253), or a Velcro thumb spica splint (p. 251).

STEP 2 (3 TO 4 WEEKS FOR MORE SEVERE OR PERSISTENT CASES) Perform a local injection of D80.

Repeat the injection at 4 to 6 weeks if the symptoms are not reduced by 50%.

Severe cases that require a second injection can be treated concurrently with either a dorsal hood splint or a short-arm cast with a thumb spica (p. 249).

STEP 3 (6 TO 8 WEEKS FOR CHRONIC CASES) Apply gentle stretching exercises of the thumb in flexion if the symptoms have improved and thumb flexibility has been impaired (p. 278).

Consider a surgical consultation for tendon release if two injections fail to control the active inflammation.

PHYSICAL THERAPY Physical therapy does not play a prominent role in the treatment of de Quervain's tenosynovitis.

PHYSICAL THERAPY SUMMARY
1. Ice 2. Phonophoresis with a hydrocortisone gel 3. Gentle stretching exercises in flexion, passively performed (prevention)

Acute Period Ice and phonophoresis are used in the treatment of active tenosynovitis. *Ice* applied to the radial styloid effectively can reduce local pain and swelling.

Phonophoresis with a hydrocortisone gel may be helpful in minor cases, but cannot take the place of a local corticosteroid injection in persistent or chronic cases.

Recovery and Rehabilitation Stretching exercises are used to prevent recurrent tenosynovitis. After the signs and symptoms of active tenosynovitis have resolved (3 to 4 weeks), gentle *passive stretching exercises* of the extensor and abductor tendons into the palm are performed. Sets of 20 stretches, each held 5 seconds, are performed daily (p. 278).

INJECTION Because most patients delay seeking medical attention for several weeks beyond the time simple immobilization would be effective (hoping the condition would improve, difficulty obtaining an appointment, or assuming this is just arthritis), corticosteroid injection is the treatment of choice.

Positioning The wrist is kept in neutral position and turned on its side, radial side up.

Surface Anatomy and Point of Entry The radial styloid is identified and marked. The point of entry is directly over the radial styloid 0.5 to 1 cm proximal to the anatomic snuffbox and halfway between the abductor pollicis longus and the extensor pollicis longus tendons as they course over the radial styloid.

Angle of Entry and Depth The needle is advanced carefully at a 45-degree angle down to the hard resistance of the radial styloid periosteum (pain). If the bone is not encountered at $^3/_8$ to $^1/_2$ inch (typical depth), the point of entry may have been too distal.

Anesthesia Ethyl chloride is sprayed on the skin. Local anesthetic is placed just above at the radius.

Technique Successful treatment involves a single passage of the needle down to the periosteum of the radius, slow dilation of the tissues with anesthesia, and injection with D80, all in one step. After freezing the skin with ethyl chloride spray, a 25-gauge needle is advanced gently down to the radial styloid, and 2 to 2.5 mL of anesthesia is injected slowly to dilate the soft tissues around the tendons gradually (a bubble should appear). Moderate pressure to injection, a poorly distensible sac, or both may indicate a chronic stenosis of the tendons (i.e., adhesions). With the needle left in place (avoid multiple punctures), the syringe containing the anesthetic is removed and replaced with the syringe containing 0.5 mL of D80. The treatment is completed by injecting the corticosteroid.

INJECTION AFTERCARE
1. *Rest* for 3 days, by avoiding all gripping, grasping, and direct pressure over the styloid.
2. Use *ice* (15 minutes every 4 to 6 hours) and *acetaminophen (Tylenol ES)* (1000 mg twice a day) for postinjection soreness.
3. *Protect* the wrist for 3 to 4 weeks with a dorsal hood splint, a thumb spica splint, or a Velcro wrist immobilizer worn during the day (optional but recommended for severe or recurrent cases).

DE QUERVAIN'S TENOSYNOVITIS

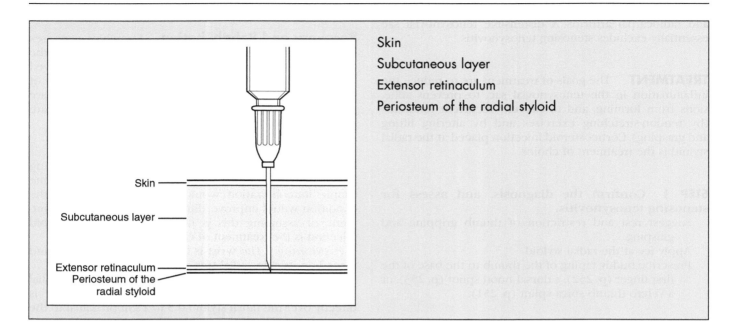

Skin
Subcutaneous layer
Extensor retinaculum
Periosteum of the radial styloid

Skin
Subcutaneous layer
Extensor retinaculum
Periosteum of the
radial styloid

4. Begin passive *stretching exercises* of the thumb in flexion at 3 weeks.
5. Repeat *injection* at 6 weeks if symptoms have not improved by 50% (*warning:* skin and subcutaneous fat atrophy may be greater or permanent with a second injection in 30% of patients).
6. To avoid recurrence, re-emphasize the need to avoid grasping and lifting with the wrist ulna deviated.
7. Obtain a *consultation* with an orthopedic surgeon if two injections in 1 year fail to resolve the condition.

SURGICAL PROCEDURE   Surgical release of the first dorsal compartment is recommended if two injections within 1 year fail to resolve the condition.

PROGNOSIS   Patients who receive treatment within 6 months of developing de Quervain's tenosynovitis have an excellent prognosis. Local injection combined with dilation of the soft tissues over the radial styloid should be effective in 95% of cases. Patients who have had symptoms for longer than 6 months are at risk for fibrosis (stenosing tenosynovitis). Local injection and dilation can be used in these patients, but the results of treatment are not as predictably successful (Table 4-1).

De Quervain's tenosynovitis can occur concomitantly with arthritis of the wrist or CMC joint or CTS. Patients with combined symptoms require x-rays of the wrist and thumb, NCV testing, or both.

4–1   CLINICAL OUTCOMES OF 55 CASES OF DE QUERVAIN'S TENOSYNOVITIS TREATED WITH METHYLPREDNISOLONE (DEPO-MEDROL 80)*

Complete resolution (single injection)	30 (58%)
Recurrence (reinjected; average 11.9 mo to recurrence)	17 (32%)
Failed to respond; chronic tendinitis	5 (10%)
Total	*52*

*Prospective follow-up of 95% of patients enrolled: 4.2 years.
Data from Anderson BL, Manthey R, Brouns ML. Treatment of de Quervain's tenosynovitis with corticosteroids. Arthritis Rheum 34:793-798, 1991.

CARPOMETACARPAL OSTEOARTHRITIS

Enter $^3/_8$ inch proximal to the base of the metacarpal bone, in the "anatomic snuffbox," adjacent to the abductor pollicis longus tendon.

Needle: $^5/_8$-inch, 25-gauge
Depth: $^1/_2$ to $^5/_8$ inch flush against the trapezium bone
Volume: 0.5 mL of anesthetic injected at $^3/_8$ inch and 0.5 mL of K40 injected flush against the trapezium

NOTE: Moderate pressure may be necessary.

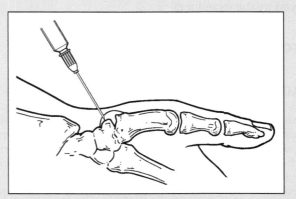

FIGURE 4–2. Carpometacarpal joint injection.

DESCRIPTION CMC joint arthritis is a common form of osteoarthritis of the base of the thumb. Repetitive gripping and grasping and excessive exposure to vibration in susceptible patients (patients with a positive family history) lead to wear and tear of the articular cartilage between the metacarpal of the thumb and the trapezium carpal bone of the wrist. Pain, swelling, bony enlargement, and loss of ROM gradually develop over many years. Advanced disease is associated with loss of articular cartilage, osteophyte formation, and subluxation of the metacarpal bone. Although this is a common form of osteoarthritis, it does not herald the onset of systemic forms of osteoarthritis.

SYMPTOMS The patient has pain, swelling, or enlargement at the base of the thumb. The patient frequently rubs over the radial side of the wrist and the base of the thumb when describing the condition. Not every patient with bony enlargement experiences symptoms.

"I've had to stop crocheting and knitting because of the constant pain in my thumbs."

"My thumbs are starting to look like the arthritis my grandmother had."

"Every time I lift my coffee cup, I get this terribly sharp pain in the base of my thumb."

"It looks like the bones in my thumb are getting bigger."

"The only way I can do my housework is if I put pressure over the thumb and hold it in place."

When an 85-year-old Russian woman, a former potato harvester from Odessa, was asked whether she needed treatment for her severely deformed and arthritic CMC joint, she replied, "No, doctor, it's past the pain part."

EXAM Each patient is examined for swelling and inflammation at the base of the thumb, the degree of subluxation of the metacarpal bone, and loss of ROM of the joint.

EXAM SUMMARY

1. Compression tenderness across the joint
2. Crepitation of the joint in circumduction
3. Pain aggravated at the extremes of thumb motion
4. Bony deformity, subluxation, or both (the shelf sign)
5. Atrophy of the thenar muscles

(1) Tenderness and swelling are present over the base of the thumb. Sensitivity is best shown by compressing the joint in the anteroposterior plane. Pressure applied from the snuffbox is usually much less painful. Swelling is best seen with the wrist turned radial side up. An accurate assessment of the enlargement of the base of the thumb is best appreciated in this position. *(2)* Crepitation is palpable when the metacarpal is rotated forcibly against the trapezium (the mortar and pestle sign). *(3)* Pain often is aggravated when the joint is passively stretched to the extremes of extension and flexion. *(4)* As the condition progresses, greater degrees of bony deformity and metacarpal subluxation contribute to the enlargement of the base. Progressive subluxation creates an abnormality called the *shelf sign.* The smooth contours of the distal radius and thumb are replaced by a bony protuberance of the metacarpal. *(5)* End-stage disease often shows atrophy of the thenar muscles.

X-RAYS X-rays of the wrist (including posteroanterior and lateral views) are often sufficient to determine the degree of osteoarthritic wear and tear in the thumb. Nearly all symptomatic cases have abnormal x-rays. Variable degrees of bony sclerosis, asymmetric joint narrowing, spur formation, and radial-side subluxation can be seen at the trapezial-metacarpal articulation. The early changes on plain x-rays are not always appreciated or commented on by the radiologist (these x-rays should be viewed by the examiner).

SPECIAL TESTING No special testing is indicated.

DIAGNOSIS The diagnosis is based on the clinical findings of local joint tenderness, joint crepitation, and painful motion of the joint coupled with the characteristic abnormalities on plain films at the trapezial-metacarpal articulation. X-rays often are used to gauge the severity of the condition and to predict the need for surgery. A regional anesthetic block occasionally is necessary to differentiate de Quervain's tenosynovitis and radiocarpal arthritis from symptomatic CMC arthritis.

TREATMENT The goals of treatment are to relieve swelling and inflammation, to reduce subluxation (allowing the joint to articulate more freely), and to assess the need for surgery. Overlap taping along with restrictions on heavy gripping and exposure to vibration are the treatments of choice for early disease. Local corticosteroid injection placed in the depths of the anatomic snuffbox is the treatment of choice for more advanced or persistent cases.

STEP 1 **Assess the joint for soft-tissue swelling, bony enlargement, and subluxation; obtain plain x-rays of the wrist (including posteroanterior and lateral views).**

Apply ice over the base of the thumb.

Suggest rest and restriction of gripping and grasping during active treatment.

Recommend oversized tools, grips, and other occupational adjustments.

Demonstrate overlap taping of the joint (p. 251) or prescribe a dorsal hood splint (p. 249) or a Velcro thumb spica splint (p. 251).

Prescribe a 3- to 4-week course of a nonsteroidal anti-inflammatory drug (NSAID) (e.g., ibuprofen [Advil, Motrin]).

STEP 2 (3 TO 4 WEEKS FOR PERSISTENT CASES)
Perform a local injection of K40.

Repeat the injection at 4 to 6 weeks if symptoms have not decreased by 50%.

STEP 3 (6 TO 8 WEEKS FOR RESISTANT CASES)
Combine fixed immobilization using a thumb spica cast (p. 251) with a local corticosteroid injection.

STEP 4 (2 TO 3 MONTHS FOR CHRONIC CASES)
Stretching exercises of the thumb in flexion and extension are used to restore the ROM followed by

active isometric toning exercises of the thumb flexors and extensors (if the patient has improved sufficiently to tolerate them).

Continue to alter or restrict gripping and grasping to prevent future arthritic flare-ups.

Consult with a hand surgeon for implant arthroplasty or tendon graft interposition if two injections, fixed immobilization, and physical therapy exercises fail to restore the function of the thumb and hand.

PHYSICAL THERAPY Physical therapy does not play a significant role in the treatment of CMC osteoarthritis. Instead the focus of therapy is on restricted use, immobilization and taping, and anti-inflammatory treatments. If significant loss of muscle tone has occurred, isometric toning of flexion, extension, abduction, and adduction is recommended. Preferential toning of extension (almost always weaker than flexion) may reduce the tendency of the joint to undergo subluxation to the radial direction.

INJECTION Local anesthetic injection is used to differentiate CMC arthritis from de Quervain's tenosynovitis or radiocarpal joint conditions. Corticosteroid injection is the anti-inflammatory treatment of choice for symptoms persisting beyond 6 to 8 weeks.

Positioning The wrist is kept in neutral position and turned on its side, radial side up.

Surface Anatomy and Point of Entry The proximal end of the metacarpal bone is identified and marked. The point of entry is $3/8$ inch proximal to the metacarpal and adjacent to the abductor pollicis longus tendon.

Angle of Entry and Depth The needle is advanced carefully at a 45-degree angle down to the hard resistance of the trapezium (typical depth is $1/2$ to $5/8$ inch).

Anesthesia Ethyl chloride is sprayed on the skin. Local anesthetic is placed in the subcutaneous fat (0.5 mL) and $1/4$ inch above the trapezium (0.5 mL).

Technique The successful injection must be placed against the trapezium in the depths of the snuffbox and at the level of the periosteum. After anesthesia in the superficial layers, the needle is advanced gently at a 45-degree angle down to the trapezium bone ($1/2$ to $5/8$ inch). If the hard resistance of bone is encountered at a superficial depth ($3/8$ inch), the needle is withdrawn and redirected. In this case, the point of entry may have been too distal, which is a common error. *Note:* The anesthesia needs to be injected above the bone, reserving the deeper site for the corticosteroid. Firm but not hard pressure may be required when injecting at the deeper site. *Caution:* The radial artery courses through the snuffbox. If the needle is advanced slowly, the artery moves to the side. If the radial artery is encountered—blood immediately entering the syringe (10% chance), withdraw completely out of the skin, hold pressure for 5 minutes, re-enter $1/4$ inch to either side, hold pressure for 5 minutes, and redirect the injection.

INJECTION AFTERCARE

1. *Rest* for 3 days, avoiding all grasping, pinching, exposure to vibration, and direct pressure.

CARPOMETACARPAL JOINT INJECTION

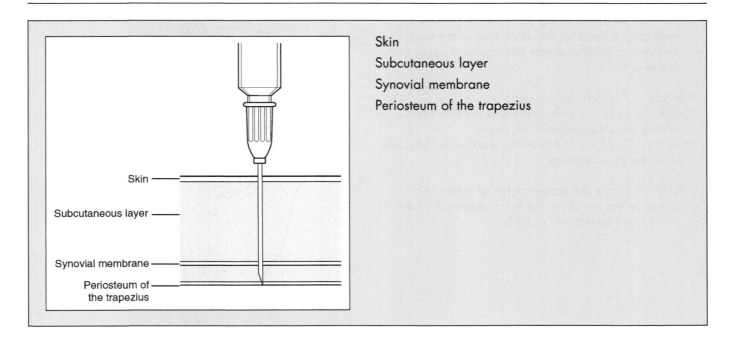

Skin
Subcutaneous layer
Synovial membrane
Periosteum of the trapezius

2. Use *ice* (15 minutes every 4 to 6 hours) and *acetaminophen* (1000 mg twice a day) for postinjection soreness.
3. *Protect* the thumb for 3 to 4 weeks by limiting grasping, pinching, and exposure to vibration or for greater protection with overlap taping the joint, a dorsal hood splint, or a thumb spica splint.
4. Re-emphasize light gripping of pens, padding of hand tools, antivibration types of gloves, and oversized grips for golf clubs and rackets.
5. Begin passive *stretching exercises* of the thumb in flexion and extension at 3 weeks if the ROM was impaired either by the condition or because of the immobilization.
6. Repeat *injection* at 6 weeks if symptoms have not improved by 50%.
7. Obtain a *consultation* with an orthopedic surgeon if two injections, immobilization, and physical therapy fail to provide at least 3 to 4 months of symptomatic relief.

SURGICAL PROCEDURE Surgery is often necessary in working or active patients who present with symptoms and range in age from 45 to 55 years old. Surgery is indicated when symptoms become refractory to treatment or when restrictions, immobilization, and two consecutive injections fail to provide months of symptom-free use. Tendon interpositional arthroplasty—interposition of the flexor carpi radialis tendon between the bones of the joints—is recommended for patients younger than age 62, and trapezial arthroplasty—replacement of the trapezium bone—is performed in patients older than 62. Both procedures are well tolerated and, more importantly, improve the overall function of the thumb in most patients.

PROGNOSIS Local injection is highly successful in the temporary relief of symptoms in most patients. A single injection can provide control of symptoms and improvement in function, especially when swelling predominates over bony enlargement. Two or three treatments over the course of several years can serve as a bridge from the symptomatic phase of the condition to the "burnt-out" phase of the condition (lessening symptoms but with persistent deformity). Because most patients eventually enter this phase of the condition, surgical referral is necessary infrequently (5% to 10% of cases) (Table 4-2). When patients fail to enter this remission phase, or when the response to injection and immobilization gradually shortens (progressive loss of cartilage, bony enlargement, joint subluxation, and persistent inflammation), surgical intervention should be considered.

4-2 CLINICAL OUTCOMES OF 50 CASES OF CARPOMETACARPAL OSTEOARTHRITIS TREATED WITH TRIAMCINOLONE (KENALOG-40)

Epidemiology	Average age 50 yr (range 34-83 yr); ratio of women to men 7:1; right side and left side equally affected
Injection results	46 of 50 (92%) responded to single or multiple treatment, averaging 10 mo of relief (range 3-19 mo)
Surgery	4 patients failed to respond and underwent surgery

Data generated between 1990 and 1996 at Sunnyside Medical Orthopedic Clinic, Portland, Oregon.

GAMEKEEPER'S THUMB

Enter ¹/₄ inch distal to the prominence of the distal metacarpal head on the ulnar side of the joint; use anesthesia to differentiate this ligament injury from acute arthritis.

Needle: ⁵/₈-inch, 25-gauge
Depth: ¹/₈ to ¹/₄ inch, just under the skin and above the ulnar collateral ligament
Volume: 0.25 mL of anesthetic (corticosteroid is not used for this condition)

NOTE: To locate the proper depth of injection, advance the needle to the hard resistance of the bone, then withdraw ¹/₈ inch.

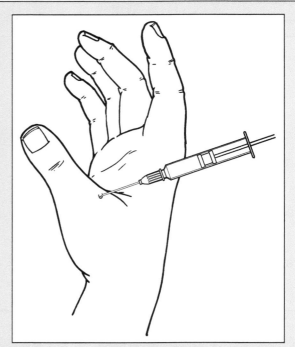

FIGURE 4–3. Gamekeeper's thumb: ulnar collateral ligament injury of the metacarpal joint.

DESCRIPTION The gamekeeper of the royal court was likely to injure the ulnar collateral ligament of the thumb (the metacarpophalangeal [MP] joint) when twisting the necks of the fowl or rabbits hunted for the king. Today, ski pole injuries are the most common cause of this condition. Whether by injury or repetitive use, the disrupted ligament leads to instability of the MP joint, poor pinching and opposition function of the thumb, and in later years degenerative arthritis.

SYMPTOMS In the acute phase, the patient complains of pain and swelling along the ulnar side of the MP joint. In the chronic phase, the patient complains of pain, weakness, or loss of stability. The patient often takes the thumb and first finger and rubs over the MP joint when describing the condition.

"I took a bad fall while skiing. My thumb got caught in my pole straps."

"It's hard for me to sew. My thumb [pointing to the MP joint] hurts when I try to thread the needle."

"My thumb hurts whenever I try to use a hammer."

"I think I dislocated my thumb when I fell down."

"I can't take the lid off my coffee thermos."

"I jammed my thumb really bad. Now it won't bend."

EXAM The MP joint is examined for acute swelling, ROM, and stability of the collateral ligaments.

EXAM SUMMARY

1. Local tenderness and swelling along the ulnar side of the MP joint
2. Pain or excessive motion with valgus stress testing of the ulnar collateral ligament
3. Impaired MP joint flexion and extension, especially when acute and swollen
4. Decreased pinching strength resulting from instability or acute pain
5. Local anesthetic block necessary to assess the extent of ligament injury fully

(1) MP joint tenderness is localized to the ulnar side of the joint. The entire joint may be swollen, or the swelling may be restricted to the ulnar side. *(2)* The MP joint is unstable to stress testing. With the examiner's thumb at the MP joint and index finger at the interphalangeal joint, valgus stability and valgus-induced pain are assessed. A comparison should be made with the stability of the contralateral thumb. *(3)* Impairment of flexion and extension of the MP joint is related directly to the extent of injury

to the ligament and joint. With severe involvement, the MP joint may not flex fully to 90 degrees, and extension may be incomplete. *(4)* The strength or holding power of thumb and first finger may be compromised. *(5)* Local anesthesia placed just over the ulnar collateral ligament allows accurate grading of the injury. Grade 1 injuries have all of the physical signs above but without laxity. Grade 2 partial tears have laxity that readily returns to the normal position. Grade 3 complete tears have looseness to the ligament that does not readily return to its anatomic position.

X-RAYS   Plain x-rays of the hand are usually normal. Late-onset degenerative changes may be present years after the initial injury. No special testing is used at this small joint.

DIAGNOSIS   A tentative diagnosis can be made based on the pain and swelling of the MP joint, the localized tenderness along the ulnar side of the MP joint, and the characteristic aggravation of symptoms with valgus stress applied across the joint. A definitive diagnosis requires anesthetic block, however, to define the extent of ligament injury; this is especially true for higher degree injuries. It is impossible to discern a second-degree from a third-degree injury without anesthesia. This discernment is a crucial step in the evaluation of this injury because third-degree tears require urgent referral to consider primary repair surgery. In addition, local anesthetic block may be necessary to differentiate symptoms arising from the CMC joint or referred from the carpal tunnel.

TREATMENT   Immobilization with a dorsal hood splint or thumb spica cast is the treatment of choice for this ligament injury. Local corticosteroid injection is reserved for cases complicated by osteoarthritis.

■ **STEP 1**   **Local anesthetic block is used to confirm the diagnosis and grade the severity of the injury, and routine x-rays of the thumb (including postero-anterior and lateral views) are obtained to exclude avulsion or bony fracture.**

Apply ice over the MP joint to reduce swelling.

Immobilize with overlap taping (p. 251), a dorsal hood splint (p. 249), or a thumb spica splint (p. 251) to be worn continuously for 4 to 6 weeks to maximize the reattachment of the ligament.

Educate the patient: "The thumb must be protected and completely rested over several weeks to allow the ligaments to reattach in their proper positions."

Immediately obtain a consultation with an orthopedic hand specialist for third-degree, complete tears of the ligament.

■ **STEP 2 (3 TO 6 WEEKS FOR RECOVERY)**   **After immobilization, begin gentle stretching exercises of the thumb in flexion and extension for first-degree and second-degree sprains.**

After flexibility is restored, begin isometric toning of thumb flexion (gripping).

Avoid heavy gripping or grasping until grip has been restored isometrically.

Avoid exposure to vibration.

■ **STEP 3 (6 TO 10 WEEKS FOR CHRONIC CASES)**   **Consider orthopedic consultation if the thumb remains unstable, and there is interference with gripping and grasping.**

Consider corticosteroid injection with D80 for grade 1 and 2 ligament injuries that fail to improve with immobilization and follow-up physical therapy.

Obtain a *consultation* with an orthopedic surgeon specializing in hand surgery if first-degree (simple stretching of the ligament) and second-degree (partial tear of the ligament) sprains fail to improve with immobilization, physical therapy, and a single corticosteroid injection.

■ **STEP 4 (YEARS)**   **Consider intra-articular injection for secondary osteoarthritic changes.**

PHYSICAL THERAPY   *Ice* provides temporary relief of pain and swelling in the acute stage of this injury. After immobilization, gentle, passive *ROM exercises* in flexion and extension are performed for several days to restore full mobility to the thumb. Subsequently, *isometric toning exercises* of thumb flexion (gripping) are begun and followed by more active exercises after ROM and baseline grip strength are restored.

PHYSICAL THERAPY SUMMARY
1. Ice over the MP joint 2. Passive ROM exercises in flexion and extension 3. Toning exercises of gripping, isometrically performed

INJECTION   The indication for injection at the MP joint is limited. Local anesthetic block is used routinely to determine the degree of ligament injury and the decision to refer to the hand surgeon urgently to consider primary repair. Corticosteroid injection is used infrequently. The principal indication is to treat secondary osteoarthritis. Occasionally, corticosteroid is used to arrest the persistent inflammation of a first-degree or second-degree sprain failing to resolve with immobilization and physical therapy.

Positioning   The hand is placed flat with the palm down, the thumb abducted, and the fingers extended.

Surface Anatomy and Point of Entry   The prominence of the MP joint is identified and marked. Enter $1/4$ inch distal to the prominence of the distal metacarpal head in the midplane of the ulnar side of the joint.

LOCAL ANESTHETIC BLOCK FOR GAMEKEEPER'S THUMB

Skin
Subcutaneous layer
Ulnar collateral ligament

Skin

Subcutaneous layer

Ulnar collateral ligament

Angle of Entry and Depth The needle is inserted perpendicular to the skin. The ulnar collateral ligament is the first tissue plane below the subcutaneous tissue, 1/4 inch in depth.

Anesthesia Ethyl chloride is sprayed on the skin. Local anesthetic is placed at the interface of the subcutaneous tissue and the ulnar collateral ligament.

Technique The depth of injection can be determined accurately by gradually advancing the needle until the rubbery resistance of the ulnar collateral ligament is felt. *Note:* A painful reaction to injection or firm resistance during injection suggests that the needle is too deep, likely within the body of the ligament (withdraw 1/8 inch). Alternatively the proper depth can be confirmed by applying traction to the overlying skin. If the needle is placed properly above the ligament, it should move freely in the dermis when applying skin traction. Conversely the needle sticks in place if the tip has penetrated the body of the ligament. In this case, the needle simply is withdrawn 1/8 inch. The local anesthetic always should be injected at the interface between the subcutaneous fat and the ligament.

SURGICAL PROCEDURE The principal indication for surgery is instability. Reattachment of the torn distal ligament, tendon graft repair, or arthrodesis (fusion) is indicated when the stability of the joint has been severely compromised (third-degree sprains). Surgery can be considered for persistent symptoms over months (second-degree sprains) or late in the course of the condition when osteoarthritis intervenes.

PROGNOSIS The outcome of treatment is related directly to the severity of the initial injury and whether or not injury to the underlying articular cartilage has occurred concomitantly. Patients with first-degree microtorn ligament with mild secondary swelling have the best prognosis. In contrast, the prognosis is less predictable for patients with second-degree and third-degree macrotorn ligaments, regardless of the amount of secondary inflammatory response. Patients who exhibit persistent swelling and impaired motion of the joint despite signs of ligament healing likely have injured articular cartilage. These patients have the greatest risk of developing future post-traumatic arthritis.

Most patients have pathology that falls between the extremes. To ensure the optimal results, immobilization must be combined with an appropriate degree of anti-inflammatory treatment when pain, swelling, and impaired flexion and extension persist.

CARPAL TUNNEL SYNDROME

Enter $^1/_2$ to $^3/_4$ inch proximal to the palmar prominence of the wrist, at the distal volar crease, and on the ulnar side of palmaris longus tendon (there is more room between the ulnar side of the tendon and the pisiform).

Needle: $^5/_8$-inch, 25-gauge
Depth: $^1/_2$ to $^5/_8$ inch
Volume: 1 to 2 mL of anesthetic and 0.5 mL of K40

NOTE: If the patient experiences nerve irritation, withdraw 1 or 2 mm or redirect to the radial or ulnar side.

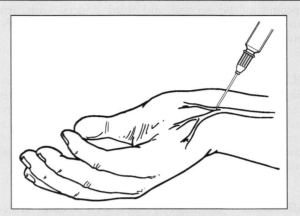

FIGURE 4–4. Carpal tunnel injection.

DESCRIPTION CTS is a compression neuropathy of the median nerve. Compression occurs under the transverse carpal ligament at the wrist, at the pronator teres muscle in the proximal forearm or, rarely, in the distal forearm after penetrating trauma. Traditionally and anatomically, the term *CTS* is used to refer to the compression at the wrist. *Compression neuropathy of the medial nerve* is a more general term that encompasses all causes of median nerve symptoms. Patients present with a variety of symptoms, including hypesthesias, dysesthetic pain in the forearm and hand, muscle weakness, and motor loss with atrophy. The stage of the condition (from sensory loss to motor loss with atrophy) correlates directly with the degree of compression and the chronicity of the symptoms. Mild to moderate CTS (sensory symptoms only) can be managed with a combination of medical treatments. Advanced CTS with motor involvement should be treated with surgical release.

SYMPTOMS The patient complains of a loss of sensation in the tips of the first three fingers, pain traveling through the forearm and wrist, weakness of grip, or all three. The variability in symptoms reflects the stage of the condition, the amount of nerve compression, and the length of time symptoms have been present. The patient often rubs the fingers across the wrist, palm, and first three fingers when describing the condition.

"My thumb and first two fingers go to sleep at night."

"After I've typed all day, I get these shooting pains up and down my arm."

"My hand keeps going numb."

"After long bike rides, my fingers go to sleep."

"My hand feels dead. I've started to drop things."

EXAM The degree of median nerve dysfunction is assessed by examining the sensation of the first three fingers, the degree of nerve irritability with provocative testing, and the integrity of the thumb muscles by inspection and by function testing of thumb opposition. If median nerve symptoms do not seem to be arising from the wrist, the exam is performed at the pronator teres muscle and then at the distal forearm.

EXAM SUMMARY

1. Sensory loss in the first three fingers
2. Loss of thumb opposition
3. Positive Tinel's sign, Phalen's sign, or both
4. Pressure over the pronator teres in the proximal forearm
5. Median nerve block confirming the diagnosis

Depending on the time of day, the amount of use, and the daily variation of symptoms, the examination of the median nerve may reveal total normality despite a clinically significant problem. (1) Two-point discrimination, light touch, and pain sensation may be decreased at the fingertips of the first three digits. (2) The strength of thumb opposition may be decreased; this is best tested by asking the patient to hold the thumb and fifth finger together. (3) Tests for Tinel's sign and Phalen's sign are performed at the wrist to test nerve irritability. The test for Tinel's sign should be performed using vigorous tapping over the transverse carpal ligament, with the wrist held in extension. The test for Phalen's sign—holding both wrists in extreme volar flexion—should be held for 30 to 60 seconds. (4) If these results are negative, compression in the forearm should be performed. Pressure is applied 1 to 2 inches distal to the antecubital fossa. This pressure can be enhanced by resisting forearm pronation. (5) Further confirmation of the diagnosis can be made by median nerve block at the wrist or short-term response to corticosteroid injection.

Median nerve distribution varies from one patient to another. Most patients experience paresthesia in the first three fingers; however, a few patients may experience symptoms in the second and third fingers, with little involvement of the thumb. Occasionally a median nerve involves the radial side of the fourth finger.

SPECIAL TESTING No characteristic changes in x-rays occur with CTS. X-rays of the wrist are unnecessary, unless there is clinical evidence of an underlying carpal or radiocarpal arthritis. NCV testing is the test of choice. The result of NCV testing is positive in approximately 70% of cases. A negative result on NCV testing does *not* totally exclude the presence of median nerve compression.

DIAGNOSIS In advanced cases, such as cases involving prolonged symptoms or motor involvement, NCV testing is the diagnostic test of choice, and it has high predictive value; however, patients with intermittent symptoms or mild sensory symptoms present a diagnostic dilemma. The result of NCV testing is often normal in these patients. When the diagnosis is suspected on clinical grounds (e.g., a characteristic pain pattern, Tinel's sign, or Phalen's sign), a regional anesthetic block plus a corticosteroid injection should be considered. Almost 90% of patients experience relief from this procedure, helping to confirm the clinical suspicion of CTS.

TREATMENT The goals of treatment are to reduce compression of the nerve, to treat concurrent flexor tenosynovitis, and to prevent a recurrence of CTS through improved ergonomics. For early disease, the treatments of choice include adjustments at the patient's workstation and wrist splinting. Advanced disease with motor involvement should be treated with surgery.

STEP 1 Evaluate the stage of the condition and the underlying cause by clinical or NCV testing. Treat the underlying cause using diuretics (if fluid retention is found), NSAIDs (if there is rheumatoid arthritis), or levothyroxine (for myxedema).
Reduce gripping, grasping, and repetitive wrist motion.
Use antivibration padded gloves (Sorbothane orthotic devices).
Make ergonomic adjustments of the wrist at the keyboard or assembly line.
Use a Velcro wrist splint with metal stay to reduce the symptoms manifesting at night; the splint is used continuously, day and night, for optimal results (p. 249).

STEP 2 (2 TO 4 WEEKS FOR PERSISTENT CASES) Re-evaluate the stage of the condition.
Order NCV testing in patients with persistent or progressive symptoms, patients with motor involvement (subjective weakness, diminished grip strength, atrophy), and patients contemplating surgery.

Order x-rays of the wrist (including posteroanterior, lateral, and carpal tunnel views) to exclude primary arthritis of the wrist and a lunate dislocation.
Perform a local injection of K40 (for sensory symptoms only).
Prescribe a Velcro wrist splint to be used day and night.
Repeat the injection in 4 to 6 weeks if symptoms have not been reduced by 50%.

STEP 3 (6 TO 8 WEEKS FOR CHRONIC SYMPTOMS): Begin stretching exercises in extension to improve flexibility of the flexor tendons if symptoms have improved (p. 278).
Re-emphasize ergonomics and proper use.
Request a neurosurgical or orthopedic consultation if two injections fail to control sensory symptoms; consultation is strongly advised if the patient shows impairment or loss of motor function.

PHYSICAL THERAPY Although surgical release is still the mainstay of treatment, more emphasis has been placed on the role of physical therapy in the management of CTS. Ergonomic adjustments can have a tremendous impact on the response to treatment and on the rehabilitation of the condition. Proper hand and wrist placement according to normal anatomic position cannot be over-emphasized. In addition, stretching exercises of the nine flexor tendons of the hand may reduce the overall recurrence rate (p. 278). These stretching exercises are especially helpful when combined with local corticosteroid injection.

INJECTION The indications for corticosteroid injection are limited to special situations. Corticosteroid injection is used for patients adamant about avoiding surgery, patients with symptoms restricted to mild to moderate CTS, and patients with CTS-compatible symptoms and normal NCV testing. Approximately 30% of patients with CTS have intermittent symptoms, equivocal signs on examination of the upper extremity and neck, and normal NCV testing. Because patients with this constellation of findings still respond to corticosteroid injection (90%), empirical treatment has been advocated as a diagnostic aid.
Positioning The wrist is placed palm up, dorsiflexed to 30 degrees.
Surface Anatomy and Point of Entry The pisiform bone and the palmaris longus tendons are located and marked. The point of entry is at the intersection of the distal volar crease and the ulnar side of the palmaris longus.
Angle of Entry and Depth The needle is advanced carefully at a 45-degree angle down to and through the transverse carpal ligament (typical depth is $^3/_8$ to $^1/_2$ inch). This angle coupled with the short $^5/_8$-inch needle makes it nearly impossible to enter the nerve.
Anesthesia Ethyl chloride is sprayed on the skin. Local anesthetic is placed in the subcutaneous fat (0.5 mL), at the firm resistance of the transverse carpal ligament

CARPAL TUNNEL INJECTION

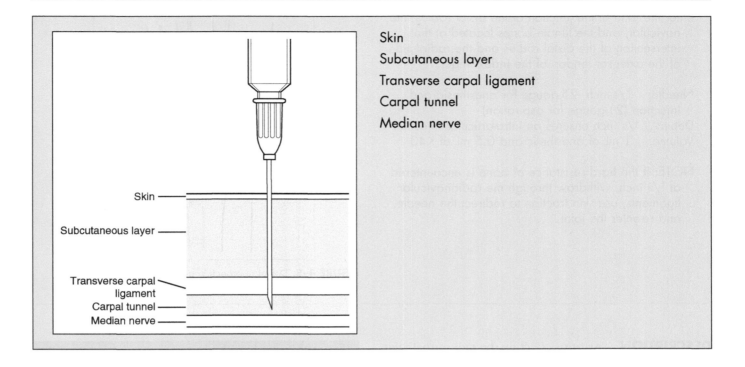

Skin
Subcutaneous layer
Transverse carpal ligament
Carpal tunnel
Median nerve

Skin
Subcutaneous layer
Transverse carpal ligament
Carpal tunnel
Median nerve

(0.5 mL), and in the carpal tunnel (0.5 to 1 mL). A median nerve block confirms the accurate placement.

Technique The successful injection must be placed just underneath the transverse carpal ligament. The proper depth can be determined by measurement, by feel as the needle is advanced, and by the flow of medication. Based on the point of entry and the 45-degree angle of entry, the proper depth of injection is $1/2$ to $5/8$ inch. As the needle is advanced through the ligament, a "popping" or a "giving-way" sensation is often felt. Lastly, the flow of medication above or within the transverse ligament requires moderate pressure as opposed to the minimum pressure that is required when injecting medication in the tunnel. The patient may experience a temporary median nerve irritation when the needle enters the tunnel. *Note:* If the patient continues to feel nerve irritation with injection, the needle is repositioned or withdrawn $1/8$ inch.

INJECTION AFTERCARE

1. *Rest* for 3 days, avoiding all wrist movement, finger motion, and exposure to vibration and direct pressure.
2. Use *ice* (15 minutes every 4 to 6 hours) and *acetaminophen* (1000 mg twice a day) for postinjection soreness.
3. *Protect* the wrist for 3 to 4 weeks with a Velcro wrist immobilizer with a metal stay and by limiting grasping, pinching, gripping, and exposure to vibration.
4. Re-emphasize the need to make ergonomic adjustments at the workstation.

5. Begin passive *stretching exercises* of the fingers in extension at 3 to 4 weeks.
6. Repeat the *injection* at 6 weeks if symptoms have not improved by 50%.
7. Obtain a *consultation* with a neurosurgeon or an orthopedic surgeon if two injections fail to provide at least 4 to 6 months of symptomatic relief or if loss of motor function intervenes.

SURGICAL PROCEDURE Release of the transverse carpal ligament is the treatment of choice for persistent symptoms and motor involvement (recurrent median nerve involvement).

PROGNOSIS Medical therapy provides long-term control of symptoms in less than half of patients. A local injection is highly effective in the short-term (months), but only 25% to 30% have long-term benefit over years. Symptoms often persist because of secondary factors, especially repetitive wrist and hand use, uncontrollable factors on the job, and unavoidable exposure to vibration.

Surgery is indicated for persistent or slowly progressive nerve dysfunction or motor loss, such as loss of grip and specific loss of thumb opposition. Surgical release of the transverse carpal ligament is successful in 90% of cases; 10% of cases fail to improve because of nerve damage, postoperative neuritis, or recurrent compression secondary to scar tissue formation.

RADIOCARPAL JOINT ARTHROCENTESIS

Enter the joint at the junction of the distal radius, the navicular, and the lunate bones located at the intersection of the distal radius and the radial side of the extensor tendon of the index finger.

Needle: 5/8-inch, 25-gauge for anesthesia and injection (21-gauge for aspiration)
Depth: 1/2 inch ensures an intra-articular injection
Volume: 1 mL of anesthetic and 0.5 mL of K40

NOTE: If the hard resistance of bone is encountered at 1/4 inch, withdraw through the radionavicular ligaments, use skin traction to redirect the needle, and re-enter the joint.

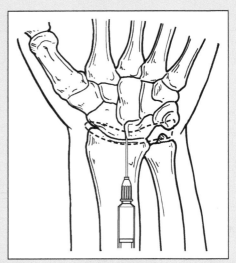

FIGURE 4–5. Dorsal approach to arthrocentesis and injection of the wrist joint.

DESCRIPTION   Arthritis affecting the radiocarpal joint is uncommon. Significant involvement of the wrist joint always should be suspected with dorsal swelling associated with loss of flexion and extension (average ROM is 90 degrees in flexion and 80 degrees in extension). Aspiration of synovial fluid and laboratory analysis are indicated to differentiate rheumatoid arthritis, post-traumatic osteoarthritis, crystal-induced arthropathy, and the uncommon septic arthritis. Radiocarpal joint involvement in rheumatoid arthritis is common. Osteoarthritis of the wrist is uncommon and nearly always results from injury (multiple wrist sprains, fracture of the navicular or distal radius, or dislocation of the carpal bones). Persistent swelling at the radiocarpal joint can lead to secondary CTS symptoms.

SYMPTOMS   The patient complains of pain, swelling, and loss of ROM at the wrist. The patient often rubs over the dorsum of the wrist when describing the condition.

"I can't bend my wrist."

"My wrist is swollen."

"I cannot perform my usual assembly job. The constant turning of my wrist has become too painful."

"I've sprained my wrist so many times that I've lost count. Over the last few years of basketball coaching, my wrist has slowly begun to stiffen."

EXAM   Each patient is examined for dorsal wrist swelling, for tenderness over the proximal navicular, and for pain and loss of ROM in dorsiflexion and volar flexion.

EXAM SUMMARY

1. Tenderness at the intersection of the navicular, radius, and extensor tendons
2. Loss of ROM and end-point stiffness or pain with forced flexion or extension
3. Swelling over the dorsum
4. Associated bony enlargement, ganglion, or prominent carpal bones over the dorsum

(1) Joint line tenderness is located at the intersection of the distal radius and to the radial side of the extensor tendon of the first finger. Firm pressure is applied over the navicular with or without passive flexion of the finger. Local tenderness also may be palpable in the proximal snuffbox. *(2)* Loss of ROM and end-point stiffness occur with passive flexion and extension of the wrist. The normal ROM is 90 degrees for flexion and 80 degrees for extension. Severe wrist involvement shows only 45 degrees of flexion and extension. *(3)* Swelling of the wrist is best appreciated over the dorsum of the wrist. Subtle swelling fills in the depression over the navicular. Moderate to severe swelling of the joint causes a visible bulging or convexity over the navicular. *(4)* Advanced osteoarthritis of the wrist may cause bony enlargement dorsally or overproduction of synovial fluid, causing a soft tissue ganglion.

X-RAYS   X-rays of the wrist (including posteroanterior, lateral, and oblique) always are recommended. The normal thickness of the articular cartilage between the radius and navicular is 2 to 3 mm. Rheumatoid arthritis causes a symmetric loss of cartilage and the characteristic thinning of the bones (juxta-articular osteoporosis). Osteoarthritis of the wrist causes an asymmetric loss of cartilage, sclerosis of the radius and navicular bones, and gradual resorption of the navicular (shrinkage).

SPECIAL TESTING   Synovial fluid analysis is indicated when septic arthritis and crystal-induced arthritis must be excluded.

DIAGNOSIS   The diagnosis of rheumatoid arthritis or osteoarthritis is strongly suggested by the physical exam findings of loss of ROM and local tenderness. The diagnosis can be confirmed by intra-articular injection of local anesthesia. If septic arthritis or gout/pseudogout is suspected, synovial fluid analysis must be performed.

TREATMENT   The goals of treatment are to reduce the inflammation and to restore the ROM of the joint. Aspiration of fluid for laboratory analysis is often unsuccessful. For mild wrist involvement, ice and a Velcro wrist immobilizer are the treatments of choice. Local corticosteroid injection is the treatment of choice for moderate to severe involvement of the nonseptic effusion. Septic arthritis is rare.

STEP 1   Measure the ROM in flexion and extension (volar flexion and dorsiflexion), and order plain x-rays of the wrist (including posteroanterior, lateral, and oblique views).

  Aspirate, flush the joint with saline, and send the fluid for diagnostic studies if septic arthritis is suspected: Gram stain and culture, uric acid crystal analysis, and cell count and differential.

  Apply ice over the dorsum of the wrist for 15 minutes several times a day.

  Avoid repetitious movement, including gripping, grasping, and bending.

  Prescribe a Velcro wrist immobilizer with a metal stay (p. 249).

  Prescribe an NSAID (e.g., ibuprofen) for 3 to 4 weeks.

  Describe ergonomic adjustments at the workstation, which include keeping repetitive work within 1 to $1^1/_2$ feet of the torso, keeping the wrists straight and aligned with the forearms, and performing most lifting with both hands.

  Prescribe glucosamine sulfate, 1500 mg/day.

STEP 2 (1 TO 3 DAYS AFTER LABORATORY ANALYSIS)   If septic arthritis is not a consideration, and the patient already has tried an oral NSAID, perform an intra-articular injection of K40 for a rheumatoid or osteoarthritic effusion.

  Continue the Velcro wrist immobilizer with metal stay.

  Begin gentle ROM stretch exercises to restore full flexion and extension.

STEP 3 (3 TO 4 WEEKS FOR PERSISTENT CASES)   Repeat the local injection of K40 if there is persistent swelling and pain.

  Continue ROM exercises to restore full flexion and extension.

STEP 4 (3 MONTHS FOR CHRONIC CASES)   If symptoms persist, and at least half of the normal ROM has been lost, consider an orthopedic consultation for diagnostic arthroscopy or joint fusion.

PHYSICAL THERAPY   Physical therapy plays a minor role in the active treatment of radiocarpal arthritis and a significant role in the prevention of future arthritic flares. *Ice* applications and phonophoresis with a hydrocortisone gel are effective for the temporary control of pain and swelling. As soon as acute symptoms have been controlled, gentle *ROM exercises* are performed passively. *Isometric toning exercises* (p. 276) of gripping and wrist flexion and extension are performed after all symptoms have resolved. Increasing the resting tone of the extensor muscles—restoring the balance between the strength of the flexor muscles and the extensor muscles—should provide the best protection against future arthritic flares.

PHYSICAL THERAPY SUMMARY

1. Ice over the dorsum of the wrist
2. Phonophoresis with a hydrocortisone gel
3. Toning exercises of gripping, isometrically performed
4. Toning exercises of wrist extension, isometrically performed

---

INJECTION   Local corticosteroid injection commonly is used when ice, restricted use, immobilization, and an oral NSAID fail to control symptoms.

Positioning   The hand and wrist are placed in the prone position. The wrist is flexed to 30 degrees and held in place with a rolled-up towel.

Surface Anatomy and Point of Entry   The extensor tendon of the index finger is identified and marked as it crosses the radius. The edge of the distal radius is palpated and marked. The point of entry is on the radial side of the tendon and the distal edge of the radius. Alternatively the exact point of entry can be found by gently placing a pen firmly against the skin between the radius, navicular, and lunate. The point of entry is determined where the pen makes the greatest indentation.

Angle of Entry and Depth   The needle is inserted perpendicular to the skin. The average depth is $^1/_2$ inch. If the firm resistance of bone or ligament is encountered at a superficial depth ($^1/_4$ to $^3/_8$ inch), the needle must be withdrawn back through the ligament and repositioned with the aid of skin traction.

RADIOCARPAL JOINT INJECTION

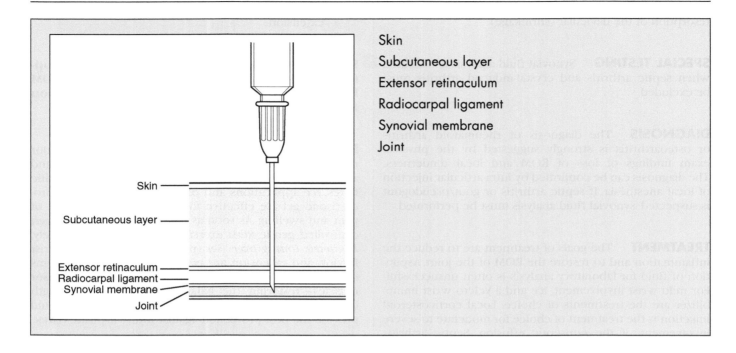

Skin
Subcutaneous layer
Extensor retinaculum
Radiocarpal ligament
Synovial membrane
Joint

Skin ⎯
Subcutaneous layer ⎯
Extensor retinaculum ⎯
Radiocarpal ligament ⎯
Synovial membrane ⎯
Joint ⎯

Technique   The *dorsal approach* is preferred. A successful injection carefully enters the ¼-inch space between the radius, navicular, and lunate at a depth of ½ inch. The 25-gauge needle is advanced perpendicularly through the radionavicular ligament and into the wrist. The needle must be redirected if bone is encountered at ¼ inch. If fluid is not obtained with the 25-gauge needle, a 22-gauge needle can be used to aspirate. If aspiration is still negative, the joint can be irrigated with 1 to 2 mL of sterile saline and sent for Gram stain and culture. For the aseptic effusion, the needle is left in place, and the joint is injected with 0.5 mL of K40.

INJECTION AFTERCARE

1. *Rest* for 3 days, avoiding repetitive motion, tension across the wrist, and direct pressure.
2. Use *ice* (15 minutes every 4 to 6 hours) and *acetaminophen* (1000 mg twice a day) for postinjection soreness.
3. *Protect* the wrist for 3 to 4 weeks with a Velcro wrist brace worn continuously for the first week (especially for advanced disease with loss of 30% to 40% of ROM).
4. Begin *isometric toning exercises* of wrist flexion and extension at 3 weeks.
5. Repeat *injection* at 6 weeks if swelling persists or chronic synovial thickening develops.
6. Advise on the long-term protection of the joint (e.g., avoid vibration exposure and heavy impact, maintain forearm muscle tone to support the joint, wear a wrist brace with heavy use).
7. Obtain a *consultation* with an orthopedic surgeon if

symptoms persist, if 50% of normal ROM has been lost, and if the patient is willing to undergo surgical fusion.

SURGICAL PROCEDURE   Patients with severe restrictions of motion (>50% loss) and persistent symptoms can be considered for fusion of the wrist (arthrodesis). The patient has to be willing to accept the loss of wrist motion in exchange for pain control. Although this surgery is effective in controlling symptoms, few patients want to sacrifice the last remaining motion of the joint.

PROGNOSIS   Rheumatoid arthritis and post-traumatic osteoarthritis—the dominant conditions affecting the radiocarpal joint—are readily diagnosed by a combination of x-ray changes and serologic abnormalities. Both conditions respond favorably, albeit temporarily, to intra-articular injection. To ensure optimal results, corticosteroid injection should be combined with fixed immobilization. Septic arthritis requires synovial fluid analysis to confirm the diagnosis and to decide on the appropriate intravenous antibiotics. Whenever joint aspiration yields small volumes of fluid (<1 mL), priority should be given to analysis of Gram stain and culture.

Patients with persistent wrist swelling, limited ROM, normal x-rays, and normal blood serologies in the setting of wrist trauma should be considered for special studies. Bone scanning and MRI may show disruption of the triangular cartilage of the separate ulnocarpal joint, carpal dissociation, intraosseous ganglion, or other subtle changes of the lunate, navicular, or radius.

DORSAL GANGLION

Enter at the base of the palpable cyst, paralleling the skin and avoiding the adjacent veins or tendons.

Needle: ⁵/₈-inch, 25-gauge for anesthesia; 1¹/₂-inch, 18-gauge for aspiration
Depth: variable, rarely below ³/₈ inch
Volume: 0.5 mL of anesthetic in the subcutaneous tissues adjacent to the cyst wall and 0.5 mL of K40

NOTE: A 10-mL syringe is necessary to obtain enough vacuum pressure to aspirate the highly viscous fluid.

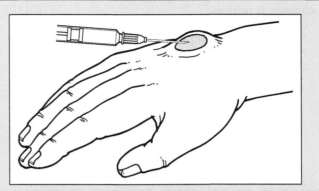

FIGURE 4–6. Dorsal ganglion aspiration and injection.

DESCRIPTION A dorsal ganglion is an abnormal accumulation of synovial or tenosynovial fluid. Subtle abnormalities in the wrist or the extensor tendon sheath cause an overproduction of fluid that leaks into the subcutaneous tissue. The fluid, rich in protein content, irritates the tissues and leads to cyst formation. The overproduction of fluid is always due to subtle abnormalities of the wrist joint or the extensor tendon sheath (e.g., old cartilaginous or tendon injury, poor muscular support, hypermobility caused by too lax supporting ligaments). Other names for this common condition include Bible cyst, wrist cyst, or dorsal tendon cyst. Volar synovial cysts, located almost exclusively at the base of the thumb, occur but are distinctly less common, occurring in a ratio of 1:20 or less.

SYMPTOMS Most patients complain of a painless lump at the wrist. Some patients have symptomatic cysts, however, when pressure is exerted on an adjacent structure (e.g., pressure on the carpal bones, neuritic complaints when pressure occurs on the superficial branch of the radial nerve).

"I noticed this swelling over my wrist. My brothers have all died of cancer, and I'm very worried about it."

"I developed this really ugly swelling over the back of my hand. I want it taken off."

"I type all day long. Over the last several months I have noticed this lump on the back of my hand."

"I've had this bump on the back of my wrist for years, but it recently has grown bigger."

EXAM The characteristics (e.g., size, mobility, and compressibility) of the cyst are evaluated, and an assessment is made of the function of the wrist joint and the dorsal tendons that cross the wrist.

EXAM SUMMARY

1. A highly mobile, fluctuant cyst overlying the wrist
2. Minimal tenderness
3. Normal wrist motion in most cases
4. A characteristic highly viscous aspirate

(1) A 1- to 2-cm, highly mobile, fluctuant-to-tense cyst is palpable in the subcutaneous tissue. It should not be grossly adherent to the underlying tissue. *(2)* Tenderness is minimal, unless the cyst is pressing against one of the cutaneous nerves (a superficial branch of the radial nerve; causes numbness or paresthesias over the back of the hand and fingers). *(3)* Wrist motion is painless and full, unless underlying carpal or radiocarpal arthritis is present. *(4)* The diagnosis is confirmed by aspirating the thick, highly viscous, nearly colorless fluid from the cyst (the consistency of Karo syrup or 90-weight lubricating oil).

X-RAYS X-rays of the wrist are unnecessary for the diagnosis. Most x-rays are normal, unless there is underlying carpal or radiocarpal arthritis.

SPECIAL TESTING No special testing is indicated.

DIAGNOSIS The diagnosis is confirmed by showing the typical thick, nonbloody aspirate.

TREATMENT The goals of treatment are to reassure the patient that this is not a serious problem, to decompress the cyst, and to prevent recurrent cyst formation. The treatment of choice is simple aspiration.

STEP 1   Determine the dimensions of the cyst, measure the motion of the wrist, and note whether the cyst moves with passive movement of the extensor tendons.

Observe the cyst, which may diminish with time.

Educate the patient: "This may resolve spontaneously."

Perform a simple aspiration.

Limit wrist motions, emphasizing keeping any repetitive work within 1 to 1½ feet directly in front, holding the wrists aligned with the forearms, and performing lifting with both hands.

Avoid vibration.

Use a Velcro wrist brace with metal stay to reduce the overproduction of fluid (p. 249).

STEP 2 (8 TO 10 WEEKS FOR PERSISTENT CASES)   Repeat aspiration, and inject with K40.

Continue using the wrist brace.

STEP 3 (≥12 WEEKS FOR CHRONIC CASES)   Consider a repeat injection with K40 (if the first treatment was partially successful).

Perform gripping and wrist-toning exercises (p. 276), especially if the ganglion is associated with a chronic or recurrent wrist condition.

Consider an orthopedic consultation for removal if the patient has pressure symptoms, radial nerve paresthesias, or a chronic wrist condition with significant loss of range of function (motion or strength).

Educate the patient: "Some cases may recur even after surgical removal, depending on whether you continue to produce too much lubricating fluid."

PHYSICAL THERAPY   The role of physical therapy is limited in the treatment and prevention of ganglia. Wrist-strengthening exercises (p. 276) are indicated if there is clinical evidence of underlying radiocarpal arthritis. Generally, isometric toning exercises are performed to strengthen wrist extension and flexion in patients who work intensively with their hands.

INJECTION   Aspiration is the treatment of choice for ganglia that fail to resolve with time. At least half of ganglia respond to simple aspiration. Corticosteroid injection is the treatment of choice for ganglia that cause pressure on a superficial branch of the radial nerve (dysesthetic pain on the dorsum of the hand and fingers) and for recurrent cysts that are larger than 1 inch in diameter.

Positioning   The hand and wrist are placed in the prone position. The wrist is flexed 30 to 45 degrees and held in place with a rolled-up towel.

Surface Anatomy and Point of Entry   Most dorsal ganglia are located directly over the navicular and are more prominent when the wrist is flexed. The point of entry is at the proximal base of the cyst away from any local vein or tendon.

Angle of Entry and Depth   The 18-gauge needle is advanced into the center of the cyst, paralleling the skin. The depth is rarely more than ¼ to ⅜ inch from the surface.

DORSAL GANGLION INJECTION

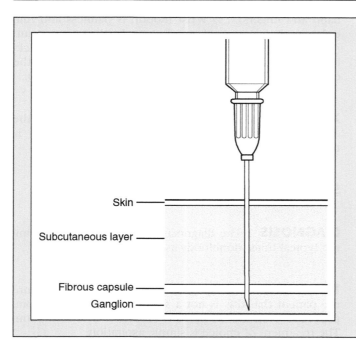

Skin
Subcutaneous layer
Fibrous capsule
Ganglion

Skin —
Subcutaneous layer —
Fibrous capsule —
Ganglion —

Anesthesia   Ethyl chloride is sprayed on the skin. Local anesthetic is placed in the subcutaneous fat adjacent to the cyst (the cyst wall has few, if any, nerve endings).

Technique   Success of injection depends on complete cyst aspiration and subsequent injection through the same needle. Optimal aspiration is at the *base* of the ganglion. An 18-gauge needle attached to a 10-mL syringe is advanced into the center of the cyst. The bevel of the needle is rotated 180 degrees, and the highly viscous fluid is removed. Manual pressure applied from either side may assist in the removal of the fluid. With the needle left in place, the cyst is injected with 0.5 mL of K40.

INJECTION AFTERCARE

1. *Rest* for 3 days, avoiding repetitious motion, tension across the wrist, and direct pressure.
2. Use *ice* (15 minutes every 4 to 6 hours) and *acetaminophen* (1000 mg twice a day) for postinjection soreness.
3. *Protect* the wrist for 3 to 4 weeks by avoiding repetitive lifting, gripping, grasping, and vibration.
4. Suggest that a Velcro wrist brace be worn if advanced wrist arthritis is present.
5. Begin *isometric toning exercises* of wrist flexion and extension at 3 weeks if the forearm muscles have weakened from disuse.
6. Repeat *injection* at 6 weeks with corticosteroid if fluid reaccumulates.
7. Consider an intra-articular injection of the radiocarpal joint to reduce the overproduction of joint fluid (especially with significant radiocarpal joint disease).
8. Obtain a *consultation* with an orthopedic surgeon if the patient has pressure symptoms, radial nerve paresthesias, or swelling that interferes with normal wrist motion.

SURGICAL PROCEDURE   Excision of the cyst and sinus tract is the surgical procedure for a ganglion.

PROGNOSIS   Without exception, patients diagnosed with a dorsal ganglion have an underlying radiocarpal joint or extensor tenosynovitis causing an overproduction of fluid. Evaluation should include a thorough examination of the wrist joint, extensor tendons, and measurement of grip and forearm muscle strength. Patients with recurrent dorsal ganglia should undergo radiographic studies to identify the subtle abnormalities involving the joint. All patients must be apprised of the relationship of the ganglion to the subtle abnormalities affecting the joint and tendons and the frequent recurrence rates based on this relationship.

The results of aspiration and injection vary. Simple aspiration is effective in 50% of cases. Aspiration must be combined with corticosteroid injection to resolve an additional 30% of cases. Approximately 20% of patients fail to respond to aspiration with corticosteroid injection because of constant overproduction of fluid (e.g., chronic arthritis, chronic tenosynovitis, tendon scarring). Surgical removal of the cyst and the sinus tract can be offered to these patients.

NAVICULAR FRACTURE AND SEVERE WRIST SPRAIN

A tentative diagnosis of navicular fracture is made if the patient has sustained a fall on an outstretched hand or has suffered a direct blow to the wrist, especially when associated with the following signs:

Dramatic tenderness over the dorsum of the wrist
Dramatic tenderness in the anatomic snuffbox
Loss of half the normal range of motion owing to pain and mechanical limitation of motion
Treatment of choice: fixed immobilization to protect against avascular necrosis, nonunion, or medicolegal entanglement

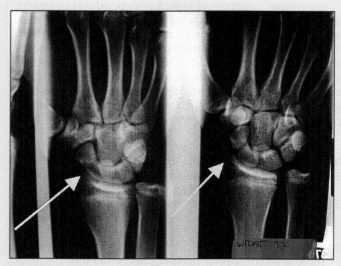

FIGURE 4–7. Traumatic navicular fracture (*arrows* point to the mid-body fracture).

DESCRIPTION Patients with an uncomplicated sprained wrist can be treated with ice, a simple wrist brace, and limited use over 7 to 10 days with uniform good results. When wrist pain is severe, snuffbox or dorsal wrist tenderness is dramatic, and the ROM of the wrist has been decreased by 50%, the health care provider must evaluate and treat for navicular fracture, lunate dislocation, or carpal avascular necrosis. Failure to recognize the fracture can result in a poor outcome for the patient and potential medicolegal issues for the health care provider.

SYMPTOMS The patient complains of pain, swelling, and loss of ROM at the wrist. The patient often supports the wrist with the contralateral hand, resisting any movement.

"I fell skateboarding, and now I can't bend my wrist."

"Any movement of my wrist hurts like hell."

"I fell several weeks ago. My doctor told me my x-rays were okay. Now I'm having more and more trouble moving my wrist."

"I've sprained my wrist again. But this seems so different. It's so much more painful and stiff."

EXAM The patient is examined for navicular tenderness, painful loss of wrist ROM in flexion and extension, and swelling over the dorsum.

EXAM SUMMARY

1. Acute navicular tenderness over the dorsum of the wrist, in the anatomic snuffbox, or both
2. Acute loss of half the normal ROM of wrist in flexion and extension, restricted by severe pain
3. Acute swelling over the dorsum
4. Chronic navicular fracture is characterized by a progressive or chronic loss of ROM and moderate local navicular tenderness

(1) The hallmark sign of navicular fracture is exquisite bony tenderness over the dorsum of the wrist, in the depths of the anatomic snuffbox, or both. Fractures of the proximal navicular may be most tender over the dorsum. Distal navicular fractures have classic tenderness in the anatomic snuffbox. *(2)* Passive flexion and extension of the wrist is exquisitely painful. Most patients guard most movement of the wrist and resist any attempts to move the wrist beyond 45 degrees of flexion and extension (loss of half the normal movement). *(3)* Swelling of the wrist is best appreciated over the dorsum of the wrist. Subtle swelling fills in the depression over the navicular. Moderate to severe swelling of the joint causes a visible bulging or convexity over the navicular. *(4)* Chronic navicular fracture, undiagnosed in the acute phase, is characterized by progressive or chronic loss of ROM

(approaching a loss of 50% of normal) and moderate bony tenderness over the dorsal navicular.

X-RAYS X-rays of the wrist (including posteroanterior, lateral, and oblique) are always recommended. Small, nondisplaced fractures may have normal initial films. Serial films over 2 to 3 weeks eventually show the fracture line as the bone heals.

SPECIAL TESTING Bone scanning and MRI are sensitive tests for navicular fracture.

DIAGNOSIS A tentative diagnosis is based on a history of wrist trauma, an exam showing local navicular tenderness either over the dorsum or within the depths of the anatomic snuffbox, and the painful loss of flexion and extension of the wrist. The diagnosis rests on showing the fracture by sequential plain x-rays of the wrist, cone-down views of the navicular, or special testing.

TREATMENT If navicular fracture is suspected, suggested either by the severity of the injury or by the dramatic changes on exam, fixed immobilization of the wrist and thumb and close follow-up are mandatory.

STEP 1 **Measure the ROM in flexion and extension (volar flexion and dorsiflexion) and order plain x-rays of the wrist (posteroanterior, lateral, and oblique views).**
  Consider local anesthetic block to distinguish de Quervain's or extensor tenosynovitis from involvement of the radiocarpal joint if equivocal signs on examination are present.
  Apply ice over the dorsum of the wrist for the acute swelling.
  Prescribe a thumb spica cast or posterior splint that incorporates immobilization of the thumb to be worn continuously until orthopedic surgeon consultation is completed (p. 251).
  Prescribe an analgesic for pain.
  Obtain an urgent orthopedic consultation to confirm the diagnosis and continue care.

STEP 2 (2 TO 4 WEEKS) **X-rays should be repeated at 2 to 4 weeks to evaluate the progress of healing and to exclude avascular necrosis or bony nonunion.**

STEP 3 (4 TO 6 WEEKS AFTER THE ACUTE MANAGEMENT) **Continue immobilization with a thumb spica cast or Velcro wrist immobilizer with metal stay.**
  Begin gentle stretching ROM exercises to restore full flexion and extension.

Begin isometric toning exercises of gripping, wrist flexion, and wrist extension.
Resume activities of daily living and sport activities gradually.

STEP 4 (3 MONTHS FOR CHRONIC CASES) **If symptoms persist, and at least half of the normal ROM has been lost, consider an orthopedic consultation for joint fusion.**

PHYSICAL THERAPY Physical therapy plays a minor role in the active treatment of navicular fracture but a significant role in the rehabilitation after immobilization or surgical intervention. *Ice* applications are effective for the temporary control of acute pain and swelling. Gentle *ROM exercises* in flexion and extension are necessary to restore full ROM to the wrist. These are begun after the active period of immobilization or surgery. *Isometric toning exercises* of gripping and wrist flexion (p. 276) and extension are begun after unequivocal progress has been made on restoring flexibility. Increasing the resting tone of the flexor and extensor muscles of the wrist—restoring the balance in strength between these muscle groups—should provide the best protection against future injury and the development of osteoarthritis.

PHYSICAL THERAPY SUMMARY

1. Ice over the dorsum of the wrist acutely
2. Gentle ROM exercises in flexion and extension
3. Toning exercises of gripping, wrist extension, and wrist flexion, isometrically performed

---

INJECTION Local injection is performed only when the unusual combination of navicular fracture and de Quervain's or extensor tenosynovitis presents to the clinician. Anesthesia placed over the radial styloid or the dorsum of the hand is used to exclude tendon involvement. There is no indication for corticosteroid injection.

SURGICAL PROCEDURE Navicular replacement (arthroplasty) and fusion (arthrodesis) are the traditional methods of surgical treatment. Proximal row carpectomy has been advocated as a salvage operation for patients with incomplete or poor healing.

PROGNOSIS Approximately 8% to 10% of navicular fractures fail to heal and develop either nonunion or avascular necrosis despite appropriate immobilization. Surgery is necessary for these complicated cases. Patients who decline surgical intervention are at the highest risk for the development of secondary osteoarthritis.

DIFFERENTIAL DIAGNOSIS OF HAND PAIN

Diagnoses	Confirmations
Osteoarthritis (most common)	
Heberden's and Bouchard's nodes	Exam; x-rays—hand series
Post-traumatic monarthric osteoarthritis	Exam; x-rays—hand series
Mucinoid cysts atop the joint	Exam; simple puncture
Erosive subtype of osteoarthritis	X-rays—hand series
Flexor tendons	
Trigger finger/flexor tenosynovitis	Exam
Fixed locked digit	Exam
Tendon cyst	Exam; simple puncture
Benign giant cell tumor	Surgical removal; pathology
Palmar fascia	
Palmar fibromatosis without contracture	Exam
Dupuytren's contracture	Exam
Limited joint mobility syndrome (in long-standing diabetes)	Exam
Extensor tendons	
Mallet finger	Exam
Dorsotenosynovitis	Exam
Reflex sympathetic dystrophy	Exam; bone scan
Rheumatoid arthritis (RA)	Synovial fluid analysis; erythrocyte sedimentation rate; rheumatoid factor
Post-traumatic metacarpophalangeal (MCP) joint arthritis	Exam; local anesthetic block; x-rays
Gamekeeper's thumb	Exam; local anesthetic block

TRIGGER FINGER

The point of entry for the *finger* is just proximal to the first volar crease in the midline, directly over the center of the tendon. The point of entry for the *thumb* is at the distal volar crease in the midline, directly over the center of the tendon.

Needle: ⁵/₈-inch, 25-gauge
Depth: ¹/₄ to ³/₈ inch, flush against the tendon
Volume: 0.5 mL of anesthetic and 0.5 mL of D80

NOTE: *Never* inject with hard pressure within the body of the tendon. If the patient experiences pain, withdraw 1 to 2 mm.

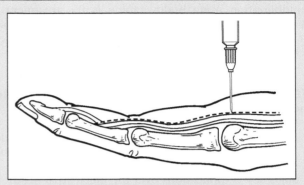

FIGURE 5–1. Trigger finger injection.

DESCRIPTION   Trigger finger is an inflammation of the two flexor tendons of the finger as they cross the metacarpophalangeal (MCP) head in the palm. Repetitive gripping and grasping or direct pressure over the MCP joint (e.g., tools, golf clubs) causes swelling of the tendon and inflammation of the tendon sheath (stage 1—tenosynovitis). As the swelling increases, the two flexor tendons lose their smooth motion through the sheath and under the A-1 pulley, the specialized ligament that anchors the tendons to the metacarpal bone (stage 2—triggering or mechanical catching). If the tendon continues to swell, an irreversible threshold is reached, the tendons no longer can pass under the A-1 pulley, and the finger remains in a locked position (stage 3—fixed locked digit).

SYMPTOMS   The patient complains of a painful finger or of loss of smooth motion of the finger when gripping or pinching. The patient rubs over the tendon in the palm or demonstrates the locking phenomenon when describing the condition.

"My finger keeps catching."

"I wake up in the morning and my finger is locked."

"My finger has started to tie up again."

"The dumb thing locks down."

"I had to stop knitting because my finger hurts all the time."

"If I use scissors or fingernail clippers, I get this sharp pain in my finger [pointing to the base of the finger in the palm]."

"I just thought that this was arthritis! I ignored the pain for the longest time. I didn't know that it could be treated."

EXAM   Each patient is examined for active tenosynovitis of the flexor tendons of the finger along with the degree of mechanical locking.

EXAM SUMMARY

1. Local tenderness at the MCP head
2. Pain aggravated by stretching the finger in extension, passively performed
3. Pain aggravated by resisting finger flexion, isometrically performed
4. Mechanical locking of the proximal interphalangeal (PIP) joint (fingers) and the interphalangeal joint (thumb)

(1) Local tenderness is present at the base of the finger, directly over the tendon as it courses over the metacarpal head. There also is subtle, palpable swelling in 10% of cases. *(2)* Pain is aggravated by stretching the tendon in extension. *(3)* Resisting the action of flexion isometrically also aggravates the pain. *(4)* Clicking or locking with active flexion may or may not be present, depending on the time of day or how long the patient has been symptomatic.

X-RAYS   Plain x-rays of the hand are unnecessary. Calcification of the tendon rarely occurs.

SPECIAL TESTING   No special tests are indicated.

DIAGNOSIS   The diagnosis is based on a history of locking and showing on exam three of the four principal signs: locking, local tenderness at the MCP head, painful stretching in extension, or isometrically resisted flexion. A regional anesthetic block rarely is necessary to make the diagnosis except in the case of tenosynovitis complicating an early presentation of Dupuytren's contracture.

TREATMENT   The goals of treatment are to reduce the swelling and inflammation in the flexor tendon sheath, to allow smoother movement of the tendon under the A-1 pulley, and to perform stretching exercises in extension to prevent recurrent tenosynovitis. In the first 4 to 6 weeks, immobilization using buddy taping is the treatment of choice. Corticosteroid injection is the treatment of choice for patients with symptoms that have been present beyond 6 weeks.

STEP 1   Assess the degree of mechanical locking and the degree of active tenosynovitis.

Restrict gripping, grasping, and pinching.

Demonstrate for the patient the technique of buddy taping to the adjacent finger (p. 252) to reduce movement of the affected finger.

Suggest ice applications over the metacarpal head.

Recommend a metal finger splint if buddy taping is poorly tolerated or unsuccessful (p. 253).

Recommend antivibration padded gloves (Sorbothane).

Discuss the typical causes of the condition: *"Trigger finger is caused either by heavy unaccustomed gripping and grasping or by direct pressure over the tendon in the palm. Trigger finger is not caused by an internal problem."*

STEP 2 (4 TO 6 WEEKS FOR PERSISTENT CASES) Perform a local injection of D80.

Repeat the injection at 6 weeks if symptoms have not improved by at least 50%.

STEP 3 (10 TO 12 WEEKS FOR CHRONIC CASES)   Recommend padded or oversized tools.

Advise reducing the tension when gripping or pinching.

Begin gentle stretching exercises in extension of the fingers (p. 278) when symptoms have improved significantly.

Consider surgical release if symptoms are not relieved by two injections within 12 months or if the patient presents with a fixed locked digit (unable to straighten).

PHYSICAL THERAPY   Physical therapy plays a minor role in the overall management of trigger finger. Stretching exercises in extension are used to prevent recurrent tenosynovitis and to rehabilitate the tendons in the postoperative recovery period. Sets of 20 gentle stretches are performed daily to maintain flexor tendon mobility and to reduce the contracture over the MCP head. Physical therapy is not appropriate for active tenosynovitis.

INJECTION   Local injection is the anti-inflammatory treatment of choice, especially if symptoms have been present for more than 6 to 8 weeks, simple immobilization has failed, or the patient presents with severe locking.

Positioning   The hand is placed flat on the exam table with the palm up and the fingers outstretched.

Surface Anatomy and Point of Entry   The proximal volar crease of the *finger* or the distal volar crease over

TRIGGER FINGER INJECTION

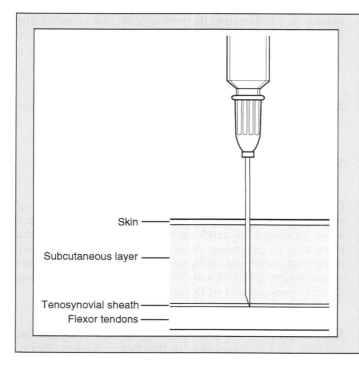

Skin
Subcutaneous layer
Tenosynovial sheath
Flexor tendons

Skin
Subcutaneous layer
Tenosynovial sheath
Flexor tendons

the MCP joint of the *thumb* is identified. The point of entry for the *finger* is just proximal to the first volar crease in the midline. The point of entry for the *thumb* is at the distal volar crease in the midline.

Angle of Entry and Depth The needle is inserted perpendicular to the skin. The depth of injection is $1/4$ to $3/8$ inch for trigger *finger* and $1/8$ to $1/4$ inch for trigger *thumb*.

Anesthesia Ethyl chloride is sprayed on the skin. Local anesthetic is placed in the subcutaneous tissue.

Technique A *volar approach* directly over the center of the tendon is preferred. After applying the ethyl chloride spray, the skin is grasped and pinched up to facilitate the entry of the needle and reduce the chance of inserting the needle directly into the superficially located tendon. Local anesthetic is placed just under the skin. Then the needle is advanced carefully down to the firm resistance of the flexor tendon, a rubbery sensation. The needle is held flush against the tendon, using just the weight of the syringe. Without advancing the needle, the corticosteroid is injected just atop the tendon and underneath the tenosynovial sheath.

INJECTION AFTERCARE

1. *Rest* for 3 days, avoiding all direct pressure, gripping, and grasping.
2. *Buddy tape* the adjacent two fingers for the first few days.
3. Use *ice* (15 minutes every 4 to 6 hours) and *acetaminophen (Tylenol ES)* (1000 mg twice a day) for postinjection soreness.
4. *Protect* the fingers for 3 to 4 weeks by avoiding repetitive gripping, grasping, pressure over the MCP heads, and vibration.
5. Begin passive *stretching exercises* of the fingers in extension at 3 weeks.
6. Repeat *injection* at 6 weeks with corticosteroid if tenosynovitis or locking persists.
7. Suggest *padded gloves* or *padded tools* for long-term prevention in recurrent cases.

8. Obtain a *consultation* with an orthopedic surgeon if two consecutive injections fail to provide at least 6 months of relief.

SURGICAL PROCEDURE Surgery is indicated when locking and tenosynovitis persist despite two consecutive local corticosteroid injections. Percutaneous release and open surgical release of the A-1 pulley ligament are equally effective.

PROGNOSIS A local injection with D80 is highly effective (Table 5-1). Two thirds of cases require only one injection for long-term benefit. One quarter of cases require reinjection within 1 year. Patients with recurrent tenosynovitis or mechanical locking need to evaluate their work and recreational habits to identify activities that cause pressure over the A-1 pulley or activities that require excessive gripping and grasping; often one activity is the inciting event causing the tendon swelling. Of patients, 10% fail medical therapy and require surgical release. This outpatient surgery is safe and effective. The fascial tissue over the tendon at the MCP head is sharply dissected. Recovery may take 3 to 4 weeks. Rarely, multiple trigger fingers can be associated with rheumatoid arthritis in its early stages (p. 100).

5-1 CLINICAL OUTCOMES OF 77 CASES OF TRIGGER FINGER TREATED WITH D80*

Resolved with 1 injection	45 (61%)
Recurrence requiring 1-3 additional injections	20 (27%)
Failed to respond completely	9 (12%)[†]
Total	*74*

*Followed prospectively for 4.2 years.
[†]Of the 9 patients, surgical release was performed in 5, and 4 declined surgery. Data from Anderson BC, Kaye S. Treatment of flexor tenosynovitis of the hand ("trigger finger") with corticosteroids. Arch Intern Med 151:153-156, 1991.

TENDON CYST

Enter directly over the palpable nodule.

Needle: ⁵/₈-inch, 21- or 25-gauge
Depth: ¹/₄ to ³/₈ inch into the cyst
Volume: 0.5 mL of anesthetic

NOTE: After treatment, apply manual pressure from either side to decompress the cyst.

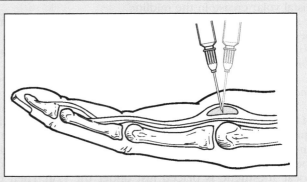

FIGURE 5-2. Tendon cyst puncture and decompression.

DESCRIPTION   A tendon cyst is an abnormal collection of tenosynovial fluid, either within the body of the tendon or adjacent to it. Direct, nonpenetrating trauma causes minor, reversible injury to the tendon or tendon sheath. This injury leads to an overproduction of fluid, which collects inside the tendon or leaks out into the subcutaneous tissues, where it incites fibrous cyst formation. Despite its size (5 to 8 mm in diameter), and in contrast to its sister diagnosis trigger finger, the nodule rarely interferes with the function of the tendons; the finger retains its normal flexion and extension, and mobility of the MCP joint is preserved.

SYMPTOMS   The patient complains of a lump in the palm of the hand, which is mildly tender to compression. The patient points to the area when describing the problem.

"I have this small knot right here (pointing to the base of the finger in the palm)."

"Feel this thing, kind of like a little marble or BB."

"When I use my little scissors and place pressure over my finger, I get a sharp pain."

"My doctor told me that I have a cyst in my tendon, but I'm not so sure that I believe her. I'm worried about it."

"Ever since I hit the countertop with my hand, I've felt this lump in my palm (pointing to the base of the finger)."

"I'm a professional percussionist. My favorite instrument is the tambourine. About 4 weeks ago, I noticed a pain along my fourth finger every time I tried to hold my tambourine. There's a small lump there now."

EXAM   The location and size of the nodule relative to the position of the tendon and metacarpal head are assessed in each patient.

EXAM SUMMARY

1. A smooth, firm nodule 5 to 8 mm in diameter that is palpable in the palm
2. Very mild tenderness to firm compression
3. Absence of mechanical locking, triggering, or palmar fascial thickening
4. Decompression with simple cyst puncture

(1) A firm nodule is palpable in the palm, usually adjacent to the distal metacarpal head. If the nodule is inside the tendon, passive motion of the finger in flexion and extension causes it to move. If the nodule is adjacent to the tendon, the nodule is less likely to move directly with passive motion. *(2)* Mild tenderness may be present over the nodule. Firm pressure exerted toward the underlying bone causes pain; it is most pronounced in the first few months. With time, this tenderness becomes less prominent. *(3)* The flexor tendons are free of mechanical catching or locking (i.e., the MCP and PIP joints should have full, smooth flexion and extension).

X-RAYS   Plain x-rays of the hand are unnecessary. Calcification of the cyst is rare. Significant underlying bony changes do not occur.

SPECIAL TESTING   No special testing is indicated.

DIAGNOSIS   A presumptive diagnosis is based on the size and location of the nodule in the palm. A simple puncture with decompression confirms the diagnosis and differentiates this kind of cyst from the solid cyst, "giant cell tumor." Patients with cysts that fail to decompress with simple puncture may need to have their diagnoses confirmed surgically.

TREATMENT   The goal of treatment is to decompress the abnormal accumulation of fluid. Simple puncture with manual decompression is the treatment of choice for cysts that are symptomatic and that have not resolved spontaneously.

STEP 1   Assess the size of the cyst and its relationship with the tendon, compare the mobility of the affected finger with its contralateral finger, and evaluate the tendon for active tenosynovitis. Observe the condition over weeks to months for spontaneous resolution.

Educate the patient: *"This is simply a cyst of the tendon. Many times this kind of cyst resolves without any specific treatment."*

Reduce vibration exposure and direct pressure (suggest gloves or an adhesive pad placed over the cyst for protection).

STEP 2 (4 TO 8 WEEKS FOR PERSISTENT CASES)   Perform simple puncture and manual decompression.

Repeat the puncture and decompression at 4 to 6 weeks, and combine with injection of 0.25 mL of K40.

Reduce gripping and grasping tension; use padded tools or antivibration gloves (Sorbothane).

STEP 3 (MONTHS FOR CHRONIC CASES)   Consider surgical decompression for tendon cysts that continue to interfere with gripping or grasping.

PHYSICAL THERAPY   Physical therapy does not have a significant role in the treatment of tendon cysts.

INJECTION   Simple puncture and manual decompression is the treatment of choice for symptomatic cysts that do not resolve on their own.

Positioning   The hand is placed flat on the exam table with the palm up and the fingers outstretched.

Surface Anatomy and Point of Entry   The course of the flexor tendon is identified. The center of the tendon is marked above and below the cyst. The cyst is palpated, and marks are placed on either side of it. The point of entry is centered directly over the cyst.

Angle of Entry and Depth   The needle is inserted perpendicular to the skin. The depth of injection is $1/4$ to $3/8$ inch.

Anesthesia   Ethyl chloride is sprayed on the skin. Local anesthetic is placed in the subcutaneous tissue.

Technique   The cyst is identified by placing a finger tip above and a finger tip below it. While holding the cyst firmly in place, the needle is centered over the nodule and passed down into the body of the cyst at least twice.

TENDON CYST PUNCTURE

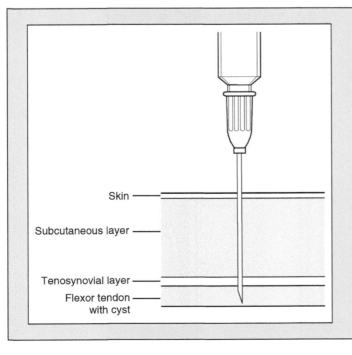

Skin
Subcutaneous layer
Tenosynovial layer
Flexor tendon with cyst

The bevel of the needle is kept parallel to the tendon fibers (separating the tendon fibers rather than cutting them). To ensure the accurate placement inside the cyst, the tendon can be passively flexed and extended; the needle should move back and forth if properly placed. Aspiration of the small amount of highly viscous fluid is usually unsuccessful. Manual pressure using the barrel of a syringe in a rolling fashion or with digital pressure decompresses most cysts. The procedure can be repeated with a 21-gauge needle if the nodule is not reduced in size. Less than 10% of cysts fail to decompress with simple puncture (cysts that have very little fluid within the cyst cavity).

INJECTION AFTERCARE

1. *Rest* for 3 days, avoiding all gripping, grasping, and direct pressure.
2. *Buddy tape* the adjacent two fingers for the first few days.
3. Use *ice* (15 minutes every 4 to 6 hours) and *acetaminophen* (1000 mg twice a day) for postinjection soreness.
4. *Protect* the fingers for 3 to 4 weeks by avoiding repetitive gripping, grasping, pressure over the MCP heads, and vibration.
5. Repeat *puncture and decompression* at 6 weeks if the cyst fluid reaccumulates.
6. Suggest *padded gloves* or *padded tools* for long-term prevention in recurrent cases.
7. *Observe* it; commonly the cyst slowly diminishes in size over several months.
8. Obtain a *consultation* with an orthopedic surgeon if two consecutive procedures and time fail to resolve

the condition; advise the patient of the possibility of postoperative scarring over the MCP joint that could adversely affect the range of motion (ROM) of the finger.

SURGICAL PROCEDURE For problem cysts that remain symptomatic (pressure pain, interference with gripping and grasping, persistent worry that this is something more serious), excision of the cyst can be considered. (Surgery performed on the hand can cause significant scarring over the tendon or adjacent joint, limiting the movement of the finger in extension.)

PROGNOSIS Simple puncture is highly effective for most tendon cysts, particularly cysts that are fluid filled. Surgical excision is indicated if the nodule persists and hand function is interfered with in a significant way. Surgery for cosmetic results is to be discouraged. Postoperative scarring may develop, which because of its size and location can limit the mobility of the finger much more than the original cyst.

Tenosynovial cysts are always the result of direct pressure or trauma over the flexor tendons as they course through the palm and down the finger. They are not a reflection of any rheumatic or systemic conditions. As such, workup is not indicated, including radiographs, which are always normal. For patients who develop recurrent cysts and patients who develop multiple cysts, the most important evaluation is to identify the inciting activities or specific tasks that cause the cyst to form (e.g., excessive gripping, vibration from a lawn mower or chain saw, leaning on a walking cane).

DUPUYTREN'S CONTRACTURE

Enter adjacent to the nodular thickening in the midline over the flexor tendon; hold the needle vertically; injection is indicated only when tenosynovitis accompanies the fibrotic process.

Needle: ⁵/₈-inch, 25-gauge
Depth: ¹/₄ to ³/₈ inch
Volume: 0.5 mL of anesthetic and 0.25 mL of K40

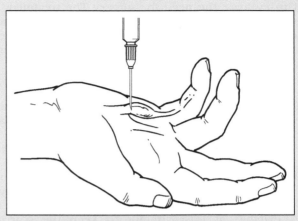

FIGURE 5–3. Dupuytren's contracture injection.

DESCRIPTION Dupuytren's contracture is a progressive fibrosis of the palmar fascia. Tissue thickening envelops the flexor tendons—typically the fourth and fifth tendons—and leads to a gradual flexion contracture of the fingers into the palm. The condition develops insidiously over decades. The initial tendon thickening often goes unnoticed and undiagnosed, gradually causing ever greater joint stiffness, palmar thickening, and finger contracture. Most cases are inherited, occurring more frequently in individuals of northern European descent. Chronic liver disease (one of the classic extrahepatic signs of advanced cirrhosis) and postoperative scarring account for a small percentage of cases.

SYMPTOMS The patient complains of finger stiffness, thickening in the palm, loss of motion of the affected finger or fingers, or all three. The patient often rubs the palm and fingers in an attempt to straighten them out as the condition is described.

"I've got these knots in my palm."

"I can't straighten my ring and little fingers."

"My fingers have slowly drawn down into my hand."

"I can't hold my hammer and small tools anymore. I can't open my hand enough."

EXAM Each patient is examined for the extent and location of the palmar fibrosis, for the impairment of flexion and extension in the affected fingers (i.e., the degree of flexion contracture of the fingers), and for any concurrent tenosynovitis.

EXAM SUMMARY

1. Puckering of the skin over the flexor tendon in the palm with forced extension of the finger
2. Painless palmar nodules
3. Fixed flexion contracture of the affected fingers (usually the fourth and fifth fingers)
4. Signs of active tenosynovitis are uncommon (tenderness, pain, or locking)

(1) Discrete nodules are visible and palpable along the course of the flexor tendons. Passive extension of the affected fingers shows the puckering of the tendon as it courses over the MCP head. The tendons of the fourth and fifth fingers are most commonly involved. *(2)* The flexibility of the MCP and PIP joints is reduced, leading to fixed flexion contractures (loss of full extension). *(3)* Signs of active inflammation are notably absent in most cases. Specifically, local tenderness, swelling, and pain with passive flexion and extension are absent, unless a concurrent tenosynovitis is present (uncommon except in the earliest cases).

X-RAYS Plain films of the hand are unnecessary. Calcification of the tendons does not occur.

DIAGNOSIS The diagnosis is based on the history of painless stiffness of the fingers and on the characteristic physical findings of peritendinous thickening and flexor tendon deformity. Rarely, Dupuytren's contracture can be painful. In the early stages, tenosynovitis can be present.

TREATMENT   The goals of treatment are to educate the patient regarding the slowly progressive nature of the condition, to improve the flexibility of the flexor tendons, and to evaluate the need for surgery. The treatment of choice for early disease is passive stretching of the flexor tendons after lanolin massage. Surgery is the treatment of choice for advanced tendon contracture that interferes with the function of the hand.

STEP 1   Assess the extent of the fibrosis, measure the loss of finger and MCP flexibility, and evaluate the tendon for active tenosynovitis.

Educate the patient: *"The process slowly worsens over many years, even over decades."*

Recommend passive stretching of the flexor tendons after heating and lanolin massage to maintain finger flexibility and ROM. If the scarring process is inevitable, at least attempt to keep the scarring process from contracting the finger.

Suggest thick-padded gloves or adhesive padding placed over the palmar thickening to protect against the aggravation of direct pressure.

STEP 2 (MONTHS TO YEARS FOR PERSISTENT OR PROGRESSIVE CASES)   If pain in the palm develops and is accompanied by local tenderness over the tendon (active tenosynovitis), local injection with K40 can be performed.

STEP 3 (YEARS FOR CASES WITH FLEXION CONTRAC-TURES)   Offer consultation with a hand surgeon to consider surgical débridement and release of the scar tissue if the contracture process progresses and causes poor function of the affected fingers.

Educate the patient: *"Surgery is effective in the short-term but it will not cure the problem, only improve function temporarily."*

PHYSICAL THERAPY   Physical therapy stretching exercises remain the treatment of choice for the early stages of this condition. Passive stretching exercises in extension are used to prevent flexion contractures and to rehabilitate the postoperative patient.

INJECTION   Fewer than 5% of cases have concomitant tenosynovitis. Local injection with corticosteroid is performed infrequently (p. 87).

SURGICAL PROCEDURE   Partial fasciectomy is the procedure of choice to débride and release the fibrotic tissue enveloping the tendon. The success of surgery depends on the complete removal of the pathologic tissue, the sparing of the normal fascial layers, the degree of postoperative bleeding, and the patient's postoperative scarring and healing. Because there are as many forms of Dupuytren's contracture as there are fascial layers (e.g., palmar, digital, intermetacarpal), this delicate surgery should be performed by a hand surgeon.

PROGNOSIS   Dupuytren's contracture is a slow, progressive scarring of the flexor tendons of the hand. All treatments are palliative. No therapy has been shown to stop the scarring process. It is important to advise the patient, however, on the proper stretching exercises to retard the development of flexion contracture. When function has been impaired significantly, surgical removal of the fascial thickening is the treatment of choice. Fasciotomy and fasciectomy are usually successful in the short-term. Despite careful technique and meticulous dissection, in many cases, the condition progresses. In the case of recurrent fibrosis and progressive contracture, long-term stretching exercises or even a second operation may be recommended.

Although Dupuytren's contracture is associated with chronic liver disease and diabetes, 95% of cases are idiopathic with no underlying systemic disease. Further workup rarely is indicated after diagnosing the condition; the scarring and contracture are typically a late manifestation of advanced cirrhosis of the liver and insulin-dependent diabetes.

METACARPOPHALANGEAL JOINT ARTHROCENTESIS

Enter over the joint line just distal to the metacarpal head, staying on the dorsal half of the joint.

Needle: $^5/_8$-inch, 25-gauge
Depth: $^1/_4$ to $^3/_8$ inch flush against the bone
Volume: 0.5 mL of anesthetic and 0.25 mL of K40

NOTE: The joint does not accept more than 0.25 mL; place the anesthetic in the subcutaneous tissue and the steroid just under the synovial membrane.

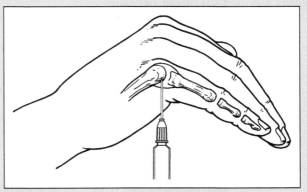

FIGURE 5–4. Arthrocentesis and injection of the metacarpophalangeal joint.

DESCRIPTION   Isolated arthritic involvement of the MCP joints is uncommon. The second and third MCP joints are the most susceptible. Swelling and inflammation of the joint are usually the result of remote and often unrecognized trauma—"post-traumatic monarthric arthritis." Involvement of multiple MCP joints, especially bilaterally, is more likely rheumatic in nature (patients with this presentation require a full workup) (p. 100). Septic arthritis of the MCP joint is rare; it usually is caused by a penetrating injury. Aspiration of the joint rarely yields synovial fluid.

SYMPTOMS   The patient complains of pain and swelling of the affected joint or of the inability to make a closed fist. The patient often attempts to make a fist when describing the condition.

"My knuckle is swollen."

"I can't close my hand."

"I can't hold onto my hammer because my knuckle hurts too much."

"When I close my hand, it feels like the tendons are slipping."

EXAM   The patient is examined for tenderness and swelling of the individual MCP joints and for loss of full flexion and extension.

EXAM SUMMARY

1. Swelling and tenderness of the affected MCP (loss of the normal hills and valleys of the knuckles)
2. A positive MCP squeeze sign
3. Inability to make a closed fist

(1) Swelling and tenderness are located over the dorsum of the affected MCP joint. With the MCP joints flexed to 90 degrees, the normal contours formed by the knuckles are obliterated. *(2)* Squeezing the MCP joints together aggravates the pain. Pressure is applied across the MCP joints while holding the joints in line with the opposite hand. *(3)* Severe swelling prevents full flexion. A full fist cannot be made. *(4)* Multiple MCP joint swelling in a symmetric pattern suggests inflammatory arthritis or other rheumatologic conditions that cause a symmetric small-joint polyarthritis.

X-RAYS   X-rays of the hand (including posteroanterior and lateral views) are unnecessary in the case of monarthric arthritis of a single MCP joint. Patients with multiple MCP joint involvement have a greater likelihood of having inflammatory arthritis, however, and should be evaluated with bilateral hand x-rays (p. 100).

DIAGNOSIS   The diagnosis is based on the characteristic swelling and loss of ROM of the MCP joint. Occasionally, local anesthetic block is required to confirm the diagnosis and distinguish this localized joint problem from flexor tenosynovitis or injury to the supporting ligaments.

TREATMENT   The goals of treatment are to reduce joint swelling and to increase the ROM. When joint swelling is moderate to severe, local corticosteroid injection is the treatment of choice for nonseptic effusion. Because of the size of the joint and the inability of the orally administered nonsteroidal anti-inflammatory drugs (NSAIDs) to penetrate the joint, the response to corticosteroid injection is much more favorable than the response to the NSAIDs.

STEP 1   **Document the number of fingers that are involved and the degree of loss of ROM, and measure the strength of gripping (dynamometer versus a rolled-up blood pressure cuff).**

Restrict gripping and grasping (limit repetitive flexion and extension).

Recommend the use of oversized tools, padding, grip tape, thick gloves, and any other occupation-oriented adjustment to protect the hands.

Ice applied directly to the joint is effective for mild swelling.

Prescribe 3 weeks of immobilization using a radial gutter splint (p. 249) for the first or second MCP joints or an ulnar gutter splint (p. 250) for involvement of the third or fourth MCP joint.

A 4-week course of an NSAID (e.g., ibuprofen [Advil, Motrin]) can be tried, but it has limited efficacy because of poor penetration into this small joint.

STEP 2 (3 TO 4 WEEKS FOR PERSISTENT CASES)
Perform a local injection of K40.

Repeat the injection after 4 to 6 weeks if symptoms have not decreased by 50%.

Perform ROM exercises in flexion and extension followed by gripping exercises to complete the treatment.

STEP 3 (2 TO 3 MONTHS FOR CHRONIC CASES)
Consider a consultation with a hand surgeon for implant arthroplasty.

PHYSICAL THERAPY   Physical therapy plays a minor role in the treatment of monarthric involvement of the MCP joint. *Ice* and *phonophoresis with a hydrocortisone gel* can provide temporary relief of pain and swelling. In the recovery phase, passively performed stretching exercises in flexion and extension are used to restore full ROM.

INJECTION   Corticosteroid injection is the preferred anti-inflammatory treatment for nonseptic effusions. The response to local corticosteroid injection depends on the extent of injury to the joint. If synovitis is accompanied by damage to the articular cartilage (pitted, fissured, or eroded articular cartilage), injection provides temporary benefit only. If the injury is simply a swollen, inflamed joint with minimal damage to the articular cartilage surface, injection appears to resolve the problem entirely. The response to treatment is often the most reliable indicator of prognosis.

Positioning   The hand is placed flat on the exam table with the palm down and the fingers outstretched.

Surface Anatomy and Point of Entry   The point of entry is adjacent to the MCP joint line. The joint line is $1/4$ inch distal to the metarcapal head (the knuckle is the distal head of the metacarpal bone). Alternatively the joint line can be identified by subluxation of the proximal phalangeal bone dorsally. For the second and fifth digits, the 25-gauge needle is inserted just above the mid-plane to avoid the neurovascular bundle. For the third and fourth digits, the point of entry is halfway between the MCP heads.

INJECTION OF THE METACARPOPHALANGEAL JOINT

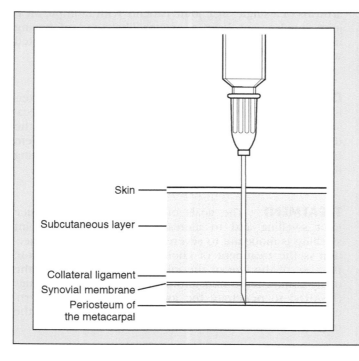

Skin
Subcutaneous layer
Collateral ligament
Synovial membrane
Periosteum of the metacarpal

Angle of Entry and Depth The needle is inserted perpendicular to the skin for the second and fifth digits and at a 45-degree angle for the third and fourth digits. The depth of injection is $1/4$ to $3/8$ inch.

Anesthesia Ethyl chloride is sprayed on the skin. Local anesthetic is placed in the subcutaneous tissue (0.5 mL).

Technique A *dorsal approach* is preferable. The needle is advanced until the firm resistance of the supporting ligament and joint capsule is encountered. Anesthesia is injected just outside this layer ($1/8$ inch). Then the needle is advanced to the hard resistance of the bone ($1/4$ inch), and 0.25 mL of K40 is injected under the synovial membrane. The small joints of the hand can accommodate only a small volume of medication. If the pressure of injection increases, withdraw $1/16$ inch. A periarticular injection is just as effective as an intra-articular injection.

INJECTION AFTERCARE

1. *Rest* for 3 days avoiding all direct pressure, gripping, grasping, extremes of motion, vibration, and cold.
2. Use *ice* (15 minutes every 4 to 6 hours) and *acetaminophen* (1000 mg twice a day) for postinjection soreness.
3. *Protect* the fingers for 3 to 4 weeks by avoiding repetitive gripping, grasping, pressure over the MCP heads, and vibration, or alternatively suggest the use of a Velcro wrist immobilizer with a metal stay for more advanced disease (e.g., dramatic swelling, lost ROM, poor grip).
4. Begin passively performed ROM *stretching exercises* in flexion and extension at 2 to 3 weeks.
5. Begin isometrically performed *gripping exercises* at 4 to 5 weeks.
6. Repeat *injection* at 6 weeks with corticosteroid if swelling persists or if ROM is still significantly impaired.
7. Suggest *padded gloves* or *padded tools* for long-term prevention in recurrent cases.
8. Obtain a *consultation* with an orthopedic surgeon if two consecutive injections fail to resolve the condition.

SURGICAL PROCEDURE MCP joint implant arthroplasty (replacement) is used in carefully selected cases. Patients with severe disease manifested by a loss of 50% of ROM and near-total loss of the articular cartilage are the optimal candidates for replacement.

PROGNOSIS Isolated involvement of one or two MCP joints uniformly is caused by trauma. Although close inspection and width measurement of the articular cartilage on plain x-rays of the hands is the best way to determine the severity and prognosis of the condition, ultimately the long-term outcome depends on how effectively treatment controls the inflammatory response and the ability of the body to smooth over any damaged cartilage.

Most patients respond favorably to a combination of immobilization and corticosteroid injection. The long-term outcome for patients with post-traumatic monarthric involvement of the MCP depends on the extent of damage sustained by the articular cartilage, the associated bony fracture with persistent deformity (poorly aligned boxer's fracture), and the physical demands placed on the joint.

Patients with symmetric involvement of the MCP joints of both hands have the classic presentation of inflammatory arthritis. These patients require a complete joint exam and laboratory testing to define the specific rheumatic condition.

OSTEOARTHRITIS OF THE HAND

Only the proximal interphalangeal joint can be injected easily; enter at the joint line, $^1/_4$ inch beyond the distal end of the proximal phalanges above the midplane.

Needle: $^5/_8$-inch, 25-gauge
Depth: $^1/_4$ to $^3/_8$ inch, flush against the adjacent bone
Volume: 0.25 to 0.5 mL of anesthetic and 0.125 mL of K40

NOTE: Use small amounts of anesthetic in the superficial layers; the joint accepts only small volumes.

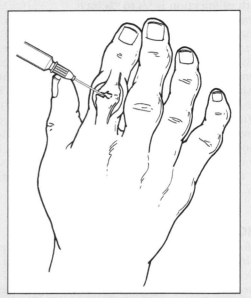

FIGURE 5–5. Proximal interphalangeal joint injection.

DESCRIPTION Osteoarthritis of the small joints of the hand is a universal problem. It occurs as a result of heredity, age, or injury. It is characterized by relatively painless bony enlargement and bony deformity of the small joints of the hand. Involvement of the distal interphalangeal (DIP) joints or the Heberden nodes is most common. Fewer patients have involvement at the PIP joints or Bouchard nodes. X-rays show variable degrees of asymmetric wear of the articular cartilage, reactive bony osteophytes at the joint margins, and subchondral sclerosis of the adjacent bones as the classic changes of this wear-and-tear arthritis. A family history, heavy use, and repeated exposure to vibratory tools all are associated with an increased susceptibility.

SYMPTOMS Most patients complain of bony enlargement of the fingers and seek confirmation of their self-diagnosis. A few patients experience acute inflammatory flares that manifest as pain and swelling in a single or in multiple joints and are known as inflammatory osteoarthritis. Many patients look at their hands, describe the deformity, and rub the individual fingers as they describe the condition.

"Am I getting what my grandma called 'old-age arthritis'?"

"I hate my hands. They're so crooked and ugly."

"Look at my hands; I'm really getting older."

"I can't make a fist anymore; my fingers won't close."

"My hands are a little stiff in the morning, but they really don't hurt that much."

"I know I have arthritis, but my middle knuckle is so much bigger than the others, and it won't bend."

EXAM Each patient is examined for bony enlargement, loss of finger flexibility, and signs of inflammation involving the DIP and PIP joints of the hand.

EXAM SUMMARY

1. Bony enlargement of the DIP and PIP joints
2. Inability to flex the fingers fully to make a fist
3. Angulation of the DIP and PIP joints
4. Relative absence of inflammatory changes (synovitis) except in the inflammatory subtype
5. Ankylosis of the joints in the advanced stages

(1) The DIP and PIP joints have bony enlargement palpable along the sides of the joints. The involvement is greater in the DIP joints in most cases. (2) As the disease progresses, the flexibility of the fingers gradually decreases, creating the typical deformities. The patient is unable to make a fist. Extension of the fingers may be impaired. (3) Subluxation of the DIP joints leads to the characteristic ulnar deviation. (4) Inflammation and synovitis are notably absent except in patients with the subtype of erosive, inflammatory osteoarthritis. This condition typically is seen in young women and presents with swelling, heat, and boggy enlargement of the DIP and PIP joints. (5) The end stage form of the disease is

characterized by large, palpable bony osteophytes, decreased ROM of the DIP and PIP joints, ankylosis of some joints, and atrophy of the intrinsic muscles of the hand.

X-RAYS   Routine x-rays of the hand (posteroanterior and lateral views) are not always necessary, but are diagnostic. Distribution among joints can be assessed accurately. Asymmetric narrowing of the articular cartilage and bony osteophyte formation on either side of the joint line are characteristic. Advanced cases show ever-increasing ulnar deviation, subchondral cyst formation, and ankylosis. The periarticular erosions so typical of RA are notably absent.

DIAGNOSIS   The characteristic changes of bony enlargement with little inflammatory reaction in the typical joint distribution suggest the diagnosis. The diagnosis is confirmed, especially in early presentations, by the typical changes seen on x-rays.

TREATMENT   The goals of treatment are to confirm the diagnosis, to advise on proper joint protection, and to reduce acute inflammation and swelling.

STEP 1   Define the joint distribution, examine for bony osteophytes, and consider ordering x-rays of the hand (posteroanterior and lateral views).

Educate the patient: *"This is wear-and-tear arthritis that results from aging."*

Advise on avoiding cold exposure, extremes of movement, repetitive gripping, and heavy grasping.

Limit exposure to vibration (vacuum cleaners, lawn mowers, and tools that vibrate).

Prescribe coated aspirin (8 to 12 per day in divided dose) or acetaminophen (1 g twice a day); use of NSAIDs is reserved for acute flare-ups.

Apply heat, including paraffin treatments (paraffin warmed in a crock pot, 10 coatings of wax on each hand every morning, gentle passive stretching of the joints to follow).

Avoid exposure to cold (gloves, wear warm enough clothing to maintain the body's core temperature in a range high enough to avoid peripheral vasoconstriction).

STEP 2 (WEEKS TO YEARS FOR ACUTE FLARES)   For inflammatory flares, recommend simple immobilization with buddy taping (p. 252) or a tube splint (p. 252).

Recommend topical applications of capsaicin cream (Zostrix) or 0.1% triamcinolone cream.

Prescribe glucosamine sulfate, 1500 mg/day.

Perform a local injection of K40 into the fingers with the most prominent swelling or loss of ROM (p. 102).

Recommend gentle ROM exercises using manual assisted movement or the time-honored Chinese chime balls to maintain overall hand function.

PHYSICAL THERAPY   Physical therapy plays a minor role in the overall treatment of osteoarthritis, simply because most patients do not seek medical treatment or experience symptoms severe enough to justify intervention. Application of heat to the affected joints in warm to hot water and avoidance of exposure to cold always are recommended, however. Gentle stretching exercises in extension and toning exercises involving gentle gripping (p. 276) are recommended to preserve function.

INJECTION   Occasionally an isolated small joint of the hand has enlargement, pain, and swelling that are disproportionate to that being experienced in the other joints of the hand (enough swelling to interfere with the full flexion of the joint). A history of trauma often is obtained. The symptoms develop gradually over weeks, as opposed to the acute presentation of a monarthric infective arthritis that occurs over hours or days. This monarthric traumatic arthritis is an acute flare of an underlying osteoarthritic joint and is often responsive to intra-articular injection.

PROGNOSIS   Arthritis affecting a single joint is nearly always a result of previous trauma (bony fracture, chondral fracture, or high-grade ligament injury causing instability). The acute flare of post-traumatic arthritis usually responds well to a combination of injection and immobilization, but only temporarily. Recurrent flare-ups are the rule depending on the patient's occupation, the patient's extracurricular activities, and the degree of arthritic changes on x-ray. Any treatment, including injection, is palliative. Surgery rarely is indicated and generally should be discouraged. Cyst removal, resection of prominent osteophytes, and osteotomy to realign the joints can cause significant periarticular scarring, joint stiffness, and joint contracture, all of which may have a greater effect on joint function than does the arthritis itself. Arthritis involving multiple joints, especially with bilateral involvement and prominent inflammatory features (e.g., swelling, heat), warrants a laboratory workup for rheumatoid, psoriatic, or lupus-based arthritis (p. 299).

RHEUMATOID ARTHRITIS

Enter at the joint line above the mid-plane.

Needle: ⁵/₈-inch, 25-gauge
Depth: ¹/₄ to ³/₈ inch
Volume: 0.125 to 0.25 mL of K40 flush against the
         bone after minimal subcutaneous anesthetic

NOTE: Do not insert the needle between the articular
  surfaces of the joint (damaging); with the needle
  held gently against the bone adjacent to the joint
  line, the medication is injected under the synovial
  membrane and flows into the joint.

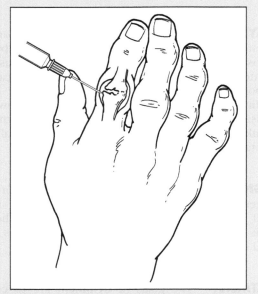

FIGURE 5–6. Proximal interphalangeal joint injection.

DESCRIPTION   RA is an inflammatory arthritis that can manifest in a variety of ways. Classic RA presents as a symmetric, polyarticular, small-joint arthritis affecting the MCP, PIP, and metatarsophalangeal joints. The affected joints exhibit moderately intense inflammation, fusiform swelling, and boggy synovial thickening. Nonclassic RA may present in a single joint (monarthric) or several medium to large joints (pauciarticular) or as a fleeting, small-joint arthritis that has the same joint distribution as classic RA (palindromic). Palindromic RA is the most difficult to diagnose because the pain and swelling typically last only a few days and often are resolved by the time the patient is examined. In all of the presentations, x-rays and serologic markers are often normal in the first few months of the disease. In most cases, an initial presumptive diagnosis of RA relies on the demonstration of inflammation and swelling in the typical pattern (classic or palindromic RA) or the demonstration of inflammatory exudates on synovial fluid analysis (monarthric or pauciarticular RA).

SYMPTOMS   Depending on the clinical presentation, the patient complains of fatigue and diffuse arthralgias; small-joint stiffness and swelling; or stiffness, swelling, and loss of mobility in a particular joint.

"My hands have been swelling at the knuckles."

"I have to put my hands in hot running water in the morning to get rid of the horrible stiffness."

"I'm losing my grip. I can't hold onto my tools any longer."

"My hands hurt so much that it's even hard to pull up the sheets on the bed."

"The balls of my feet are so tender, I can't wear my shoes any longer."

"Every time I go up the stairs, the balls of my feet hurt."

"My knee is swollen and feverish."

"I can't straighten my elbows all the way."

EXAM   The patient is examined for joint inflammation, swelling, and deformity, and involvement of the small, medium, and large joints of the skeleton is documented carefully.

EXAM SUMMARY

1. Early—a normal exam and subtle swelling in the MCP, PIP, or metatarsophalangeal joints
2. The MCP or metatarsophalangeal joint squeeze signs create dramatic pain
3. Joint enlargement secondary to synovial thickening
4. Loss of joint mobility
5. Deformity—ulnar deviation, subluxation, and hammer toes

(1) The earliest findings in RA may be so subtle or so evanescent (depending on the time of day) as to escape detection by the examiner. *(2)* As the condition advances, swelling and localized tenderness appear. Recreating the patient's pain by squeezing the MCP or

metatarsophalangeal joints together from side to side is a useful, quick screening sign for hand and foot involvement. (3) Otherwise, individual joints are inspected and palpated for localized tenderness, swelling, and thickening. For the PIP joints, this inspection is best accomplished by alternating compression of the joint with four fingers. One finger is placed above the joint and one below, and a finger is placed along each side of the joint. Pressure is alternated back and forth to feel for synovial thickening. (4) As the condition progresses, finger flexibility becomes impaired, the hand becomes doughy and loose owing to ligamentous laxity, and the intrinsic muscles of the hand begin to waste. (5) Ulnar deviation of the MCP joints eventually develops. The hand generally loses its strength.

Early involvement of the wrist is associated with subtle swelling dorsally and dramatic degrees of pain when passively moving the joint to the extremes of full dorsiflexion and volar flexion. Involvement of the elbow is associated with a loss of full extension and lateral joint line swelling (the "bulge sign" appears halfway between the olecranon process and the lateral epicondyle). Early involvement of the ankle is associated with general swelling anteriorly, loss of the contours around the medial and lateral malleoli, and pain at the extremes of full plantar flexion and dorsiflexion. Knee involvement almost always is associated with a moderate suprapatellar effusion, warmth anteriorly, and loss of full flexion.

X-RAYS   X-rays of the hand (posteroanterior and lateral views) are always indicated. Early plain x-rays are often normal or show only subtle juxta-articular osteoporosis. As the condition progresses, osteoporosis becomes more obvious, symmetric loss of articular cartilage develops, and joint erosions form close to the lateral margins of the joints, usually the MCP and PIP joints.

DIAGNOSIS   The diagnosis of RA may be elusive early in the course of the disease. In the first few months (up to 1 year), the diagnosis rests on the clinical findings of a symmetric, small-joint pattern of stiffness, pain, and swelling (classic RA) or on the demonstration of an inflammatory effusion (pauciarticular or monarthric RA). In some cases, re-examination and re-evaluation may be necessary at 1- to 2-month intervals until the case "blossoms." As the months pass, plain films of the hand are useful in determining the extent and severity of the disease, but cannot replace the more accurate clinical information obtained from an accurate history and comprehensive exam. The rheumatoid factor should *not* be relied on as a screening test for patients presenting with arthralgia or arthritis. It may take 6 to 9 months for this serologic marker to become positive, and at least 15% of patients with a clinical diagnosis of RA are seronegative.

TREATMENT   The goals of treatment are to confirm the diagnosis, to stage the extent of the disease, and to begin step-by-step care to reduce pain and inflammation. Systemic treatment with oral medication is the treatment of choice.

STEP 1   **Define the distribution among joints, examine for acute synovitis, order x-rays of the hand (posteroanterior and lateral views), and obtain baseline values of complete blood count and erythrocyte sedimentation rate.**

If a large or medium-sized joint is swollen, obtain synovial fluid for laboratory analysis.

Ice applied directly to the joints can reduce pain and swelling.

Reduce repetitive, fine finger motions and heavy gripping and grasping.

Appropriate immobilization is applied to the most involved joints: buddy taping for the PIP joints, radial or ulnar gutter splint for MCP joints, or Velcro wrist immobilizer with metal stay.

Modify the work schedule, adding rest periods in between periods of repetitive handwork.

Encourage the patient to remain active, balancing periods of rest with activity.

Recommend gentle, passive stretching exercises (p. 278).

Avoid exposure to vibration (vacuum cleaners, lawn mowers, and tools that vibrate).

Prescribe salicylates, acetaminophen, or an NSAID for moderate disease.

Recommend heat to reduce stiffness (e.g., warm water, shower, paraffin treatments).

Minimize the use of narcotics.

STEP 2 (MONTHS TO YEARS FOR PERSISTENT OR PROGRESSIVE DISEASE)   **Alternate between chemical classes of the NSAIDs to maintain efficacy.**

Perform a local injection for flares in isolated joints (always perform synovial fluid analysis to exclude infection if one joint is disproportionately inflamed).

Consider a consultation with a rheumatologist in the case of progressive disease, especially for the appropriate use of the disease-modifying drugs.

Perform an intramuscular injection of 2 mL of K40 to reduce mild to moderate flares.

Prescribe gold salts, hydroxychloroquine (Plaquenil), penicillamine, or methotrexate for progressive or advanced cases.

Use a moderate dose of oral prednisone for 1 to 2 months, with a slow taper to reduce the intensity of a moderate to severe flare (30 to 40 mg/day, tapering by 5 mg until 10 to 15 mg is reached, then by 1- to 2-mg increments until the course is completed; when tapering, never reduce the dose by >10% to 15%).

Limit narcotics to severe flare-ups and to a specified number per week or month.

Avoid long-term use of oral corticosteroids.

STEP 3 (YEARS FOR CHRONIC ARTHRITIS)   **Obtain an orthopedic consultation for joint replacement when severe deformity accompanies dramatic functional impairment.**

PHYSICAL THERAPY   Physical and occupational therapy play a crucial role in the overall management of RA, especially in the late stages.

PHYSICAL THERAPY SUMMARY

1. Ice for any acutely inflamed joint
2. Phonophoresis with a hydrocortisone gel applied to the small joints of the hands
3. Heating to reduce morning stiffness
4. Gentle, passively performed stretching exercises to preserve ROM
5. Isometrically performed toning exercises, especially for large and medium-sized joints
6. Occupational therapy (specialized splints, occupational aids)
7. Low-impact aerobic exercises as tolerated

Acute Period   *Ice* and *phonophoresis* using a hydrocortisone gel provide temporary relief of pain and swelling. Immobilization (e.g., wrist splinting, buddy tape) enhances the effectiveness of these treatments.

Recovery and Rehabilitation   *Heating,* often discovered and used regularly by the patient, is used to reduce the gel phenomenon and morning stiffness. *ROM* exercises are mandatory to preserve joint flexibility and to guard against tendon contracture. Medium-sized and large joints must be supported by well-toned muscles. If the patient has lost significant motor function because of chronic arthritis or deformity, *isometric toning exercises* must be used as a substitute for regular activities. *Occupational therapy* consultation should be considered if chronic arthritis or deformity interferes with the activities of daily living. Low-impact *aerobic exercise* is recommended for general conditioning.

INJECTION   Many patients with early presentations of RA, especially the monarthric and pauciarticular forms, can be managed successfully with local corticosteroid injection.

Positioning   The hand is placed flat with the palm down and the fingers extended.

Surface Anatomy and Point of Entry   The distal head of the proximal phalanges is located and marked. The joint line of the PIP joint is 1/4 inch distal to the most prominent portion of the head of the proximal phalanges. The point of entry is adjacent to the joint line and above the midplane.

Angle of Entry and Depth   The needle is inserted perpendicular to the skin. The depth of injection is 1/4 to 3/8 inch.

Anesthesia   Ethyl chloride is sprayed on the skin. Because the depth of the synovial membrane is so superficial, injection of local anesthetic in the subcutaneous tissue (0.25 mL) is optional. The tissues surrounding the small joints of the hand can accommodate only a small volume, so anesthetic should be kept to a minimum.

PROXIMAL INTERPHALANGEAL JOINT INJECTION

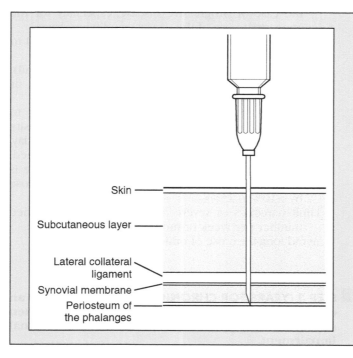

Skin
Subcutaneous layer
Lateral collateral ligament
Synovial membrane
Periosteum of the phalanges

Technique This technique uses an *indirect method* of injecting cortisone into the joint, taking advantage of the anatomic attachment of the synovial membrane to the adjacent bone. The synovial membrane is approximately 1 cm in length (p. 100). Instead of attempting to perform the injection into the center of the joint, which is difficult, painful, and potentially dangerous (cartilage damage), the 25-gauge needle is advanced through the synovial membrane and down to the bone adjacent to the joint line. The center of the joint is *not* entered directly. With the needle held flush against the bone, the medication is injected under the synovial membrane. Moderate pressure may be needed. If excess pressure or pain is experienced with injection, the needle is withdrawn $^1/_{16}$ inch.

INJECTION AFTERCARE

1. *Rest* for 3 days, avoiding all direct pressure, gripping, grasping, pinching, extremes of motion, vibration, and cold.
2. Use *buddy taping* to the adjacent PIP joint or a *finger splint* for the first few days.
3. Use *ice* (15 minutes every 4 to 6 hours) and *acetaminophen* (1000 mg twice a day) for postinjection soreness.
4. *Protect* for 3 to 4 weeks by limiting repetitive gripping, grasping, and pinching.
5. Begin passive ROM *stretching exercises* in flexion and extension at 2 to 3 weeks.
6. Begin isometrically performed *gripping exercises* at 4 to 5 weeks.
7. Repeat *injection* at 6 weeks if swelling persists or if ROM is still affected.
8. Suggest *padded gloves* or *padded tools* for long-term prevention in recurrent cases.

9. Obtain a *consultation* with a rheumatologist for advice on systemic medication for recurrent or progressive cases.

SURGICAL PROCEDURE Patients with poor response to systemic treatment, severe loss of articular cartilage, progressive deformity, or dramatic functional impairment should be offered surgical consultation. Procedures most often recommended include synovectomy for the large joints; arthroscopic débridement for medium-sized and large joints; arthroplasty for the shoulder, hip, and knee; and implant arthroplasty (replacement) for the small joints.

PROGNOSIS Most patients with early presentations of RA, especially the monarthric and pauciarticular forms, can be managed successfully with local corticosteroid injection. As the disease progresses to multiple joint involvement (especially multiple small joint involvement), however, systemic treatment with oral medication should be initiated. The decision to start sulfasalazine, hydroxychloroquine, gold, penicillamine, methotrexate, or a cytotoxic drug should not be delayed. These slow-acting antirheumatic drugs may take weeks or months to have an appreciable clinical effect. Patients with long-standing disease with progressive deformity and severe functional impairment should be evaluated by an orthopedic surgeon for synovectomy (large joints), arthroscopic débridement (medium-sized and large joints), arthroplasty (shoulder, hip, and knee), or implant arthroplasty (small joints).

DIFFERENTIAL DIAGNOSIS OF CHEST PAIN

Diagnoses	Confirmations
Rib cage (most common)	
Costochondritis	Local anesthetic block
Sternochondritis	Local anesthetic block
Tietze's syndrome	Exam
Endemic pleurodynia	Exam; local anesthetic block
Rib fracture, nondisplaced	Chest compression sign; chest x-ray or bone scan
Rib fracture, displaced	Chest compression sign; chest x-ray
Xiphodynia	Exam
Sternum	
Sternoclavicular joint strain	Local anesthetic block
Inflammatory arthritis of sternoclavicular joint	Local anesthetic block; abnormal erythrocyte sedimentation rate; exam correlations
Septic sternoclavicular joint (intravenous drug abuse)	Aspiration and culture
Referred pain to the chest wall	
Hiatal hernia	Gastrointestinal cocktail taken orally; barium swallow; endoscopy
Cholelithiasis	Liver chemistries; ultrasound
Splenic flexure syndrome	Exam; abdominal x-ray
Coronary artery disease	Electrocardiogram; creatine phosphokinase; troponin; angiogram
Aortic aneurysm	CT scan of chest; angiogram
Pneumonia	Chest x-ray; complete blood count; cultures
Pulmonary embolism	Oxygen saturation; D dimer; lung scan; CT scan; angiogram

STERNOCHONDRITIS/COSTOCHONDRITIS

Enter atop the center of the rib; angle the syringe
   perpendicular to the skin.

Needle: ⁵/₈-inch, 25-gauge
Depth: ¹/₂ to 1 inch, depending on the site
Volume: 1 to 2 mL of local anesthetic and 0.5 mL
   of either D80 or K40

NOTE: The injections should be placed flush against
   the cartilage adjacent to the costochondral
   junction using mild pressure.

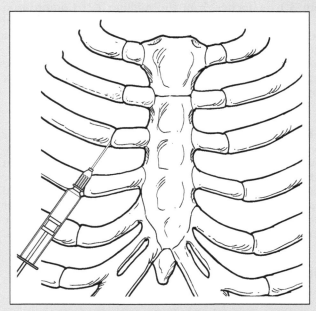

FIGURE 6–1. Costochondritis injection.

DESCRIPTION   *Costochondritis* is the term most clinicians use when referring to inflammation of the cartilage
of the chest wall. Specifically, costochondritis is the
inflammation that occurs at the junction of the rib and
the costal cartilage. *Sternochondritis* is the term applied
to the inflammation that occurs at the junction of the
sternum and the costal cartilage. Most cases have no
proven cause (idiopathic), although rarely cases follow
open heart surgery. Tietze's syndrome, often used
synonymously with costochondritis, is a distinct form of it.
This rare disorder is characterized by dramatic bulbous
swelling in addition to the local inflammatory changes.
Local tenderness of the chest wall and pain with chest
compression are the hallmark findings on exam. The diagnosis is confirmed with local anesthetic block placed at
the junction of the cartilage and bone. Most cases resolve
spontaneously over several weeks. Corticosteroid injection is occasionally necessary for uncommon persistent
cases.

SYMPTOMS   Most patients complain of anterior chest
pain or anterior chest pain overshadowed by the classic
symptoms of anxiety (patients are likely to confuse this
pain with coronary pain, especially if they have a positive
family history of heart disease). Patients often rub the
anterior chest wall when describing the condition.

"I think I'm having a heart attack!"

*"It hurts right here (pointing to the parasternal area
with one or two fingers) whenever I cough or take a
deep breath."*

*"I can't sleep on my left side at night … whenever I roll
over onto my side, I get this sharp pain in my chest."*

*"Ever since my bypass, I've had this sharp pain along the
side of my incision."*

"Coughing just kills me."

*"It's like there is sandpaper between the ends of my ribs.
It feels like the flesh has pulled away from the bone."*

EXAM   The patient is examined for localized tenderness
and swelling at the costochondral or the sternochondral
junctions and for pain aggravated by chest wall
compression.

EXAM SUMMARY

1. Localized tenderness either 1 inch from the
   midline of the sternum or at the costochondral
   junctions
2. Pain reproduced by chest wall compression (rib
   compression test)
3. Pain relief with regional anesthetic block just over
   the cartilage

(1) Chest wall tenderness—localized to the size of a
quarter—is palpable at the junction of the sternum and
the costal cartilage or at the junction between the rib and

the costal cartilage. The intercostal spaces should be nontender. The sternochondral junctions are $3/4$ to 1 inch lateral to the midline. The costochondral junctions vary from 3 to 4 inches from the midline. *(2)* Compression of the rib cage usually reproduces the patient's local chest wall pain. Pressure applied in the anteroposterior direction or from either side reproduces the discomfort. Similarly, a deep cough should recreate the pain. *(3)* The diagnosis is confirmed by a regional anesthetic block just atop the junction of the cartilage and bone.

X-RAYS   The patient's expectations for x-rays or special studies are always high with this condition. Routine chest x-rays and plain films of the ribs are often ordered, but they are normal in most cases. No specific changes are seen. Similarly, special testing is often ordered (e.g., bone scan, MRI) to exclude bony pathology or disease inside the chest. No specific abnormalities are seen that would assist in the diagnosis of costochondritis.

SPECIAL TESTING   Local anesthetic block is diagnostic.

DIAGNOSIS   The diagnosis is suggested by a history of localized chest pain and by an exam showing local tenderness over the bony rib cage aggravated by chest compression. The diagnosis can be confirmed by regional anesthetic block. The rapid control of chest pain with this simple, superficially placed injection is particularly useful in an anxious patient.

TREATMENT   The goals of treatment are to reassure the patient that this is not a life-threatening heart problem and to reduce the local inflammation. Observation and restriction of chest expansion and direct pressure are the treatments of choice for patients with mild symptoms that have been present only 4 to 6 weeks. Corticosteroid injection is the treatment of choice for patients with persistent or dramatic symptoms.

STEP 1   Perform a careful exam of the chest wall, heart, and lungs; identify the chondral junctions that are most involved; and order a chest x-ray and ECG to allay the concern of an anxious patient.
> Educate the patient: *"This is not a heart pain." "Most cases resolve on their own."*
> Reassure the patient that the condition is benign.
> Perform a regional anesthetic block to confirm the diagnosis or to reassure a severely anxious patient.
> Observe for 2 to 3 weeks.
> Prescribe a cough suppressant when indicated.
> Prescribe a rib binder or a neoprene waist wrap or a snug-fitting bra (do not use for a debilitated patient or for a patient >65 years old).
> Restrict chest expansion, lying on the sides, lifting, reaching, pushing, and pulling.

STEP 2 (4 TO 6 WEEKS FOR PERSISTENT CASES)   Perform a local anesthetic block and inject 0.5 mL of D80.
> Continue the restrictions.

STEP 3 (3 TO 4 WEEKS FOR PERSISTENT CASES)   Repeat the injection in 6 weeks if pain continues.
> Combine the injection with a rib binder.
> Continue the restrictions.

PHYSICAL THERAPY   Physical therapy does not play a significant role in the treatment of costochondritis. Phonophoresis with a hydrocortisone gel has questionable value.

INJECTION   Local anesthetic injection is used to differentiate the pain arising from the chest wall from coronary artery chest pain, pleuritic chest pain, or other causes of anterior chest pain. Corticosteroid injection is used to treat symptoms that persist beyond 6 to 8 weeks.
Positioning   The patient is placed in the supine position.
Surface Anatomy and Point of Entry   The point of maximum chest wall tenderness is carefully palpated. The center point of the cartilage is identified by placing one finger above and one finger below the cartilage in the intercostal spaces. The point of entry for *sternochondritis* is 1 inch from the midline of the sternum, directly over the center of the rib. The point of entry for *costochondritis* is over the point of maximum tenderness along the course of the rib.
Angle of Entry and Depth   The needle is inserted perpendicular to the skin. The depth of injection is $1/2$ inch for sternochondritis and $1/2$ to 1 inch for costochondritis.
Anesthesia   Ethyl chloride is sprayed on the skin. Local anesthetic is placed in the subcutaneous tissue (0.5 mL) and just above the firm resistance of the cartilage or the hard resistance of the bone.
Technique   Successful treatment depends on the identification of the most involved costal cartilage and the accurate localization of the junction of the cartilage and the bone. The most seriously affected costal cartilage is identified either by careful palpation of the most painful junction or by local anesthetic block. After anesthesia, an *indirect method* of injection is used to place the corticosteroid. This method takes advantage of the anatomic attachment of the synovial membrane to the rib and costal cartilage. The synovial membrane is approximately 1 cm in length. Instead of attempting to inject into the center of the joint, which is difficult, painful, and potentially damaging, the 25-gauge needle is advanced through the synovial membrane and down either to the hard resistance of the bone or to the firm resistance of the cartilage adjacent to the joint line. The center of the joint is *not* entered directly. With the needle held flush against the bone or cartilage, 0.5 mL of K40 or D80 is injected under the synovial membrane.

COSTOCHONDRITIS INJECTION

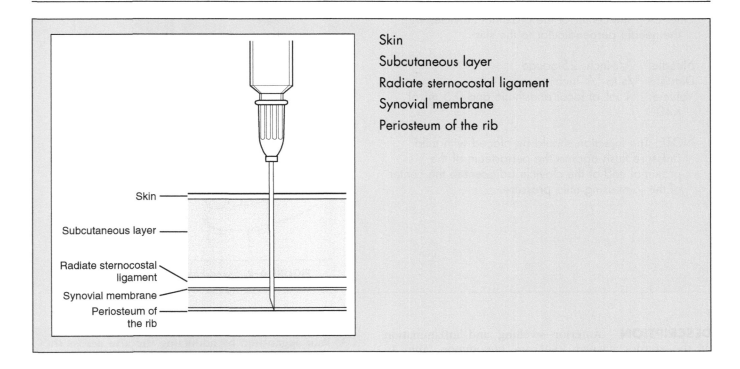

Skin

Subcutaneous layer

Radiate sternocostal ligament

Synovial membrane

Periosteum of the rib

Skin

Subcutaneous layer

Radiate sternocostal ligament

Synovial membrane

Periosteum of the rib

INJECTION AFTERCARE

1. *Rest* for 3 days, avoiding lying on the sides, lifting, strenuous activities, and direct pressure.
2. Combine the injection with a *rib binder* (or wide bra) for the first few days (especially for persistent or recurrent cases).
3. Use *ice* (15 minutes every 4 to 6 hours) and *acetaminophen (Tylenol ES)* (1000 mg twice a day) for postinjection soreness.
4. *Protect* the chest wall for 3 to 4 weeks by limiting lying on the sides, lifting, and strenuous activities and by aggressively treating coughing and sneezing.
5. Repeat *injection* at 6 weeks if local irritation continues.

SURGICAL PROCEDURE No surgical procedure is available.

PROGNOSIS Because most cases resolve spontaneously within 4 to 6 weeks, specific treatments may be unnecessary. Few cases require corticosteroid injection. In the few cases that persist beyond 4 to 6 weeks, local injection can provide excellent palliation of symptoms. Further workup is unnecessary in most cases. If symptoms are only partially controlled with local anesthesia, corticosteroid, or both, continued search for a second cause of chest pain is warranted.

STERNOCLAVICULAR JOINT SWELLING

Enter atop the center of the proximal clavicle, with the needle perpendicular to the skin.

Needle: ⁵/₈-inch, 25-gauge
Depth: ³/₈ to ¹/₂ inch
Volume: 1 mL of local anesthetic and 0.5 mL of K40

NOTE: The injection should be placed with mild pressure flush against the periosteum of the proximal end of the clavicle adjacent to the center of the joint using mild pressure.

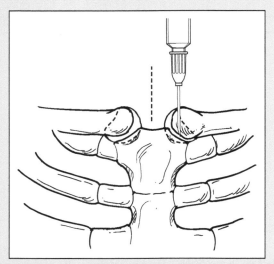

FIGURE 6–2. Sternoclavicular joint injection.

DESCRIPTION   Anterior swelling and inflammation of the sternoclavicular joint are uncommon. Mild to moderate swelling of the joint and pseudoenlargement of the proximal end of the clavicle occur most commonly as a consequence of either acute or remote trauma. Moderate inflammatory change can occur in the spondyloarthropathies, especially Reiter's disease. Septic arthritis with severe swelling, redness, and pain is an unusual complication of intravenous drug abuse.

SYMPTOMS   The patient complains of pain, swelling, or enlargement of the joint. The patient rubs over the swollen joint when describing the condition.

"My bone is growing."

"I can't sleep on my right side. The pain over my breast bone wakes me up."

"My breast bone is sore and swollen."

"I hate those stupid shoulder belts. I had a mild head-on collision and ever since the accident, my collar bone has been swollen."

EXAM   The patient is examined for swelling, tenderness, and subluxation of the sternoclavicular joint.

EXAM SUMMARY

1. Tenderness and swelling over the joint
2. Pseudoenlargement of the proximal end of the clavicle

3. Pain aggravated by adducting the arm across the chest, passively performed
4. Local anesthetic block to confirm the diagnosis

(1) The sternoclavicular joint is tender and swollen ³/₄ to 1 inch lateral to the midline, directly across from the sternal notch. *(2)* The proximal end of the clavicle often appears enlarged; this is the pseudoenlargement of the clavicle caused by swelling of the joint. Swelling of the joint not only gives the appearance of bony enlargement, but also contributes to anterior subluxation of the clavicle. *(3)* Pain arising from the sternoclavicular joint predictably is aggravated by passive adduction of the arm across the chest. This movement forces the clavicle against the sternum, compressing the joint. *(4)* Local anesthesia placed at the joint confirms the diagnosis.

X-RAYS   Apical lordotic x-rays of the upper chest adequately assess the clavicle and sternum bones. Careful comparison of the contours of the sternum and the size and relative shape of the proximal ends of the clavicles should not disclose any asymmetry.

SPECIAL TESTING   Because of the obvious enlargement of the joint and the appearance of enlargement of the proximal end of the clavicle, many patients are evaluated with bone scan, CT scan, or MRI. None of these tests diagnoses sternoclavicular arthritis.

DIAGNOSIS   The diagnosis is suggested by the typical findings of exam (local tenderness and swelling at the joint) and is confirmed by local anesthetic block placed just atop the joint. X-rays and special testing are used to rule out infection and tumor.

TREATMENT   The goal of treatment is to reduce the local swelling that has led to the pseudoenlargement of the joint. For a patient with mild symptoms that have been present only 4 to 6 weeks, direct application of ice is combined with restrictions on shoulder adduction and sleeping on the affected side. For a patient with persistent or dramatic symptoms, local anesthetic block combined with corticosteroid injection is the treatment of choice.

STEP 1   Order apical lordotic x-rays of the chest, confirm the diagnosis with local anesthesia, and reassure the patient that this is simply an enlargement of the joint resulting from swelling and subluxation.

Recommend ice over the joint to reduce pain and swelling temporarily.

Advise avoiding to-and-fro motions of the upper arm, reaching, and direct pressure.

Avoid sleeping on the affected shoulder.

Prescribe an antitussive if an acute cough develops.

STEP 2 (4 TO 6 WEEKS FOR PERSISTENT CASES)
Perform a local injection of K40.

Re-emphasize the restrictions.

STEP 3 (8 TO 10 WEEKS FOR PERSISTENT CASES)
Repeat the local injection of K40 if the first injection does not reduce swelling and pain by 50%.

Combine the injection with a shoulder immobilizer for 2 to 3 weeks.

To complete the recovery, recommend general shoulder conditioning, excluding exercises that involve reaching at or above the shoulder.

PHYSICAL THERAPY   Physical therapy does not play a significant role in the treatment or rehabilitation of this condition. Ice can be applied directly over the top of the joint for temporary control of symptoms. *General shoulder conditioning* is recommended after the acute symptoms have resolved. To avoid aggravating the joint, military press, bench press, and pectoralis exercises should be limited.

INJECTION   Local anesthetic injection is used to identify the sternoclavicular joint as the source of anterior chest wall swelling and pain. This procedure is especially necessary when the patient complains that the "bone is growing"—the pseudoenlargement of the proximal clavicle. Corticosteroid injection is used to treat symptoms that have persisted beyond 6 to 8 weeks.

Positioning   Enter directly over the center of the proximal clavicle.

Surface Anatomy and Point of Entry   The midline, the sternal notch, and the center of the proximal clavicle

STERNOCLAVICULAR JOINT INJECTION

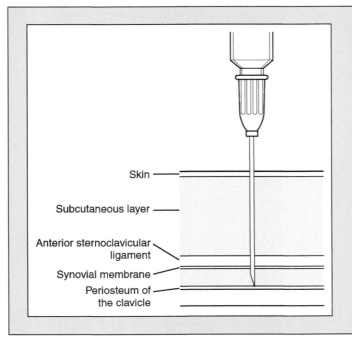

Skin
Subcutaneous layer
Anterior sternoclavicular ligament

Skin
Subcutaneous layer
Anterior sternoclavicular ligament
Synovial membrane
Periosteum of the clavicle

are identified and marked. The point of entry is $^3/_4$ to 1 inch from the midline, directly over the center of the proximal clavicle.

Angle of Entry and Depth The needle is inserted perpendicular to the skin. The depth of injection is $^3/_8$ to $^1/_2$ inch.

Anesthesia Ethyl chloride is sprayed on the skin. Local anesthetic is placed in the subcutaneous tissue (0.25 mL) and just above the firm to hard resistance of the periosteum of the bone (0.25 mL).

Technique The success of treatment depends on the accurate localization of the point of entry. After confirming the diagnosis with local anesthetic, the syringe containing the anesthetic is replaced with the second syringe containing 0.5 mL of K40. The needle is advanced down to the hard resistance of the clavicle. With just the weight of the syringe against the periosteum, the corticosteroid is injected flush against the bone. This is another example of the *indirect method* of injection of a small joint. Taking advantage of the 1-cm-long synovial membrane that attaches to the adjacent clavicle and sternum, the 25-gauge needle is held flush against the clavicle, and the medication is injected under the synovial membrane and into the joint.

INJECTION AFTERCARE

1. *Rest* for 3 days, avoiding sleeping on the affected side, reaching, lifting, and all strenuous activities.

2. Use *ice* (15 minutes every 4 to 6 hours) and *acetaminophen* (1000 mg twice a day) for postinjection soreness.

3. *Protect* for 3 to 4 weeks by limiting sleeping on the affected side, reaching, lifting, and all strenuous activities.

4. Combine the injection with a *shoulder immobilizer* for 3 to 7 days for persistent or recurrent cases.

5. Repeat the *injection* at 6 weeks if swelling persists or if range of motion is still affected.

SURGICAL PROCEDURE No surgical procedure is available.

PROGNOSIS Most patients who present with swelling in the sternoclavicular joint are concerned that the bone is growing. Apical lordotic views confirm the normal size of the proximal clavicles. CT and MRI of the chest are unnecessary. Local anesthetic block is an integral part of the diagnosis and is helpful in allaying the patient's anxiety: *"The bone appears larger because of the swelling in the joint that pushes the bone outward."* Corticosteroid injection is effective in palliating the local inflammation and pain.

DIFFERENTIAL DIAGNOSIS OF LOW BACK PAIN

Diagnoses	Confirmations
Lumbosacral back strain (most common)	
Unaccustomed or improper use	Exam: local tenderness; Schober's measurement
Reactive lumbosacral back strain	
Osteoarthritis	X-ray—routine back series
Scoliosis	X-ray—standing scoliosis views
Spondylolisthesis	X-ray—routine back series and oblique views
Herniated disk	CT or MRI
Compression fracture	X-ray—lateral view of the back; bone scan; MRI
Epidural process	MRI
Lumbosacral radiculopathy ("sciatica")	
Herniated disk	CT or MRI
Osteoarthritis—spinal stenosis	CT or MRI
Intra-abdominal process	Ultrasound or CT
Wallet sciatica	History
Sacroiliac (SI) joint	
Strain	Local anesthetic block
Sacroiliitis	X-ray—standing anteroposterior pelvis, oblique views of SI joints; bone scan
Referred pain	
Kidney (e.g., pyelonephritis, stones)	Urinalysis; intravenous pyelogram; ultrasound
Aorta	Ultrasound
Colon (e.g., appendicitis, cecal carcinoma, rectal carcinoma)	Hemoccult; barium enema
Pelvis (e.g., tumor, pregnancy)	Exam; ultrasound

LUMBOSACRAL STRAIN

Occasionally a patient presents with very localized tenderness in the erector spinae muscle; dramatic relief with local anesthesia is the best indication for corticosteroid injection.

Needle: 1¹/₂-inch, 21-gauge
Depth: 1¹/₄ to 1¹/₂ inches
Volume: 2 to 3 mL of anesthetic and 1 mL of D80

NOTE: Place the anesthesia at the first tissue plane—the erector spinae fascia—then enter the muscle three times to cover an area of approximately 1 inch horizontally.

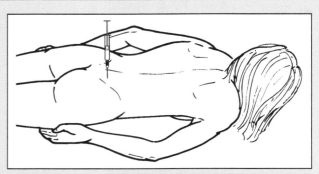

FIGURE 7–1. Acute lumbosacral back muscle injection.

DESCRIPTION   Lumbosacral strain is a spasm and irritation of the supporting muscles of the lumbar spine and is the end result of many different conditions. Although lumbosacral strain commonly occurs as an isolated problem—the overuse of improperly stretched and toned muscles—a significant proportion of cases are the result of an underlying cause. Pathologically, lumbosacral stain is the body's natural reaction to the threat of injury to the spinal column—spinal nerve, root, or cord. The most common causes of this reactive muscle spasm are poor posture, scoliosis, spondylolisthesis, advanced osteoarthritis (spinal stenosis), compression fracture, and radiculopathy from any cause. Severe and persistent muscle spasm can lead to secondary problems, including acquired scoliosis (reversible), a loss of the normal lumbosacral kyphotic curve, "sensory" sciatica (common and reversible), and trochanteric or gluteus medius bursitis (the principal cause of these conditions).

SYMPTOMS   The patient complains of a well-localized lower back pain and muscle stiffness. The patient often rubs the lower back and flank when describing the condition.

"Oh, my aching back."

"My back is so stiff in the morning I can hardly straighten up ... I have to take a long hot shower to loosen up."

"I used to be able to touch my toes."

"I get these terrible back spasms right here (using the hand to rub the side of the lower back)."

"I can't find a comfortable chair to sit in anymore ... I've tried everything from hardbacks to recliners."

"I can't bend forward without my back killing me."

"I can't find a comfortable position in bed, let alone a comfortable mattress."

"I don't want to end up like my father, all hunched over and unable to bend over."

EXAM   The patient is examined for the degree of paraspinal muscle spasm and tenderness, and an assessment is made of the loss of range of motion of the back.

EXAM SUMMARY

1. Paraspinal muscle tenderness and spasm
2. Straightening of the lumbosacral curve
3. Decreased lumbosacral flexion (abnormal Schober's measurement) and lateral bending
4. Normal neurologic exam, unless there is concomitant radiculopathy

(1) The maximum paraspinal muscle tightening is 1¹/₂ inches off the midline, adjacent to L3-L4. A second common trigger point is at the origin of the erector spinae, just above the sacroiliac (SI) joint. *(2)* The normal lumbosacral lordotic curve is straightened in the case of severe muscle spasm. If the strain is unilateral, the back may tilt to the affected side (an "acquired," or reversible, scoliosis). *(3)* Measurements of lumbosacral flexion and lateral bending are impaired. Schober's test, measuring lumbosacral flexion, is abnormal in most cases. With the patient standing as erect as possible, two lines, 10 cm apart, are marked in the midline just above a line drawn between the iliac crests. The patient is asked to flex forward at the waist. At full lumbosacral flexion, the marks are remeasured. A 50% increase to 15 cm is normal. The patient is asked to report any symptoms when flexing forward. In addition, measurements of lateral bending add to the objective measurement of back mobility. Two lines, 20 cm apart, are marked along the flank above the lateralmost point of the iliac crest and should increase

to 26 cm (a 33% increase) when bending to the side. (4) The neurologic exam of the lower extremity should be normal, unless concomitant radiculopathy is present.

X-RAYS Lumbosacral spine x-rays with oblique views can be helpful in defining the degree of spondylolisthesis, the severity of the scoliosis, the degree of degenerative disk disease, or the presence of advanced osteoarthritis or in estimating the degree of osteoporosis. Uncomplicated cases of lumbar strain—cases unassociated with scoliosis and old compression fractures—should have normal x-rays.

SPECIAL TESTING Special testing with CT or MRI is indicated when the local back symptoms are accompanied by moderate to severe radicular symptoms, particularly when neurologic symptoms and signs are prominent, and the motor system is involved (p. 116).

DIAGNOSIS The diagnosis of uncomplicated lumbosacral strain is based on the presence of pain, tenderness, and spasm localized to the lower back and on the absence of any other significant underlying back processes, such as acute compression fracture, radiculopathy, or epidural processes. If the lumbar strain presentation is atypical (e.g., severity of symptoms, intermittent but severe radicular symptoms and signs, unusual injury), a workup for an underlying process should not be delayed.

TREATMENT The goals of therapy are to reduce the acute erector spinae muscle spasm, to reduce the tendency of recurrent muscle spasm by stretching and toning exercises, and to treat any underlying structural back condition. Bed rest combined with physical therapy exercises and a muscle relaxant are the treatments of choice.

STEP 1 Examine the back thoroughly and perform a complete lower extremity neurologic exam; perform Schober's measurements, order plain x-rays of the lumbosacral spine with oblique views, and order a CT scan or MRI if radicular symptoms are prominent and involve the motor system (p. 116).
>   Recommend 3 to 4 days of bed rest for acute, severe cases.
>   Use crutches if pain and spasm are severe.
>   Apply ice, alternating with heat, to the low back.
>   Prescribe a muscle relaxant in a dosage sufficient to cause mild sedation, and recommend taking it only when the patient is recumbent.
>   Prescribe a nonsteroidal anti-inflammatory drug (NSAID), but note that the drug may have limited benefit because inflammation is not a significant part of the process.
>   Use an appropriate amount of narcotics for the first week, but limit their use thereafter.
>   Order therapeutic ultrasound from a physical therapist for deep heating. Avoid twisting and extremes of bending and tilting.

>   Advise on proper lifting: Hold the object close to the body, bend at the knee and not with the back, never lift in a twisted position, carry heavier objects as close as possible to the body.
>   Reinforce the importance of correct posture; suggest a lumbar support for the office chair and vehicle.
>   Begin gentle stretching exercises to maintain flexibility (p. 281).

STEP 2 (2 TO 4 WEEKS FOR PERSISTENT CASES) Re-evaluate the neurologic exam and back motion.
>   Begin strengthening exercises (p. 283).
>   Begin water aerobics, low-impact walking, or swimming to re-establish general conditioning without stressing the recovering back muscles.
>   Reduce the use of medication.
>   Resume normal activities gradually, but with continued attention to proper care of the back.

STEP 3 (6 TO 8 WEEKS FOR CHRONIC CASES) If symptoms are chronic, use a lumbosacral corset for external support (p. 254).
>   Order a transcutaneous electrical nerve stimulation (TENS) unit.
>   Consider the use of a tricyclic antidepressant.
>   Refer to a pain clinic.

PHYSICAL THERAPY

Physical therapy is a fundamental part of the treatment of acute and chronic low back strain and is the main treatment for rehabilitation and prevention.

PHYSICAL THERAPY SUMMARY
1. Ice alternating with heat
2. Low-impact aerobic exercises
3. Stretching exercises for erector spinae, the SI joint, and the gluteus muscles, passively performed
4. Toning exercises of the back and abdominal muscles, performed with minimal movement of the back
5. Lumbar traction

Acute Period Cold, heat, and gentle stretching exercises are used in the early treatment of lumbar strain to reduce acute muscular spasm and to increase lumbar flexibility. *Cold, heat, and cold alternating with heat* are effective in reducing pain and muscular spasm. Recommendations are based on individual clinical responses. *Stretching exercises* are fundamental for maintaining flexibility, especially in patients with structural back disease. Side-bends, knee-chest pulls, and pelvic rocks—Williams' flexion exercises—are designed to stretch the paraspinal muscles, the gluteus muscles, and the SI joints (p. 281). These exercises should be started after hyperacute symptoms have resolved. Stretching is performed after heating the body. Initially, these exercises should be performed while the patient is lying down. As pain and muscular spasm ease, stretching can be performed while the patient is standing. Each exercise is performed in sets of 20. Stretching should never exceed the patient's level of mild discomfort.

Recovery and Rehabilitation   To continue the recovery process and to reduce the possibility of a recurrence, toning exercises are added at 3 to 4 weeks. *Toning exercises* are performed after the acute muscular spasms have subsided. Modified sit-ups, weighted side-bends, and gentle extension exercises (p. 281) are performed after heating and stretching. Aerobic exercise is one of the best ways to prevent recurrence. Swimming, cross-country ski machine workouts, low-impact water aerobics, fast walking, and light jogging are aerobic fitness exercises that are unlikely to aggravate the back.

Traction is used infrequently for acute lumbosacral strain. Patients with acute facet syndrome or persistent acute lumbar strain (despite home bed rest, medication, and physical therapy) may respond dramatically to 25 to 35 lb of lumbar traction in bed. In addition, traction can be used at home in combination with traditional stretching exercises (p. 282). *Vertical traction* can be achieved by suspending the legs between two bar stools, leaning against a countertop, or using inversion equipment. The weight of the body is used to pull the lumbar segments apart. Traction is used primarily for prevention. It is not appropriate for hyperacute strain. Chronic back strain

unresponsive to traditional physical therapy may require a TENS unit for control of chronic pain.

INJECTION   Local injection of the paraspinal muscles or the lumbar facet joints is performed infrequently and is of questionable overall value. Occasionally a patient presents with localized tenderness in the erector spinae and responds to local anesthesia. Dramatic relief with anesthesia is the best indication for corticosteroid injection.

Positioning   The patient is placed in the prone position, completely flat.

Surface Anatomy and Point of Entry   The spinous processes of the lumbosacral spine are marked. The point of entry is $1^1/_2$ inches from the midline, directly at the point of maximum muscle tenderness at the convexity of the paraspinous muscle.

Angle of Entry and Depth   The needle is inserted perpendicular to the skin. The depth of injection is $1^1/_4$ to $1^1/_2$ inches.

Anesthesia   Ethyl chloride is sprayed on the skin. Local anesthetic is placed in the subcutaneous tissue (0.5 mL), just above the moderate resistance of the outer fascia of the muscle (1 mL), and in the muscle belly itself (1 to 2 mL).

Technique   The success of treatment depends on accurate *intramuscular* injection. A 22-gauge $1^1/_2$-inch needle is passed vertically down to the firm, rubbery resistance of the outer fascia of the muscle, approximately 1 to $1^1/_4$ inches deep. The muscle is entered three times

ERECTOR SPINAE MUSCLE INJECTION

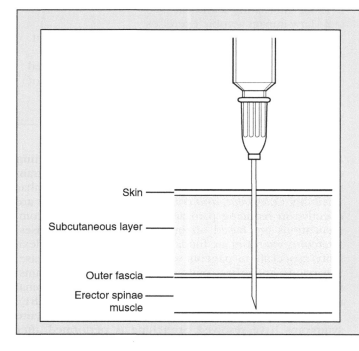

Skin
Subcutaneous layer
Outer fascia
Erector spinae muscle

Skin
Subcutaneous layer
Outer fascia
Erector spinae muscle

in an area the size of a quarter; 2 to 3 mL of local anesthetic is injected. The needle is withdrawn, and the local tenderness, range of motion, or both are re-evaluated. If pain and function are improved, the muscle can be injected with 1 mL of D80. Local anesthetic injection, either to confirm the diagnosis or to treat the acute case of lumbosacral strain, can be used alone, however.

INJECTION AFTERCARE

1. *Rest* for 3 days, avoiding all direct pressure, walking, standing, bending, and twisting.
2. Strongly recommend *bed rest for 3 days* and crutches with touch-down weightbearing for severe cases.
3. Use *ice* (15 minutes every 4 to 6 hours) and *acetaminophen (Tylenol ES)* (1000 mg twice a day) for postinjection soreness.
4. *Protect* the back for 3 to 4 weeks by limiting prolonged standing, unnecessary walking, repetitive bending, lifting, and twisting.
5. Prescribe a *lumbosacral corset* for the first 2 to 3 weeks for recurrent or severe cases.
6. Begin passive *stretching exercises* in flexion (Williams' exercises) when the acute pain has begun to resolve (knee-chest pulls, pelvic rocks, and side-bends).
7. Repeat *injection* at 6 weeks with corticosteroid if pain and muscle spasm persist.
8. Begin active *toning exercises* of the abdominal and lower back muscles when flexibility has been restored.
9. Obtain *plain x-rays, CT scans, or MRI* to identify subtle disk, progressive spondylolisthesis, or other correctable conditions in a patient with chronic symptoms.

SURGICAL PROCEDURE   Surgery is not indicated for a patient with an uncomplicated lumbosacral strain. If a correctable, underlying cause is identified (e.g., subtle disk, spondylolisthesis, scoliosis) and the chance of substantial overall improvement is likely, surgery should be considered.

PROGNOSIS   Most episodes of lumbosacral strain resolve completely with a combination of rest, stretching exercises, and 7 to 10 days of a muscle relaxant. Because lumbosacral muscle spasm can be a reaction to an underlying threat to the spinal column, however, any patient with recurrent or severe strain must be evaluated for underlying structural back disease, lumbar radiculopathy, and spinal stenosis. Plain films of the lumbar spine, CT, MRI, or electromyography is required for these more involved cases. Surgery is indicated when a correctable underlying condition is uncovered.

LUMBAR RADICULOPATHY, HERNIATED DISK, AND SCIATICA

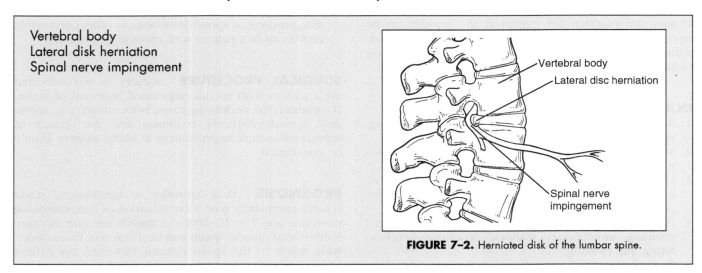

Vertebral body
Lateral disk herniation
Spinal nerve impingement

Vertebral body
Lateral disc herniation
Spinal nerve impingement

FIGURE 7–2. Herniated disk of the lumbar spine.

DESCRIPTION   *Sciatica* is the term commonly used to describe pain associated with the abnormal function of the lumbosacral nerve roots or of one of the nerves of the lumbosacral plexus. Pressure on the nerve from a herniated disk, from bony osteophytes (narrowed lateral recess or spinal stenosis), a compression fracture, or any other extrinsic pressure (e.g., epidural process, pelvic mass, or "wallet sciatica") causes progressive sensory, sensorimotor, or sensorimotor visceral loss.

Sensory-only sciatica—relatively minor degrees of nerve compression—is more likely to improve with conservative management (p. 113). Sensorimotor sciatica—significant pressure affecting the motor nerves—requires early radiographic study, more aggressive treatment, and surgical intervention, especially when neurologic function gradually deteriorates. Sciatica-associated motor or bowel and bladder symptoms—sensorimotor visceral sciatica, the most severe degree of neurologic dysfunction—are an emergent problem that requires immediate study, surgical consultation, and aggressive surgical treatment.

Patients with long-standing symptoms—chronic sciatica, nearly always sensory only—are approached separately. Treatment emphasizes physical therapy stretching, proper care of the back, and long-term restrictions, but can include epidural injection of an anesthetic and corticosteroid. This procedure should be performed by an anesthesiologist or interventional radiologist.

SYMPTOMS   The sciatica pain pattern varies considerably depending on the degree of nerve compression. The patient may complain of pain in the buttock area, pain radiating a variable distance down the lateral or posterior leg, or pain in an isolated part of the lower leg. The patient also may describe a loss of feeling or an abnormal sensation in the feet (sensory sciatica), weakness or clumsiness of the lower leg (sensorimotor sciatica), or loss of control of bowel or bladder function (visceral involvement).

"I have this shooting pain down my leg. It starts in my hip and goes all the way to my toes."

"My feet feel like they're coming out of Novocain, they're tingling."

"I'm dragging my leg."

"My leg feels weak."

"If I cough, I get this electric shock down my leg."

"If I sit too long, my toes go numb."

"It feels as if I have this burning steel rod in the center of my calf."

EXAM   The patient is examined for the degree of lower extremity neurologic impairment (sensory, sensorimotor, or sensorimotor visceral), and an evaluation of its underlying cause is conducted.

EXAM SUMMARY

1. Abnormal straight-leg-raising
2. Percussion tenderness over the spinous processes
3. Abnormal neurologic exam: sensory loss, loss of deep tendon reflex, motor weakness, loss of bowel or bladder control
4. Signs of lumbosacral strain
5. Signs reflecting the underlying cause

(1) The hallmark sign of sciatica is pain with the straight-leg-raising maneuver. The maneuver should be reproducible in a given position and angle and should reproduce the patient's radicular symptoms in the lower extremity. Forced dorsiflexion of the ankle may be necessary to bring out a subtle case. *(2)* Percussion tenderness over

the spinous processes may be present in cases of acute herniated disks, epidural processes, and other acute vertebral bony processes; however, it is an unreliable sign in spinal stenosis or any process that is outside the vertebral column. (3) Neurologically, loss of sensation in a radicular pattern is the most subtle and earliest sign of nerve dysfunction. Light touch, pinprick, and 2-point discrimination are lost early. Advanced conditions also may show loss of deep tendon reflexes, loss of strength of involved muscle groups (most commonly foot dorsiflexion and plantar flexion), or loss of bowel and urinary control (cauda equina syndrome). (4) Signs of lumbosacral muscular strain may accompany sciatica (p. 112). Local paraspinous muscle tenderness and spasm and loss of normal lumbosacral flexibility may be present. (5) Signs reflecting the underlying process must be sought if the primary process is not readily evident at the spinal level.

X-RAYS Lumbosacral spine x-rays with oblique views can be helpful in determining the integrity of the vertebral bones, the degree of spondylolisthesis, the presence of compression fractures, and an estimation of the degree of osteoarthritis (exuberant osteophytes or extreme degrees of facet joint sclerotic bone can provide a strong clue to the presence of spinal stenosis. Plain x-rays of the spine are not effective, however, in determining the specific cause of sciatica.

SPECIAL TESTING Defining the exact cause of lumbar radiculopathy requires a CT scan or MRI. These imaging techniques are mandatory when considering the diagnosis of epidural metastasis or abscess. They provide accurate anatomic measurements of the diameter of the spinal canal (spinal stenosis), the width of the lateral recess exit foramina, the degree of disk herniation along with the presence of nerve compression or spinal cord indentation, the presence of scar tissue from previous laminectomy, the integrity of the vertebral bodies, and the presence of fibrotic tissue associated with spondylolisthesis. Patients who present with intermediate symptoms and signs and inconclusive imaging may require electromyography for evaluation of specific nerve root dysfunction.

DIAGNOSIS The diagnosis of sciatica often is based solely on the description of a radicular pain provided by the patient. One of the best neurologic correlates is the patient's description of the location of the pain: down the posterior leg (L5-S1) or down the lateral leg (L4-L5). The neurologic examination is used to stage the severity of the problem (i.e., sensory, sensorimotor, or sensorimotor visceral). Definitive diagnosis requires specialized testing, however.

TREATMENT The goals of treatment are to confirm the diagnosis, to reduce the pressure over the nerve, to improve neurologic function, to reduce any accompanying low back strain, and to evaluate for the need for surgery.

The treatments of choice vary according to the neurologic findings. Three days of bed rest combined with physical therapy exercises and a muscle relaxant is the treatment of choice for patients with sensory radiculopathy and patients with mild motor involvement. Patients with dramatic motor signs can be managed similarly, but should undergo early imaging and neurosurgical consultation. Patients with sensorimotor visceral involvement should be hospitalized, seen by the neurosurgeon, and imaged the day of admission.

STEP 1   Examine the back thoroughly, perform Schober's measurement, and assess the neurologic function of the lower extremities.

Perform lumbosacral spine x-rays or order a CT scan or MRI, depending on the severity of the signs and symptoms.

Apply ice to the lower back muscles for analgesia and to reduce muscle spasm.

Order bed rest for 3 to 5 days for acute symptoms.

Limit walking and standing to 30 to 45 minutes each day.

Advocate the use of crutches to avoid pressure on the back (from bed to the bathroom and back).

Prescribe a muscle relaxant—strong enough to cause mild to moderate sedation—and an appropriate dose of a potent narcotic.

Hospitalize the patient and consult with a neurosurgeon if the patient has bilateral symptoms, extreme motor weakness, incontinence of stool or urine, or urinary retention.

STEP 2 (7 TO 14 DAYS ACUTE FOLLOW-UP)   Reevaluate the patient's neurologic and back exams.

Begin gentle stretching exercises while the patient is still on bed rest (p. 281).

Use hand-held weights in bed to keep the upper body toned.

Liberalize the amount of time spent out of bed, still relying on crutches.

Use a simple lumbosacral corset while out of bed (p. 254).

Consider an injection of the erector spinae muscle with local anesthetic, corticosteroid, or both for muscle spasms or an epidural injection of D80 for persistent nerve irritation.

STEP 3 (2 TO 3 WEEKS FOR PERSISTENT CASES)   Reevaluate the patient's neurologic and back exams.

Consider a moderate dose of oral corticosteroid for persistent sensory sciatica (prednisone, 30 to 40 mg for several days, followed by a rapid taper).

Reduce the use of medications.

Begin muscle-toning exercises of the lower back (p. 283).

Advise swimming to tone muscles and recondition the cardiovascular system.

Use crutches to assist in ambulation until the patient has recovered sufficient muscle tone.

Emphasize proper care of the back.

STEP 4 (3 TO 6 WEEKS FOR PERSISTENT CASES OR WORSENING SYMPTOMS)   Order a neurosurgical consultation if motor symptoms intervene, persist, or progress.

Refer the patient to an anesthesiologist for an epidural steroid injection in the case of persistent sensory sciatica.

Resume normal activities gradually, but with continued attention to proper care of the back.

If symptoms are chronic, use a lumbosacral corset for external support (p. 254), order a TENS unit, consider the use of a tricyclic antidepressant, or refer to a pain clinic.

Passive stretching exercises of the lower back in flexion are performed after heat applications (knee-chest pulls, side-bends, and pelvic rocks) and combined with the McKenzie extension exercises as tolerated.

PHYSICAL THERAPY   Physical therapy plays an integral part in the active treatment and prevention of recurrent sciatica. Greater emphasis is placed on bed rest for hyperacute symptoms, on crutches to assist in ambulation, and on general muscular toning while on bed rest.

INJECTION   Local injection of the paraspinal muscles or of the lumbar facet joints is performed infrequently and is of questionable overall value. Occasionally a patient presents with localized tenderness in the erector spinae and responds dramatically to local anesthesia, corticosteroid injection, or both (p. 114).

SURGICAL PROCEDURE   Large disk herniation, fragmented disk herniations, or osteoarthritic changes causing persistent pressure on the spinal nerve, root, or cord should be considered for diskectomy, decompression laminectomy (spinal stenosis), or surgical fusion (unstable vertebral body). Surgery is not indicated for intermittent sciatic pain, minor disk bulges, or radicular symptoms that do not correlate directly with scan results.

PROGNOSIS   To determine the most appropriate treatment and to ensure the best outcome, it is imperative that the patient's symptoms and signs correlate exactly with the anatomic abnormalities on x-ray or imaging studies. The history and neurologic exam are used to define which neurologic level is affected and the degree of neurologic impairment. Imaging studies are used to define the anatomy and distinguish herniated nucleus pulposus from spinal stenosis, spondylolisthesis, and epidural abscess. Electromyography is used to confirm the extent of neurologic impairment and identify the most involved nerve root when more than one spinal level is affected. The outcome of lumbar radiculopathy depends on the degree of neurologic impairment on exam, the length of time the nerve has been under pressure, the underlying process (e.g., herniated nucleus pulposus, spinal stenosis, epidural abscess), and the age and general medical condition of the patient. Patients with sensory complaints only or with minimal motor findings do well with medical treatment. Most patients (75% to 80%) respond to nonsurgical conservative therapy. Surgical consultation always is indicated for progressive neurologic deficits, large disk herniations associated with dramatic motor loss or incontinence, and fragmented disks with fragments lodged in the neuroforamina.

SACROILIAC STRAIN

Enter 1 inch caudal to the posterior superior iliac spine and 1 inch lateral to the midline; advance at a 70-degree angle to the firm resistance of the posterior supporting ligaments.

Needle: 1¹/₂-inch or 3¹/₂-inch, 22-gauge
Depth: 1¹/₂ to 2¹/₂ inches
Volume: 1 to 2 mL of local anesthetic and 1 mL of K40

NOTE: The injection should be placed flush against the periosteum at the junction of the sacrum and the ileum at the maximum depth.

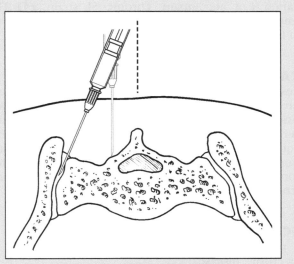

FIGURE 7–3. Sacroiliac joint injection.

DESCRIPTION SI strain and sacroiliitis are the two most common diagnoses affecting the articulation between the sacrum and the ileum. SI strain results from the mechanical irritation of improper lifting, twisting injuries, seat belt injuries, or direct trauma. Rheumatic inflammation of the joint is referred to as *sacroiliitis* and is associated most often with the spondyloarthropathies, including Reiter's disease, ankylosing spondylitis, and ulcerative colitis–associated arthritis. Septic arthritis of the SI joint is rare. Regardless of etiology, symptoms of this unique cause of low back pain are generally well localized to the lower back. With increasing severity, symptoms can be referred into the gluteal area or down the back of the leg, mimicking sciatica.

SYMPTOMS The patient complains of a well-localized pain and stiffness in the bottom of the lumbosacral spine or of pain referred to the gluteal area or down the leg. The patient often rubs the iliac crest and gluteal area when describing the symptoms.

"I have this sharp pain in my buttock every time I twist."

"I'm losing the flexibility in my lower back."

"Sitting has become very painful down here on my left side (pointing to the left lower buttock)."

"It feels like an ice pick is being shoved into my lower back."

"I can't climb into bed very easily, let alone find a comfortable position for any length of time."

"My back gets so stiff after sitting for prolonged periods that I have to push myself up with my hands (the patient demonstrates how he walks his hands up the anterior thigh to arise out of his chair)."

EXAM The patient is examined for local irritation of the SI joint, for flexibility of the lumbosacral spine, and for secondary inflammation of the trochanteric or gluteus medius bursa.

EXAM SUMMARY

1. Local tenderness directly over the SI joint
2. Tenderness aggravated by compression or by pelvic torque (fabere maneuver)
3. Stiffness to the lumbosacral spine (abnormal Schober's measurement)
4. Secondary trochanteric or gluteus medius bursa tenderness
5. Dramatic relief with local anesthetic block

(1) SI joint tenderness is best identified with the patient lying prone. A quarter-sized area of tenderness is located 1 inch medial and 1 inch inferior to the posterior superior iliac spine (PSIS). Because the joint is hidden under the iliac bone, firm pressure must be directed laterally. Contrast this with the more accessible tenderness of the erector spinae muscle located superior to the PSIS and extending well up into the lumbosacral curve. *(2)* SI pain should be aggravated by pelvic compression or by the application of torque across the joint. Compression can be accomplished by pushing down on the lateral aspect of the pelvis when the patient is lying in the lateral decubitus position. Torque can be applied to the joint by placing the hip in a figure-of-four position (p. 285) and simultaneously pushing on the contralateral anterior superior iliac spine and the ipsilateral knee—the Patrick, or *fabere* (*f*lexion, *ab*duction, *e*xternal *r*otation, and

extension) test. *(3)* As with lumbosacral strain, a patient with SI irritation may have an abnormal Schober test (p. 112). *(4)* Trochanteric and gluteus medius bursal irritation can accompany chronic SI strain. *(5)* The diagnosis is complete when dramatic relief is achieved with local anesthetic block.

X-RAYS   A standing anteroposterior pelvis x-ray is an excellent screening test for sacroiliitis, leg-length discrepancy, osteoarthritis of the hip joint, bony abnormalities of the pelvis and femur, and conditions of the lower lumbosacral spine. If sacroiliitis or SI strain is likely, oblique views of the pelvis should be obtained for greater anatomic detail. A lumbosacral spine series is indicated if concurrent scoliosis, spondylolisthesis, or other cause of structural back disease is suspected.

SPECIAL TESTING   Nuclear medicine joint scans or MRI provides more detailed information of synovitis or bony erosive disease.

DIAGNOSIS   The diagnosis of SI joint disease requires a history of localized lower back pain and an exam showing SI joint tenderness. The specific diagnosis of SI strain requires confirmation by local anesthetic block. The specific diagnosis of sacroiliitis requires an elevated erythrocyte sedimentation rate combined with typical changes on plain x-rays (erosive disease) or an abnormal nuclear medicine joint scan. A ratio of radionuclide uptake of the SI joint to the surrounding iliac bone greater than 1.3 is highly suggestive of sacroiliitis.

TREATMENT   The goals of treatment are to reduce local inflammation in the SI joint and to increase the flexibility of the lumbosacral spine and SI areas. Rest and physical therapy exercises are the treatments of choice for unilateral localized SI strain. NSAIDs are the treatment of choice for patients with inflammatory sacroiliitis. Corticosteroid injection is the treatment of choice for patients with persistent or dramatic symptoms of SI strain.

STEP 1   **Examine thoroughly the SI joint, the lumbosacral spine, and the two large bursae at the hip; perform Schober's measurement of lumbosacral flexibility; and order a standing anteroposterior pelvis x-ray.**

Ice placed over the lower sacrum can be tried, but is only partially effective because of the depth of the joint.

Avoid twisting and extremes of bending and tilting.

Advise on proper lifting involving the knees: Hold the object close to the body, bend at the knee and not with the back, never lift in a twisted position, carry heavier objects particularly close to the body.

Reinforce the need to maintain correct posture; suggest a lumbar support for the office chair and vehicle.

Suggest an SI belt to be worn during the day (p. 254).

Begin Williams' flexion exercises to maintain muscle flexibility (p. 281).

Recommend a muscle relaxant at night in a dosage sufficient to cause mild sedation, if concurrent lumbosacral muscle spasm is present.

Limit pain medication to 7 to 10 days.

Prescribe an NSAID if sacroiliitis is suspected.

Recommend 3 to 4 days of bed rest for an acute, severe case.

Use crutches if pain and spasm are severe.

STEP 2 (2 TO 4 WEEKS FOR PERSISTENT CASES)   **Perform a local anesthetic block to confirm the diagnosis or distinguish symptoms arising from the SI joint from symptoms arising from the lower back, and inject with 1 mL of K40 if the SI joint is the primary source.**

Recommend 3 to 4 days of bed rest after the injection. Continue the restrictions.

Begin flexion stretching exercises (knee-chest pulls, side-bends, and pelvic rocks) after the pain and inflammation have been substantially controlled.

STEP 3 (6 TO 8 WEEKS FOR PERSISTENT CASES)   **Repeat corticosteroid injection if symptoms have not improved by at least 50%.**

Begin strengthening exercises, including modified sit-ups and weighted side-bends (p. 283).

Begin general conditioning of the back, and gradually increase water aerobics, low-impact walking, or swimming.

Resume normal activities gradually, but with continued attention to proper care of the back.

STEP 4 (10 TO 12 WEEKS FOR CHRONIC CASES)   **Use a Velcro lumbosacral corset or SI belt for external support if symptoms are recurrent or become chronic (p. 254).**

Order a TENS unit.

Consider the use of a tricyclic antidepressant.

Refer to a pain clinic.

PHYSICAL THERAPY   Physical therapy plays a fundamental role in the treatment of conditions affecting the SI joint and is essential for rehabilitation and prevention.

PHYSICAL THERAPY SUMMARY
1. Ice over the SI joint
2. Williams' flexion exercises (knee-chest, side-bends, and pelvic rocks), performed passively
3. Toning exercises of erector spinae and abdominal muscles, performed with minimal motion of the lower spine

Acute Period   Cold, heat, and gentle stretching exercises are used in the early treatment of SI strain to reduce the acute muscular spasm that accompanies this localized lower back irritation. *Cold, heat, and cold alternating with heat* are effective in reducing pain and muscular spasm. Recommendations are based on individual clinical responses. *Stretching exercises* are fundamental to maintaining SI and lower back flexibility. Side-bends, knee-chest pulls, and pelvic rocks—Williams' flexion exercises—are designed to stretch the paraspinal muscles, the gluteus muscles, and the SI joints (p. 281). These exercises should be started after hyperacute symptoms have resolved. Stretching is performed after the body is heated. Initially, these exercises should be performed while the patient is lying down. As pain and muscular spasm ease, stretching can be performed while the patient is standing. Each exercise is performed in sets of 20. Stretching should never exceed the patient's level of mild discomfort.

Recovery and Rehabilitation   To continue the recovery process and to reduce the possibility of a recurrence, toning exercises are added at 3 to 4 weeks. *Toning exercises* are performed after the acute muscular spasms have subsided. Modified sit-ups, weighted side-bends, and gentle extension exercises (p. 283) are performed after heating and stretching. Aerobic exercise is one of the best ways to prevent recurrence. Swimming, cross-country ski machine workouts, low-impact water aerobics, fast walking, and light jogging are excellent low-impact exercises that are unlikely to aggravate the back. Chronic pain arising from the SI joint unresponsive to traditional physical therapy may require a TENS unit for control of chronic pain.

INJECTION   Local injection with anesthesia can be used to differentiate conditions affecting the SI joint from the local irritation and spasm of the paraspinal muscles (the origin of erector spinae), pain arising from the lumbosacral spine, or pain arising from the lower lumbosacral roots. Corticosteroid injection is used to treat the persistent inflammation of the SI joint that fails to respond to rest, physical therapy exercises, and bracing.

Positioning   The patient is placed in the prone position, perfectly flat.

Surface Anatomy and Point of Entry   The PSIS is identified and marked. A line is drawn in the midline. The point of entry is 1 inch caudal to the PSIS and 1 inch lateral to the midline.

Angle of Entry and Depth   The angle of entry is 70 degrees with the needle directed outward. The depth of injection is $1^1/_2$ to $2^1/_2$ inches, depending on the weight of the patient.

Anesthesia   Ethyl chloride is sprayed on the skin. Ideally, 1 mL of local anesthetic is placed at the joint (i.e., the greatest possible depth). Depending on the sensitivity of the patient, however, 0.5-ml volume increments may need to be injected along the periosteum of the ileum or sacrum as the needle is advanced to the posterior aspect of the joint.

Technique   The successful injection of the SI joint requires a careful passage of the needle to the maximum depth allowable between the ileum and sacral bones

---

SACROILIAC JOINT INJECTION

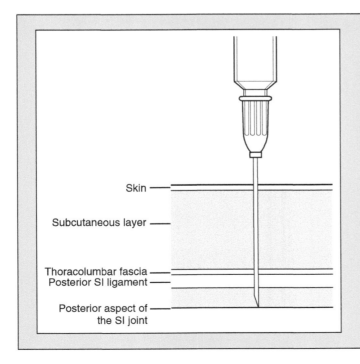

Skin

Subcutaneous layer

Thoracolumbar fascia

Posterior sacroiliac ligament

Posterior aspect of the sacroiliac joint

(the sacrum and ileum form the sides of an inverted cone with the SI joint representing the apex). The needle is advanced until the firm resistance of periosteum is encountered. If bone is encountered at $1^1/_2$ inches, the needle is withdrawn 1 inch and redirected approximately 5 degrees and advanced until the maximum depth is achieved. If the injection is placed accurately, the local anesthetic effect should permit improved flexibility and decreased pain.

INJECTION AFTERCARE

1. *Rest* for 3 days, avoiding all direct pressure, walking, standing, bending, and twisting.
2. Advise *bed rest for 3 days* and crutches with touch-down weightbearing for severe cases.
3. Use *ice* (15 minutes every 4 to 6 hours) and *acetaminophen* (1000 mg twice a day) for postinjection soreness.
4. *Protect* the joint for 3 to 4 weeks by limiting prolonged standing, unnecessary walking, and repetitive bending, lifting, and twisting.
5. Prescribe a Velcro *lumbosacral corset or sacral belt* for the first 2 to 3 weeks for severe cases.
6. Begin passive *stretching exercises* in flexion (Williams' exercises) when the acute pain has begun to resolve (knee-chest pulls, pelvic rocks, and side-bends).
7. Repeat *injection* at 6 weeks with corticosteroid if pain, inflammation, and secondary muscle spasm persist.
8. Begin active *toning exercises* of the abdominal and lower back muscles when flexibility has been restored or at 4 to 6 weeks.
9. Obtain *plain x-rays* of standing posteroanterior pelvis for leg-length discrepancy and nuclear medicine bone scan, CT scan, or MRI to identify sacroiliitis and short leg.

SURGICAL PROCEDURE   No surgical procedure is available.

PROGNOSIS   Isolated SI strain—unassociated with back or hip disease—has a favorable prognosis and responds well to local corticosteroid injection and physical therapy exercises. Patients with recurrent episodes of SI strain disease respond to treatment less predictably; the response often depends on the underlying back or hip condition. Patients with multiple episodes of SI strain or poor response to treatment require a thorough exam of the lumbosacral spine and hip, plain films of the pelvis and lower back, and CT or MRI of the lumbosacral spine. Patients with suspected sacroiliitis require blood work and a bone scan to determine the inflammatory activity. Patients with recurrent SI strain or sacroiliitis require maintenance stretching and toning exercises to reduce the possibility of recurrence.

COCCYGODYNIA

Enter 1 inch caudal to the sacrococcygeal junction in the midline; the needle is advanced at a 70-degree angle to the firm resistance of the posterior supporting ligaments or the hard resistance of bone.

Needle: 1½-inch, 22-gauge
Depth: 1 to 1½ inches
Volume: 1 to 2 mL of local anesthetic and 1 mL of D80

NOTE: The injection should be placed flush against the supporting ligaments or the periosteum of the sacrum.

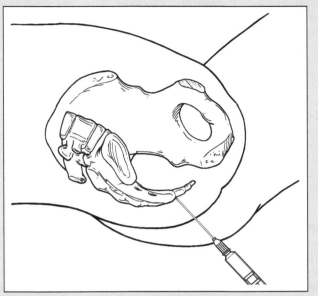

FIGURE 7–4. Injection of the sacrococcygeal junction for coccygodynia.

DESCRIPTION   Coccygodynia, or painful coccyx, is an inflammation of the articulation between the lowest sacral elements and the coccyx. Most cases result either from blunt trauma (falls directly onto the edge of a stair, the edge of a chair, or an object on the ground) or as an aftermath of childbirth. The latter cause explains why nearly 90% of cases are seen in young women. Patients complain of buttock pain aggravated by sitting or pain over the tailbone from any direct pressure. Exam shows exquisite focal tenderness at the tail end of the spinal column in the midline. Patients older than 50 years whose chief complaint is buttock or tailbone area pain must undergo rectal and pelvic exams to exclude anorectal or pelvic pathology.

SYMPTOMS   Every patient complains of buttock pain that is aggravated by direct pressure. This pain invariably is described as a well-localized area of tenderness in the midline of the gluteal crease. Occasionally the pain is described as radiating into the lateral gluteal area or down the leg, mimicking sciatica.

"Ever since I had my baby, it has become impossible for me to sit for very long."

"Sitting has become impossible. The only way I can sit is to roll onto the side of my cheek."

"It feels like I'm sitting on a tack."

"I can't ride my bicycle any longer. Even the extra padding on the seat doesn't prevent that awful butt pain."

"I'm tired of sitting on that stupid hemorrhoidal donut pad."

EXAM   The exam focuses on distinguishing tenderness arising from the sacrococcygeal joint from tenderness arising from the adjacent bones or colorectal area. In addition, the mobility of the joint is assessed, neurologic testing of the perineum is performed if there is any suspicion of a lower back condition, and a thorough exam of the rectum and pelvis is performed if the findings at the sacrococcygeal joint are equivocal.

EXAM SUMMARY

1. Sacrococcygeal joint tenderness
2. Angulation and abnormal mobility of the coccyx
3. Normal perineal sensation, rectal tone, and continence of urine and stool
4. Normal rectal and pelvic exam

(1) Localized tenderness is the hallmark feature of coccygodynia. The patient is placed in the lateral decubitus position with the hips and knees flexed to 90 degrees. The sacrum is palpated in the midline, beginning at the promontory and working down to the sacrococcygeal articulation. Maximum tenderness—the size of a dime—can be elicited by palpating in an inward and superior direction (toward the umbilicus). *(2)* The angle and

mobility of the coccyx is determined by digital rectal exam. The coccyx is grasped between the index finger in the rectum and the thumb on the outside. The coccyx is manipulated carefully. *Caution:* This manipulation often reproduces the patient's discomfort. Any anterior angulation is noted. *(3)* The exam of the sacral divisions of the spinal cord is normal in an uncomplicated case of coccygodynia. *(4)* The rectal and pelvic exams are performed if signs of joint irritation are equivocal.

X-RAYS Plain films of the sacrum and coccyx are unnecessary in the average case. The lateral views of the coccyx and a standing anteroposterior pelvis x-ray can be obtained to confirm any abnormal angulation of the joint. Plain films always are indicated if the clinical findings are nondiagnostic for sacrococcygeal joint irritation

SPECIAL TESTING Special testing is not indicated in uncomplicated cases. A nuclear medicine bone scan or MRI of the pelvis is indicated if bony tenderness extends beyond the margins of the joint, typically beyond 1 cm. Sigmoidoscopy, colonoscopy, pelvic ultrasound, and CT of the abdomen are indicated when local sacrococcygeal symptoms are accompanied by colorectal or pelvic symptoms or signs.

DIAGNOSIS The diagnosis is based on the clinical criteria of a history of localized pain over the coccyx and focal tenderness at the sacrococcygeal joint. Local anesthetic block is used to confirm the diagnosis in patients with equivocal or atypical symptoms and signs.

TREATMENT The goals of treatment are to reduce local inflammation at the sacrococcygeal joint and to protect the coccyx from future irritation.

STEP 1 Examine the sacrococcygeal joint thoroughly. Obtain plain films or order a nuclear bone scan if local tenderness extends beyond the margins of the joint. Evaluate the patient for colorectal and pelvic pathology if the exam of the joint is equivocal.
   Avoid all direct pressure and unnecessary sitting.
   Local applications of ice may afford temporary relief, but application of ice is impractical.
   Recommend a soft pillow, a cushion, or a hemorrhoidal donut pad to reduce pressure.
   Perform local anesthetic block to confirm the diagnosis if symptoms are atypical.

STEP 2 (2 TO 4 WEEKS FOR PERSISTENT CASES) Perform a corticosteroid injection with D80 for symptoms persisting beyond 4 to 6 weeks.
   Continue to avoid direct pressure and unnecessary sitting.

Continue the use of a soft pillow, cushion, or hemorrhoidal donut pad.

STEP 3 (2 TO 3 MONTHS FOR PERSISTENT CASES) Repeat the corticosteroid injection with D80 if the first injection provided only partial relief.
   Recommend gluteus muscle leg extension exercises to increase the size and tone of the buttocks and reduce the direct pressure over the coccyx.
   Consider consultation with an orthopedic surgeon for persistent symptoms.

INJECTION Local injection with anesthesia can be used to differentiate conditions affecting the sacrococcygeal joint from the referred pain arising from the SI joint, rectum, lower colon, or pelvis. Corticosteroid injection is the anti-inflammatory medication of choice to treat the persistent inflammation of the saccrococcygeal joint that failed to respond to rest, protection, and time.
   Positioning The patient is placed in the lateral decubitus position with the hips and knees flexed to 90 degrees, exposing the tail of the spine.
   Surface Anatomy and Point of Entry The sacral prominence is identified, and the gluteal crease is followed down to the inferiormost portion of the sacrum. Digital rectal exam can be used to define the exact location, degree of sensitivity, and mobility of the saccrococcygeal joint. The point of entry is $^1/_2$ to 1 inch inferior to the joint in the midline.
   Angle of Entry and Depth The angle of entry is 70 degrees with the needle directed upward toward the sacrococcygeal joint. The depth of injection is $^1/_2$ to 1 inch, depending on the thickness of the subcutaneous layer.
   Anesthesia Ethyl chloride is sprayed on the skin. Local anesthetic is placed just under the skin (0.5 mL) and just adjacent to the joint (0.5 to 1 mL).
   Technique The successful injection of the sacrococcygeal joint requires a careful passage of the needle to firm resistance of the supporting ligaments or the hard resistance of the sacrum. The assistant is asked to place upward traction on the buttock to expose the gluteal crease. The examiner places one finger firmly against the lowest aspect of the sacrum. The point of entry is $^1/_2$ to 1 inch below the placement of the examiner's finger. After placing anesthetic in the subcutaneous tissue, the needle is advanced down to the supporting ligament or sacrum. The joint is not actually entered. A second 0.5 mL of anesthetic is injected just outside this area. If the injection is placed accurately, the local anesthetic effect should reduce the pressure pain immediately. D80 (1 mL) is injected flush against the ligament or bone.

INJECTION AFTERCARE
1. *Rest* the sacrococcygeal joint for the first 3 days, avoiding direct pressure and all unnecessary sitting.
2. Recommend 3 days of *bed rest* coupled with the use of *crutches* with touch-down weightbearing for severe cases.

COCCYGODYNIA INJECTION

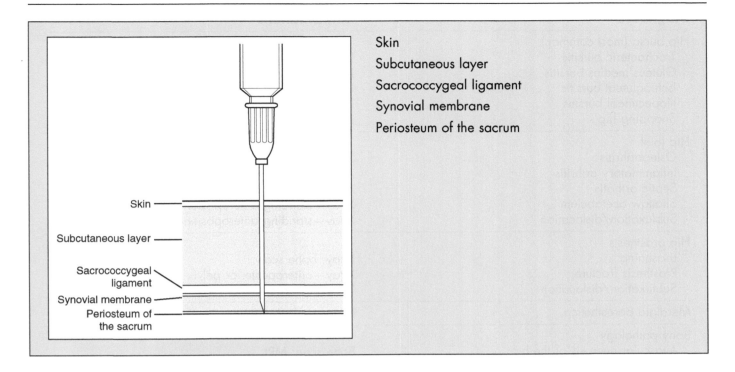

Skin
Subcutaneous layer
Sacrococcygeal ligament
Synovial membrane
Periosteum of the sacrum

Skin
Subcutaneous layer
Sacrococcygeal ligament
Synovial membrane
Periosteum of the sacrum

3. Use *acetaminophen* (1000 mg twice a day) for postinjection soreness.
4. *Protect* the joint for 3 to 4 weeks by limiting direct pressure and unnecessary sitting.
5. Encourage the use of *padding* whenever seated (a soft pillow, a cushion, or a hemorrhoidal donut pad) to avoid direct pressure.
6. *Repeat* the injection with corticosteroid at 6 weeks if pain and inflammation persist.
7. Begin active *toning exercises* of the gluteus muscles after pain and inflammation have significantly improved.
8. Obtain *plain x-rays* of the sacrum to evaluate the angulation and irregularities of the joint and a *consultation* with an orthopedic surgeon for persistent pain and inflammation that failed to improve with two consecutive injections.

SURGERY Coccygectomy is indicated if treatment fails, if symptoms persist, and especially if the sacrococcygeal junction has been fractured or otherwise altered from its normal round curvature.

PROGNOSIS Most patients with coccygodynia experience months of relief when treated with the combination of restrictions of direct pressure, padding, and local corticosteroid injection. Recurrence is common, however, secondary to reinjury or irritation caused by prolonged sitting. Patients with refractory symptoms or three or more recurrences can be considered for coccygectomy. Patients considering surgery must be warned about the possibility of postoperative infection and persistent perineal pain.

DIFFERENTIAL DIAGNOSIS OF HIP PAIN

Diagnoses	Confirmations
Hip bursa (most common)	
Trochanteric bursitis	Local anesthetic block
Gluteus medius bursitis	Local anesthetic block
Ischiogluteal bursitis	Local anesthetic block
Iliopectineal bursitis	Local anesthetic block
Snapping hip	Exam
Hip joint	
Osteoarthritis	X-ray—standing anteroposterior pelvis
Inflammatory arthritis	Aspiration/synovial fluid analysis
Septic arthritis	Aspiration/synovial fluid analysis
Shallow acetabulum	X-ray—standing anteroposterior pelvis
Subluxation/dislocation	X-ray—standing anteroposterior pelvis
Hip prosthesis	
Loosening	X-ray; bone scan
Prosthesis fracture	X-ray—anteroposterior pelvis
Subluxation/dislocation	X-ray—anteroposterior pelvis
Meralgia paresthetica	History; sensory exam
Bony pathology	
Avascular necrosis of the hip	Bone scan; MRI
Occult fracture of the femoral neck	Bone scan; MRI
Malignancy	Bone scan; MRI
Referred pain	
Lumbosacral spine	Neurologic exam; CT
Sacroiliac (SI) joint	X-ray; bone scan
Vascular occlusive disease	Exam; Doppler study
Inguinal hernia	Exam

TROCHANTERIC BURSITIS

Enter over the mid-trochanter in the lateral decubitus position; lightly advance the needle to the firm resistance of the gluteus medius tendon, then ¹/₂ inch further to the periosteum of the femur.

Needle: 1¹/₂-inch standard or 3¹/₂-inch spinal needle, 22-gauge
Depth: 1¹/₂ to 3 inches, down through the gluteus medius tendon to the periosteum
Volume: 1 to 2 mL of local anesthetic and 1 mL of K40

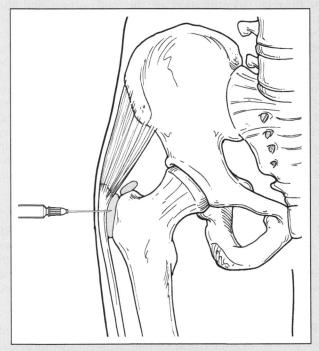

FIGURE 8–1. Trochanteric bursa injection.

DESCRIPTION   Trochanteric bursitis is an inflammation of the lubricating sac located between the mid-portion of the trochanteric process of the femur and the gluteus medius tendon/iliotibial tract. Repetitive flexing of the hip and direct pressure aggravate this condition. A disturbance in gait causes 95% of the cases of trochanteric bursitis. Abnormal patterns of walking and standing lead to increased friction and uneven contraction of the gluteus medius tendon, resulting in irritation of the bursa. Common causes of altered gait include underlying lumbosacral back disease (75%), leg-length discrepancy (10%), sacroiliac (SI) joint disorders (5%), or a lower leg gait disturbance (10%). Direct trauma to the outer thigh and osteoarthritis of the hip with decreased hip motion are relatively rare causes of this condition.

SYMPTOMS   The patient complains of hip pain over the outer thigh or difficulty with walking. The patient often rubs the outer thigh when describing the condition.

"Whenever I roll over onto my right side, this sharp pain in my hip wakes me up."

"I get this achy pain in my hip (pointing to the upper outer thigh) when I walk too much in the mall."

"I can't stand lying on either side, I just toss and turn all night long. My husband now sleeps in the other room."

"I have this sharp pain in my hip (rubbing the outer thigh) that I feel clear down the outside of my leg to my knee."

"I can't squat anymore. Climbing up the stairs has become impossible. Any bending of the hip is just too painful."

"My back has hurt me for years. Lately, I've had a sharper pain right here (pointing to the upper outer thigh) whenever I lie on a hard surface."

EXAM   The patient is examined for the degree of local tenderness at the greater trochanter, and an assessment is made of the gait, the flexibility of the lower back, and the degree of involvement of the SI joint.

EXAM SUMMARY

1. Local mid-trochanteric tenderness
2. Aggravation of pain at the extremes of hip rotation (mild)
3. Pain aggravated by resisted hip abduction (25% of cases), isometrically performed
4. Normal range of motion (ROM) of the hip
5. Associated gait disturbance, leg-length discrepancy, back or SI disease

(1) Local tenderness is present at the mid-portion of the greater trochanter. This tenderness is best identified in the lateral decubitus position with the knees flexed to 90 degrees (identification of the mid-portion and the superior portion of the trochanteric process is easier in this position). The maximum tenderness is $1^1/_2$ inches below the superior portion of the trochanter, directly over the maximum lateral prominence. *(2)* Stiffness or mild discomfort may be experienced at the extremes of internal or external rotation of the hip, but true loss of ROM is not seen. This is present in approximately 50% of cases, but is not as specific as the site of local tenderness. *(3)* Isometrically resisted hip abduction may aggravate the pain in 25% of cases. *(4)* The ROM of the hip in an uncomplicated case should be normal. *(5)* Signs of an underlying back condition, an underlying leg-length discrepancy, or a SI condition should be sought.

X-RAYS   X-rays of the hip are strongly recommended. A standing anteroposterior pelvis x-ray and specific views of the hip and back are used to evaluate for leg-length discrepancy, disease affecting the SI joint, and structural back disease. Plain films show calcification in 5% of cases.

SPECIAL TESTING   Bone scanning, CT, or MRI is used to evaluate for underlying conditions at the lumbosacral spine, the SI joint, the femur, or the pelvic bones.

DIAGNOSIS   The diagnosis of an uncomplicated case of trochanteric bursitis is based on the clinical findings of outer thigh pain, local tenderness at the mid-trochanter, and pain relief with regional anesthetic block. Regional anesthetic block may be helpful in differentiating the pain of trochanteric bursitis from referred pain from the gluteus medius bursa (p. 131) or the lumbosacral spine and from the dysesthetic pain of meralgia paresthetica (p. 138). Complicated cases with a suspected underlying cause require specialized testing for a definitive diagnosis.

TREATMENT   The goals of treatment are to reduce the inflammation in the bursa, to correct any underlying disturbance of gait, and to prevent recurrent bursitis by proper hip and back stretching exercises. The treatment of choice is the cross-leg stretching exercise of the gluteus medius combined with specific treatment of the primary gait disturbance.

STEP 1   Define the site of local tenderness, order a standing anteroposterior pelvis x-ray, and evaluate and correct any underlying gait disturbance (e.g., a shoe lift, low back stretching exercises, a knee brace, high-top shoes for ankle support, custom-made foot orthotics for ankle pronation).

Reduce weightbearing (e.g., a lean bar, sitting versus standing, crutches temporarily, weight loss for chronic cases).

Restrict repetitive bending (e.g., climbing stairs, getting out of a chair).

Advise on avoiding direct pressure.

Recommend daily stretching exercises for the gluteus medius tendon to lessen the pressure and friction over the bursa (p. 287).

Suggest sitting and sleeping with the leg moderately abducted and externally rotated to lessen the pressure over the bursa.

Prescribe a nonsteroidal anti-inflammatory drug (NSAID) (e.g., ibuprofen [Advil, Motrin]) for 4 weeks at full dose.

STEP 2 (6 TO 8 WEEKS FOR PERSISTENT CASES)   Re-evaluate for an underlying cause (e.g., CT scan of the back, bone scan).

Obtain a standing anteroposterior pelvis x-ray to evaluate for leg-length discrepancy.

Inject the bursa with K40.

Repeat the injection in 4 to 6 weeks if symptoms have not decreased by 50%.

For a patient with severe pain or a severe disturbance of gait, touch-down weightbearing with crutches or a walker can be used for 5 to 7 days.

With improvement, emphasize stretching exercises of the hip.

For patients with underlying back stiffness, the flexion stretching exercises of the back (knee-chest pull, pelvic rocks, and side-bends) are combined with general aerobic conditioning.

Avoid direct pressure.

STEP 3 (10 TO 12 WEEKS FOR CHRONIC CASES)   Perform a more thorough search for or treat the underlying gait disturbances.

Use deep ultrasound for persistent cases.

Recommend a transcutaneous electrical nerve stimulation (TENS) unit for chronic pain.

Long-term restrictions of direct pressure and repetitive bending are recommended for refractory cases.

PHYSICAL THERAPY   Physical therapy plays an important role in the active treatment of trochanteric bursitis and a major role in preventing recurrent bursitis.

PHYSICAL THERAPY SUMMARY

1. Heat
2. Stretching exercises for the gluteus medius tendon and muscle, passively performed
3. Stretching exercises for the lumbosacral spine and SI joint, passively performed
4. Ultrasound for deep heating
5. A TENS unit for chronic pain

Acute Period Heat treatments and passive stretching exercises are used in the first few weeks to reduce the pressure over the bursal sac. *Heat* is applied to the outer thigh for 15 to 20 minutes to prepare the area for stretching. *Stretching exercises of the gluteus medius tendon* are recommended to reduce the pressure over the bursa. While in the sitting position, cross-leg pulls are performed in sets of 20 (p. 287). The maximum amount of stretch is obtained when the buttocks—both ischial tuberosities—are kept flat on a hard surface. These exercises are followed by *low back and SI stretches* (p. 281). Stretching all three areas increases flexibility through the lower spine, the SI joints, and the hips. *Therapeutic ultrasound* provides deep heating to the area and can be combined with stretching. A *TENS unit* may be necessary for patients with chronic bursitis secondary to structural back disease or chronic neurologic impairment.

Recovery and Rehabilitation Several weeks after the local symptoms have resolved, daily stretching exercises are cut back to three times a week. Maintaining low back, SI, and hip flexibility reduces the chance of recurrent bursitis.

INJECTION For an uncomplicated case of bursitis—one that is not associated with a correctable underlying gait disturbance—local injection is the preferred anti-inflammatory treatment.

Positioning The patient is placed in the lateral decubitus position with the affected side up and the knees flexed to 90 degrees (the trochanter is most prominent in this position).

Surface Anatomy and Point of Entry The superior, posterior, and anterior edges of the trochanteric process are palpated and marked. The point of entry is directly over the center point of the trochanter—$1^1/_2$ inches below the superior trochanter. Alternatively the point of entry is at the crown of the trochanter, viewed tangentially in the anteroposterior and cephalad directions.

Angle of Entry and Depth The needle is inserted perpendicular to the skin. The depth is 1 to $2^1/_2$ inches to the gluteus medius tendon and $1^1/_2$ to 3 inches to the periosteum of the femur (the gluteus medius tendon/iliotibial band is $3/_8$ to $1/_2$ inch thick).

Anesthesia Ethyl chloride is sprayed on the skin. Local anesthetic is placed at the gluteus medius tissue plane (1 mL) and at the periosteum of the femur (0.5 mL).

Technique Treatment success depends on an accurate injection of the bursa at the level of periosteum of the femur. The needle is held lightly and advanced through the low resistance of the subcutaneous fat to the firm, rubbery resistance of the gluteus medius tissue plane. After anesthesia at this level, the needle is advanced (firm pressure) $1/_2$ to $5/_8$ inch farther to the periosteum of the femur. *Caution:* The patient usually experiences sharp pain as soon as the needle touches the periosteum. Injection at this deeper level requires firm pressure. If excessive pressure is encountered, the needle should be

TROCHANTERIC BURSA INJECTION

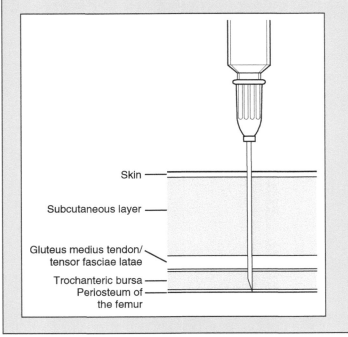

Skin

Subcutaneous layer

Gluteus medius tendon/tensor fasciae latae

Trochanteric bursa

Periosteum of the femur

rotated 180 degrees or withdrawn ever so slightly. If the trochanter tenderness is significantly relieved, 1 mL of K40 is injected through the same needle.

INJECTION AFTERCARE

1. *Rest* for 3 days, avoiding direct pressure and repetitive bending.
2. Advise 3 days of bed rest and crutches (touch-down weightbearing) for severe cases.
3. Use *ice* (15 minutes every 4 to 6 hours) and *acetaminophen (Tylenol ES)* (1000 mg twice a day) for postinjection soreness.
4. *Protect* the hip for 3 to 4 weeks by limiting direct pressure, repetitive bending, prolonged standing, and unnecessary walking.
5. Begin cross-leg *stretching exercises* for the gluteus medius on day 4.
6. For patients with accompanying structural back disease, begin flexion *stretching exercises* of the lower back (Williams' exercises) after the acute pain has begun to resolve.
7. The *injection* can be repeated at 6 weeks with corticosteroid if pain persists.
8. Obtain standing anteroposterior pelvis *x-rays* for leg-length discrepancy and *CT* or *MRI* to identify a short leg, a subtle disk, spondylolisthesis, or other condition altering the patient's gait.
9. Advise *long-term restrictions* of weightbearing and direct pressure for patients with chronic bursitis (5%).

SURGICAL PROCEDURE Iliotibial tract release is performed for chronic bursitis that has failed to improve with exercise, gait correction, and two or three injections performed over the course of the year. Bursectomy rarely is performed. The bursa probably re-forms if lateral hip friction and pressure persist.

PROGNOSIS Uncomplicated cases of bursitis—cases unassociated with a chronic or fixed gait disturbance—usually respond dramatically to one or two corticosteroid injections 6 weeks apart. Patients with short-term benefits to treatment either have developed a fibrotic thickening of the bursa or have an undiscovered, underlying cause, such as chronic conditions affecting the lumbosacral spine or SI joint, leg-length discrepancy, or functional or neurologic causes of high tension in the gluteus medius tendon (e.g., Parkinson's disease, spasticity from a previous stroke). The prognosis for recovery depends greatly on the underlying cause, the patient's steadfastness in performing the stretching exercises, and the degree of obesity. Chronic bursitis most often develops in patients who have a severe, fixed gait disturbance.

GLUTEUS MEDIUS BURSITIS/PIRIFORMIS SYNDROME

Enter 1 inch above the superior edge of the trochanteric process in the lateral decubitus position; advance the needle at a 45-degree angle down to the gluteus medius tendon, then to the periosteum of the femur.

Needle: 1¹/₂-inch to 3¹/₂-inch spinal needle, 22-gauge
Depth: 1¹/₂ to 3¹/₂ inches (down to the periosteum)
Volume: 1 to 2 mL of local anesthetic and 1 mL of K40

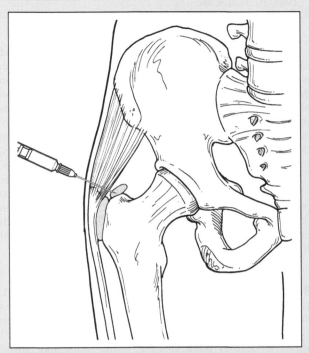

FIGURE 8–2. Injection of the gluteus medius bursa.

DESCRIPTION Gluteus medius (also referred to as the *deep trochanteric bursa*) bursitis is an inflammation of the bursal sac that is located between the superior portion of the trochanteric process and the gluteus medius tendon. Its function is to lubricate and reduce the friction between the gluteus medius tendon and the piriformis muscle insertion and the lateral aspect of the femur. It is identical to trochanteric bursitis in symptoms, presentation, underlying cause (primary gait disturbance), and treatment. The only significant differences between the two are the location of the local tenderness and the tendency of the gluteus medius bursitis to refer pain in a retrograde direction into the buttock area. It accompanies trochanteric bursitis in 30% of cases. The piriformis muscle attaches to the medial aspect of the superior trochanter (an abductor of the hip). Piriformis syndrome—a distinct clinical entity—consists of pain about the hip, muscle spasm of the piriformis muscle, and pain pattern that mimics sciatica (buttock pain that radiates down the leg caused by compression of the nerve as it courses through the muscle). Injection of the gluteus medius bursa seems to treat this syndrome effectively as well. As with trochanteric bursitis, gluteus medius bursitis and osteoarthritis of the hip rarely coexist. (The lack of mobility associated with advanced osteoarthritis prevents the development of bursitis.)

SYMPTOMS The patient complains of hip pain or difficulties in walking identical to the difficulties that occur in trochanteric bursitis.

"Whenever I roll over onto my right side, this sharp pain in my hip wakes me up."

"I get this achy pain in my hip (pointing to the upper outer thigh) when I walk too much in the mall."

"I can't stand very long."

"I have this sharp pain in my hip (rubbing the outer thigh) that I feel deep in my butt cheek."

"Climbing up the stairs has become impossible."

"I've lost my mobility in my spine from my scoliosis. But what really hurts is the sharp pain right here (pointing to the upper outer thigh)."

EXAM The patient is examined for local tenderness at the superior portion of the greater trochanter; the ROM of the hip and lumbosacral spine is measured, gait is assessed, and the SI joints are evaluated.

EXAM SUMMARY

1. Local tenderness directly over the superior portion of the trochanteric process
2. Pain aggravation at the extremes of hip rotation
3. Pain aggravated by resisted hip abduction (75% of cases), isometrically performed

Continued

4. Normal ROM of the hip
5. Associated gait disturbance, leg-length discrepancy, back or SI disease

4. Ultrasound for deep heating
5. A TENS unit for chronic bursitis

(1) Maximum tenderness is located just superior to the trochanteric process of the femur, directly in the midline. This is best identified in the lateral decubitus position with the knees flexed to 90 degrees (the superior portion of the trochanteric process is more prominent in this position). *(2)* Stiffness or mild discomfort may be experienced at the extremes of internal or external rotation of the hip. This is present in approximately 50% of cases, but is not as specific as the local point of tenderness. *(3)* Isometrically resisted hip abduction may aggravate the pain in 75% of cases. *(4)* The ROM of the hip in an uncomplicated case should be normal. *(5)* Signs of an underlying lumbosacral back condition, leg-length discrepancy, lower extremity gait disturbance, or SI condition are present in most cases.

X-RAYS   X-rays of the hip are strongly recommended. A standing anteroposterior pelvis x-ray and specific views of the hip and back are used to evaluate for the underlying cause—leg-length discrepancy, disease affecting the SI joint, or structural back disease. Plain films may show calcification in fewer than 5% of cases.

SPECIAL TESTING   Bone scanning, CT, and MRI are used to evaluate for underlying conditions at the lumbosacral spine, SI joint, femur, and pelvic bones.

DIAGNOSIS   The diagnosis of an uncomplicated case of gluteus medius bursitis is based on the clinical findings of outer thigh pain, local tenderness at the superior portion of the greater trochanter, and pain relief with regional anesthetic block. Regional anesthetic block may be helpful in differentiating the pain of gluteus medius bursitis from pain referred from the trochanteric bursa (p. 127) or the lumbosacral spine and the dysesthetic pain of meralgia paresthetica (p. 138). Complicated cases with a suspected underlying cause require specialized testing for a definitive diagnosis.

PHYSICAL THERAPY   Physical therapy plays an important role in the active treatment of gluteus medius bursitis and a major role in preventing recurrent bursitis.

PHYSICAL THERAPY SUMMARY

1. Heat
2. Stretching exercises for the gluteus medius tendon and muscle, passively performed
3. Stretching exercises for the SI joint and the lumbosacral spine, passively performed

Acute Period   Heat treatments and passive stretching exercises are used in the first few weeks to reduce the pressure over the bursal sac. *Heat* is applied to the outer thigh for 15 to 20 minutes to prepare the area for stretching. *Stretching exercises of the gluteus tendon* are recommended to reduce the pressure over the bursa. While in the sitting position, cross-leg pulls are performed in sets of 20 (p. 287). The maximum amount of stretching is obtained when the buttocks—both ischial tuberosities—are kept flat on a hard surface. These are followed by *low back and SI stretches* (p. 281). Stretching all three areas provides flexibility through the lower spine, the SI joints, and the hips. *Therapeutic ultrasound* provides deep heating to the area and can be combined with stretching. A *TENS unit* may be necessary for patients with chronic bursitis secondary to structural back disease or chronic neurologic impairment.

Recovery and Rehabilitation   Several weeks after the local symptoms have resolved, daily stretching exercises are cut back to three times a week. Maintaining low back, SI, and hip flexibility reduces the chance of recurrent bursitis.

TREATMENT   The goals of treatment are to reduce the inflammation in the bursa, to correct any underlying disturbance of gait, and to prevent recurrent bursitis by teaching proper hip and back stretching exercises. The initial treatment of choice for most patients is the cross-leg stretching exercise of the gluteus medius combined with specific treatment of the primary gait disturbance. Local corticosteroid injection is the treatment of choice for patients presenting with severe symptoms and signs.

STEP 1   Define the site of local tenderness, order a standing anteroposterior pelvis x-ray, and evaluate and correct any underlying gait disturbance (e.g., a shoe lift, low back stretching exercises, a knee brace, high-top shoes for ankle support, custommade foot orthotics for ankle pronation).

Reduce weightbearing (e.g., a lean bar, sitting versus standing, crutches temporarily, weight loss for chronic cases).

Restrict repetitive bending (e.g., climbing stairs, getting out of a chair).

Advise on avoiding direct pressure.

Recommend daily stretching exercises for the gluteus medius tendon to lessen the pressure and friction over the bursa (p. 287).

Suggest sitting and sleeping with the leg moderately abducted and externally rotated to lessen the pressure over the bursa.

Prescribe an NSAID (e.g., ibuprofen) for 4 weeks at full dose.

STEP 2 (6 TO 8 WEEKS FOR PERSISTENT CASES) Re-evaluate for an underlying cause (e.g., CT scan of the back, bone scan).

Obtain a standing anteroposterior pelvis x-ray to evaluate for leg-length discrepancy.

Inject the bursa with K40.

Repeat the injection in 4 to 6 weeks if symptoms have not decreased by 50%.

For a patient with severe pain or a severe disturbance of gait, touch-down weightbearing with crutches or a walker can be used for 5 to 7 days.

With improvement, emphasize the stretching exercises of the hip.

For patients with underlying back stiffness, the flexion stretching exercises of the back (knee-chest pull, pelvic rocks, and side-bends) are combined with general aerobic conditioning.

Avoid direct pressure.

STEP 3 (10 TO 12 WEEKS FOR CHRONIC CASES) Perform a more thorough search for or treat the underlying gait disturbances.

Use deep ultrasound for persistent cases.

Recommend a TENS unit for chronic pain.

Long-term restrictions of direct pressure and repetitive bending are recommended for refractory cases.

INJECTION For an uncomplicated bursitis—one not associated with a correctable underlying cause, such as mechanical low back stiffness, short leg, or gait disturbance—local injection is the preferred treatment. *Note:* If the gluteus and the trochanteric bursa are involved, the trochanteric bursa should be treated first (the trochanteric bursa is the dominant bursa at the hip).

Positioning The patient is placed in the lateral decubitus position with the affected side up and the knees flexed to 90 degrees (the trochanter is most prominent in this position).

Surface Anatomy and Point of Entry The superior, posterior, and anterior edges of the trochanteric process are palpated and marked. The point of entry is $3/4$ to 1 inch above the mid-point of the superiormost portion of the trochanter. Alternatively, if the trochanteric process cannot be palpated directly, the superior point of entry can be identified by viewing the crown of the trochanter tangentially in the anteroposterior and cephalad directions.

Angle of Entry and Depth The needle is inserted at a 45-degree angle in direct alignment with the femur. The depth is 1 to $2^{1}/_{2}$ inches to the gluteus medius tendon and $1^{1}/_{2}$ to 3 inches to the superior trochanter (the tendon is $1/2$ to $5/8$ inch thick).

Anesthesia Ethyl chloride is sprayed on the skin. Local anesthetic is placed at the gluteus medius tendon (1 mL) and at the periosteum of the femur (0.5 mL).

Technique The success of treatment depends on an accurate injection of the bursa at the level of the periosteum of the femur. The needle is held lightly and advanced through the low resistance of the subcutaneous fat to the firm rubbery resistance of the gluteus medius tissue plane. After anesthesia at this level, the needle is advanced (firm pressure) $1/2$ to $5/8$ inch farther to the periosteum of the femur. *Caution:* The patient usually

---

GLUTEUS MEDIUS BURSA INJECTION

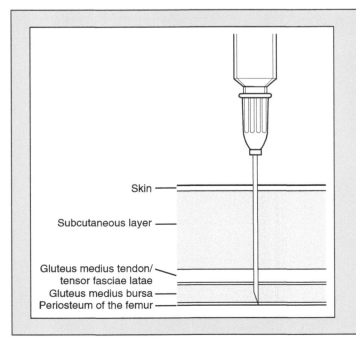

Skin

Subcutaneous layer

Gluteus medius tendon/tensor fasciae latae

Gluteus medius bursa

Periosteum of the femur

experiences sharp pain as soon as the needle touches the periosteum. Injection at this deeper level requires firm pressure. If excessive pressure is encountered, the needle should be rotated 180 degrees or withdrawn ever so slightly. If the local tenderness over the trochanter is significantly relieved, 1 mL of K40 is injected through the same needle.

INJECTION AFTERCARE

1. *Rest* for 3 days, avoiding direct pressure and repetitive bending.
2. Advise 3 days of bed rest and crutches (touch-down weightbearing) for severe cases.
3. Use *ice* (15 minutes every 4 to 6 hours) and *acetaminophen* (1000 mg twice a day) for postinjection soreness.
4. *Protect* the hip for 3 to 4 weeks by limiting direct pressure, repetitive bending, prolonged standing, and unnecessary walking.
5. Begin cross-leg *stretching exercises* for the gluteus medius on day 4.
6. For patients with accompanying structural back disease, begin flexion *stretching exercises* of the lower back (Williams' exercises) after the acute pain has begun to resolve.
7. The *injection* can be repeated at 6 weeks with corticosteroid if pain persists.
8. Obtain standing anteroposterior pelvis *x-rays* for leg-length discrepancy and a *CT* or *MRI* to identify a short leg, a subtle disk, spondylolisthesis, or other condition altering the patient's gait.
9. Advise long-term restrictions of weightbearing and direct pressure for a patient with chronic bursitis (5%).

SURGICAL PROCEDURE Iliotibial tract release is performed for chronic bursitis that has failed to improve with exercise, gait correction, and two or three injections performed over the course of the year. Bursectomy rarely is performed. The bursa probably re-forms if lateral hip friction and pressure persist.

PROGNOSIS Uncomplicated cases of bursitis—cases unassociated with a chronic or fixed gait disturbance—usually respond dramatically to one or two corticosteroid injections 6 weeks apart. Patients with short-term benefits to treatment either have developed a fibrotic thickening of the bursa or have an undiscovered, underlying cause, such as chronic conditions affecting the lumbosacral spine or SI joint, leg-length discrepancy, or functional or neurologic causes of high tension in the gluteus medius tendon (e.g., Parkinson's disease, spasticity from a previous stroke). The prognosis for recovery depends greatly on the underlying cause, the patient's steadfastness in performing the stretching exercises, and the degree of obesity. Chronic bursitis most often develops in patients who have a severe, fixed gait disturbance.

OSTEOARTHRITIS OF THE HIP

The indications for surgical replacement of the hip are:

Intractable pain

Functional loss ("I cannot put my socks on or tie my shoes")

Greater than 50% loss of internal and external rotation

Medical suitability for a 2- to 2^1/$_2$-hour operation; ideally, this operation should be considered after age 60.

The average prosthesis lasts 10 to 15 years.

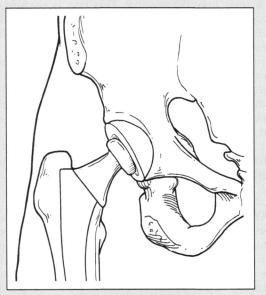

FIGURE 8-3. Hip prosthesis.

DESCRIPTION   Osteoarthritis of the hip results from wear and tear of the articular cartilage between the head of the femur and the acetabulum. Obesity, a family history of osteoarthritis, a history of systemic arthritis, and a history of severe gait disturbance are predisposing factors. Osteoarthritis is the second most common cause of pain around the hip, second only to hip bursitis.

SYMPTOMS   The patient complains of groin or thigh pain or both or loss of flexibility. The patient often pushes deep into the groin or grabs the upper thigh when describing the condition.

"I can't get my socks on anymore ... and there's absolutely no way I can tie my shoelaces."

"My hip is getting stiffer and stiffer."

"My right hip is beginning to hurt just like the left hip did before I had it replaced."

"I can't get down to do my gardening. If I squat, I would need a crane to get me back up."

"I get so aggravated. I used to be able to walk 5 miles. Now I can only go 200 feet before my hip starts to really ache."

"I can't take my usual constitutional around the golf course any longer without having to stop two or three times (because of hip pain)."

"I've had this deep, achy pain (pointing to the anterior hip area) whenever I walk a certain distance."

"I can't believe that I have arthritis in my hip. My hip has never hurt me. I feel pain in my lower thigh and knee. I thought I had arthritis in my knee."

EXAM   The patient's gait, the general function of the hip, and the ROM of the hip joint are examined in each patient.

EXAM SUMMARY

1. Impaired function: loss of normal gait, inability to remove socks, cross the legs, and so forth
2. Loss of internal and external rotation with endpoint stiffness and pain
3. A positive fabere maneuver (abnormal Patrick test)
4. Tenderness 1^1/$_2$" below the inguinal ligament

(1) General hip function can be assessed by observing the patient's gait, the move from chair to exam table, the removal of shoes and socks, and the crossing of the legs. As arthritis advances, these basic functions become more difficult to accomplish. *(2)* The ROM of the hip is restricted. Early disease shows a common pattern of loss of rotation and end-point stiffness. Classically, internal rotation is impaired first, followed by a gradual loss of external rotation and abduction. Normally a 50-year-old patient should have 45 degrees of internal and external rotation. By comparison, a young woman with supple hips

may have 60 to 70 degrees of rotation in each direction. *(3)* The result of the *fabere (flexion, abduction, external rotation,* and *extension)* maneuver (also known as the Patrick test) may be positive. This test is performed by placing the hip in flexion, abduction, and external rotation (in a figure-of-four position), and pressure is applied to the anterior superior iliac spine (ASIS) and the knee. This pressure stretches the anterior capsule of the hip, resulting in pain. This maneuver is associated with moderate pain in cases of acute synovitis and with extreme pain in cases of septic arthritis. *(4)* Tenderness may be found $1^1/_2$ inches below the mid-portion of the inguinal ligament, very close to the femoral artery. *Note:* All of these findings on exam are exaggerated with inflammatory arthritis, severe with avascular necrosis of the hip, and extreme with acute septic arthritis.

X-RAYS   Specific x-rays (including standing antero-posterior, lateral, and frog-leg views) to evaluate the extent of primary disease of the hip joint are always indicated. The most useful view for screening and evaluating hip disease is the standing anteroposterior pelvis view. This single x-ray exposure allows simultaneous comparison of both hips, screens for SI disease, and assesses leg-length discrepancy. In addition, the standing anteroposterior pelvis x-ray is useful in determining the position of the hips. This view can be used to assess for shallow acetabulum, a form of hip dysplasia, and for an unusual complication of hip disease, protrusio acetabuli, a pathologic migration of the femoral head into the pelvis. The early changes of osteoarthritis of the hip include a loss of joint space between the superior acetabulum and the femoral head (normally 4 to 5 mm), increased bony sclerosis of the superior acetabulum, variable degrees of osteophyte formation along the superior acetabulum, and subchondral cyst formation.

SPECIAL TESTING   MRI is not necessary in routine cases. If subjective pain and pain with rotation of the hip on exam are extreme, MRI may be necessary to evaluate for avascular necrosis, occult fracture, or complicating primary bone disease.

DIAGNOSIS   The diagnosis is based on the loss of hip rotation coupled with characteristic changes on plain films of the hip.

TREATMENT   The goals of treatment are to relieve pain, to preserve function, and to stage for surgery. A 3- to 4-week course of an NSAID and mild restrictions on weightbearing activities are the treatments of choice for mild disease. Total hip replacement surgery is the treatment of choice for advanced disease.

■ **STEP 1**   Measure the patient's loss of internal and external rotation (normally 40 to 45 degrees in a 50-year-old person), obtain a standing anteroposterior

pelvis x-ray, and determine the patient's functional status.

Restrict jogging, aerobics, and other impact exercises.
Suggest padded insoles to reduce impact pressure (p. 262).
Advise on passive hip-stretching exercises (p. 285) to preserve ROM.
Prescribe an NSAID (e.g., ibuprofen) at full dose. Emphasize the need to take it regularly for at least 2 to 3 weeks for its anti-inflammatory effect.
Prescribe glucosamine sulfate, 1500 mg/day.

■ **STEP 2 (MONTHS TO YEARS FOR REASSESSMENT)** Assess hip rotation and evaluate functional status.

Repeat the standing anteroposterior pelvis x-ray if rotation has decreased by more than 20% or if function has changed dramatically.
Consider switching to another chemical class of NSAIDs if the current medication has lost its effectiveness.
If the patient has become tolerant or intolerant of NSAIDs, a 3-week tapering dose of prednisone is usually temporarily effective. Starting doses range from 30 to 40 mg, tapering by 5 mg every 3 to 4 days.
Use narcotics cautiously.

■ **STEP 3 (MONTHS TO YEARS FOR PROGRESSIVE CASES)**   Assess hip rotation and functional status.
Consider orthopedic consultation when (1) pain is intractable, (2) function is severely limited, (3) internal rotation has declined to 10 to 15 degrees, or (4) protrusio acetabuli has developed.
Assess the patient's medical status and appropriateness of undergoing a 1- to 2-hour operation.

PHYSICAL THERAPY   Physical therapy plays an adjunctive role in the overall management of osteoarthritis of the hip.

PHYSICAL THERAPY SUMMARY

1. Stretching exercises of the adductors, rotators, and gluteus muscles and tendons, passively performed
2. Toning exercises of the iliopsoas and gluteus muscles, isometrically performed
3. Occupational therapy consultation for practical aids for daily activities

Acute Period, Recovery, and Rehabilitation
Stretching and toning exercises are recommended to maintain hip flexibility and to preserve muscular tone around the hip. Figure-of-four, Indian-style sitting, and knee-chest pulls are performed daily in sets of 20 to stretch the adductors, rotators, and gluteus muscles (p. 285). Toning exercises of the iliopsoas and the gluteus

muscles follow the stretching exercises. Initially, straight-leg-raising is performed without weights in the supine and prone positions (p. 289). With improvement, 5- to 10-lb weights are added to the ankle to increase the tension. Patients with advanced osteoarthritis and functional impairment may benefit from an occupational therapy assessment.

INJECTION   Intra-articular injection is limited to nonsurgical candidates with advanced disease. For optimal results, injection should be performed under fluoroscopy by an orthopedic surgeon or radiologist.

SURGICAL PROCEDURE   Patients who meet the criteria for operation should be considered for total joint replacement, or arthroplasty.

PROGNOSIS   Uncomplicated osteoarthritis of the hip is a slowly progressive disease. The patient should be educated about the slow progression over years, the nature of the course of arthritic flare, and the efficacy of surgery when indicated. Local injection should be restricted to the palliation of symptoms in nonsurgical candidates. By contrast, osteoarthritis may progress rapidly in the presence of congenital shallow acetabulum, avascular necrosis, or previous femoral neck fracture. Patients with these associated conditions should be followed closely at 2- to 4-month intervals.

MERALGIA PARESTHETICA

Enter 1 inch below and 1 inch medial to the anterior superior iliac spine; advance the needle at a 90-degree angle down to the interface of the subcutaneous fat and the fascia of the quadriceps.

Needle: 1¹/₂-inch, 22-gauge
Depth: 1 to 1¹/₂ inches (down to the fascia)
Volume: 1 to 2 mL of local anesthetic and 1 mL of K40

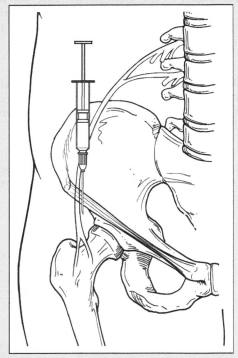

FIGURE 8–4. Injection of the lateral femoral cutaneous nerve.

DESCRIPTION   Meralgia paresthetica is a compression neuropathy of the lateral femoral cutaneous nerve as the nerve exits the pelvis, traverses the groin, and enters the thigh. The nerve penetrates the quadriceps fascia and enters the subcutaneous fat approximately 1 inch medial and 1 inch distal to the ASIS. This is the anatomic area where it is most vulnerable to the compressive forces of an overlying panniculus, tight garments worn around the waist, and scar tissue in and around the lateral aspect of the inguinal ligament.

On the exam of the lower extremity, neurologic abnormalities are restricted to sensory changes only (the nerve is a pure sensory nerve without a motor component). The degree of hypesthesia (numbness and tingling) or hyperesthesia (burning quality pain) over the anterolateral aspect of the thigh varies according to the degree of nerve compression. In contrast to the spectrum of findings accompanying lumbar radiculopathy, the remainder of the neurologic exam (lower extremity reflexes, motor strength, muscle tone and bulk) and the lower back exam are normal.

SYMPTOMS   The patient has neuritic pain in a very specific area of the anterolateral thigh. The patient often rubs the outer thigh back and forth while describing the condition.

"I have this burning pain in my thigh."

"It feels funny (pointing to the outer upper thigh) when my jeans rub over the skin."

"My skin feels numb and tingly (rubbing the skin of the outer upper thigh)."

"I think I have a pinched nerve. My leg is numb right here."

"My leg has some dead spots."

EXAM   The sensory function of the upper outer thigh is examined, and a lower extremity neurologic exam is performed in each patient.

EXAM SUMMARY

1. Hypesthetic or dysesthetic pain in the upper outer thigh
2. Lower extremity neurologic exam is normal
3. Hip, back, and SI joints are normal

(1) Pinprick and light touch are abnormal in a 10-inch × 6-inch, oval-shaped area on the anterolateral thigh. The distribution of the lateral femoral cutaneous nerve is not strictly lateral. It is not unusual for the nerve to provide sensation to a portion of the anterior thigh. (2) The neurologic exam of the lower extremity is otherwise normal. The straight-leg-raising sign is negative, and the deep tendon reflexes and distal motor strength are preserved. (3) There is no evidence of a hip, back, or SI joint abnormality.

X-RAYS Plain x-rays of the hip and pelvis are unnecessary. No characteristic changes are seen on these films. When the clinical findings are equivocal, radiographs of the lower lumbar spine often are used to exclude spondylolisthesis, spinal stenosis, or disk disease.

SPECIAL TESTING No special tests are indicated.

DIAGNOSIS The diagnosis is based on the unique description of the pain, its characteristic location, the sensory abnormalities on exam, and the conspicuous absence of neurologic abnormalities in the lower leg.

TREATMENT The treatment of choice comprises education of the patient (reassurance that *"This isn't a pinched nerve."*) combined with measures to reduce the pressure in the groin. Local corticosteroid injection is used infrequently and is reserved for patients with refractory symptoms and signs.

STEP 1 Educate the patient of the benign nature of the condition: *"This is not a serious back problem; it is not a pinched nerve. The nerve controlling the sensation of the thigh has been under pressure. As soon as the pressure is relieved, the feeling or irritative symptoms will gradually improve over several weeks."*

Avoid tight garments.

Bending at the waist must be limited, especially in a patient who has a large abdomen, and repetitive flexing of the hip should be avoided.

Avoid any exercising that involves repetitive hip extension (lunges, certain positions in yoga, leg extensions).

Apply ice over the upper outer thigh for 20 to 30 minutes three times a day.

Suggest abdominal toning exercises (e.g., half sit-ups, crunches, weighted side-bends) to tighten the inguinal area, which can reduce pressure over the nerve.

Discuss the need for weight loss.

STEP 2 (MONTHS FOR PERSISTENT SYMPTOMS) Reexamine the dysesthetic area to confirm the local nature of the problem.

Consider carbamazepine (Tegretol) or phenytoin (Dilantin) to reduce the dysesthetic pain (advise the patient: *"This relatively minor problem should not be treated with harsh and potentially harmful medications."*).

NSAIDs provide little benefit for this condition, which is mostly mechanical in nature with little accompanying inflammation.

Consider a consultation with an anesthesiologist for a local nerve block.

STEP 3 (MONTHS TO YEARS FOR CHRONIC SYMPTOMS) Consider a neurosurgical consultation for intractable dysesthetic cases.

PHYSICAL THERAPY Physical therapy does not play a significant role in the treatment of meralgia paresthetica. Abdominal muscle–toning exercises may reduce the pressure over the lateral femoral cutaneous nerve, but are of unproven value. It is important to avoid exercises that cause irritation (repetitive hip extension such as lunges, certain positions in yoga, and leg extension exercises or machinery).

INJECTION TECHNIQUE Local injection of anesthetic is used to confirm the diagnosis, especially when lower back or SI conditions coexist with this entrapment neuropathy. Because inflammation plays only a minor role, corticosteroid injection has limited benefit. Injection of a long-acting corticosteroid preparation most often is used "as a last resort" when patients are reluctant to undergo surgical intervention.

Positioning The patient is placed in the supine position with the legs kept straight.

Surface Anatomy and Point of Entry The ASIS is identified and marked. The inguinal ligament is identified as it courses to the lateral aspect of the pubic bone. The point of entry is $3/4$ to 1 inch medial to the ASIS and an equal distance below it.

Angle of Entry and Depth The needle is inserted at a perpendicular angle and advanced down to the firm tension of the fascia of the quadriceps femoris muscle. If an anesthetic block is not achieved at this point, the angle of entry is changed to a medially directed 45-degree angle, and the needle is advanced back to the fascia. If anesthetic block is still not achieved, the angle of entry is changed to a laterally directed 45-degree angle, and the needle is advanced back to the fascia.

Anesthesia Owing to the variable entry point of the nerve into the anterior thigh—most enter medially to the ASIS, and a few enter either at the ASIS or just lateral to it—anesthetic is fanned out above the fascia to define its exact location. Precise corticosteroid injection requires an accurate localization of the lateral cutaneous femoral nerve. Corticosteroid (1 mL) is placed just above the fascia of the quadriceps femoris muscle until anesthesia is achieved.

Technique The success of treatment depends as much on the accurate localization of the lateral femoral

MERALGIA PARESTHETICA INJECTION

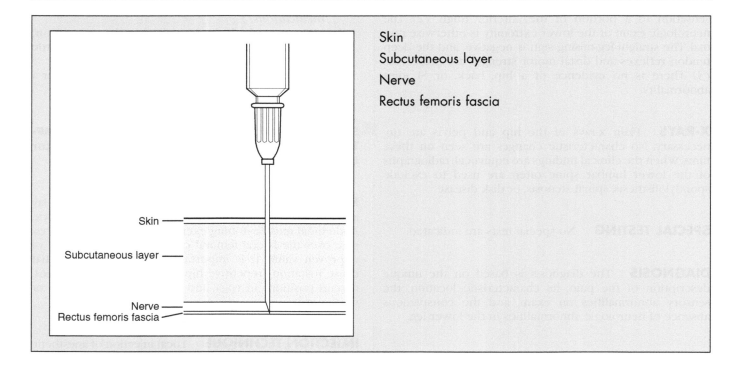

Skin
Subcutaneous layer
Nerve
Rectus femoris fascia

Skin
Subcutaneous layer
Nerve
Rectus femoris fascia

cutaneous nerve by stepwise anesthetic block as on the placement of the corticosteroid just above the fascia and adjacent to the nerve. First, the level of the quadriceps muscle fascia is identified by gradually advancing the needle down until the firm resistance of the fascia is felt at the needle tip. If the fascia is not readily identified, applying skin traction in a back-and-forth manner assists in defining the interface of the subcutaneous fat and the fascia. If the needle is above the fascia, the needle moves readily as skin traction is applied. If the needle has penetrated the fascia, the needle will not move in any direction when skin traction is applied. If injecting above the fascia does not reproduce the patient's symptoms, the needle is withdrawn close to the surface of the skin and reinserted at a 45-degree angle laterally or medially until an anesthetic block has been achieved. Anesthetic (1 or 2 mL) is placed at each location, and the patient is re-examined to evaluate its effectiveness. When the location of the nerve has been identified, 1 mL of K40 is injected through the same needle.

INJECTION AFTERCARE
1. *Rest* the affected leg and hip for the first 3 days, avoiding direct pressure, repetitive bending at the waist, and repetitive flexing of the hip.
2. Use *ice* (15 minutes every 4 to 6 hours), *acetaminophen* (1000 mg twice a day), or both for postinjection soreness.
3. *Protect* the leg and hip for an additional 3 to 4 weeks by limiting direct pressure and repetitive bending at the waist and repetitive flexing of the hip.

4. Avoid *constricting garments* at the waist, and continue weight loss efforts.
5. Repeat the *injection* at 6 weeks with corticosteroid if pain and inflammation persist.
6. *CT or MRI* is ordered if patient symptoms suggest a concomitant disk process in the upper lumbosacral spine area.
7. Obtain a *consultation* with a neurosurgeon for patients with intractable pain and patients failing two injections over several months.

SURGICAL PROCEDURE   Because most cases resolve with conservative treatment measures or time (91%), surgery is rarely necessary (J Neurosurg 74:76-80, 1991). Neurolysis of the constricting tissue, neurolysis and transposition of the nerve, or neurectomy can be considered if dysesthetic pain persists for months despite conservative care. Patients must be informed of the loss of sensation over the area after definitive neurectomy.

PROGNOSIS   Meralgia paresthetica is a self-limited, benign disease in most patients. Neurologic symptoms are restricted to sensory changes only (the nerve does not contain motor fibers). The most troublesome cases involve dysesthetic pain. If oral medication does not control symptoms, local anesthetic block can be considered. A rare case of severe and disabling dysesthetic pain can be considered for neurolysis.

AVASCULAR NECROSIS OF THE HIP

Ligamentum teres (blood supply to the proximal one third of the head of the femur)
Femoral head
Developing fracture line
Femoral neck
Haversian canals in the femoral neck (blood supply to the distal two thirds of the head of the femur)

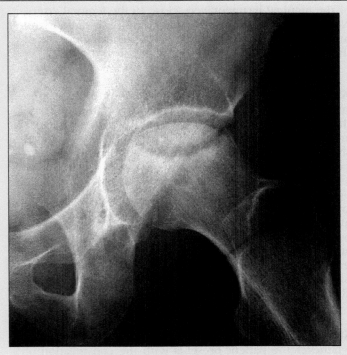

FIGURE 8–5. Avascular necrosis of the hip.

DESCRIPTION Avascular necrosis of the hip results from an interruption of the normal blood supply to the proximal portion of the femoral head. Common causes include trauma, diabetes, alcoholism, high-viscosity hematologic states, and oral corticosteroids (especially in patients with asthma, rheumatoid arthritis, or systemic lupus erythematosus). Early diagnosis is crucial, but often elusive owing to the lack of local tenderness, the lack of a high index of suspicion by the primary care provider, and the lack of abnormalities on initial radiographs of the hip (x-rays of the hip may remain normal for 1 to 2 weeks until the fracture becomes impacted or bony repair begins and a fracture line develops). The diagnosis should be suspected if (1) the patient has significant risk factors, (2) the patient describes acute and severe anterior groin pain, (3) weightbearing causes severe pain, and (4) rotation of the hip is restricted and poorly tolerated by the patient.

EXAM The exam assesses the patient's ability to bear weight and to walk, the general function of the hip, and the ROM of the hip joint.

EXAM SUMMARY

1. Severely impaired function—dramatic favoring of the hip, inability to bear weight, the patient arrives using crutches or a wheelchair
2. Severely restricted internal and external rotation with severe end-point pain
3. Barely tolerated fabere maneuver (abnormal Patrick test)
4. Dramatic tenderness 1$^{1}/_{2}$ inches below the inguinal ligament

(1) General hip function is severely compromised. All patients who attempt walking display a dramatic antalgic gait, unable to bear weight fully on the affected side. Some patients present to the clinic on crutches or in a wheelchair. Others refuse to bear any weight at all. Many patients require assistance just to move from chair to exam table. *(2)* The ROM of the hip is severely restricted. Similar to osteoarthritis of the hip joint, internal rotation is restricted to a greater degree than external rotation and abduction. Most patients with osteonecrosis are unable to rotate more than 25 to 30 degrees in either direction (half of the average 45 degrees of internal and external rotation expected in patients in their fourth or fifth decades. *(3)* Most patients are unable to tolerate the fabere maneuver, or the Patrick test. Even if patients can be placed in the figure-of-four position (*f*lexion, *ab*duction, *e*xternal *r*otation, and *e*xtension), they cannot tolerate the pressure applied to the ASIS and the knee, placing tension over the anterior capsule of the hip and creating torque through the femoral head and neck. This

maneuver causes moderate pain in cases of acute synovitis and extreme pain in cases of septic arthritis. (4) Tenderness typically is located $1^1/_2$ inches below the mid-portion of the inguinal ligament, very close to the femoral artery. *Note:* All of these findings on exam are exaggerated with inflammatory arthritis, severe with avascular necrosis of the hip, and extreme with acute septic arthritis.

X-RAYS Specific x-rays (including anteroposterior, lateral, and frog-leg views) to evaluate the hip joint and the integrity of the femur are mandatory. These views are performed lying down. If the patient can tolerate short intervals of weightbearing safely, a standing anteroposterior pelvis x-ray is also obtained. This single x-ray exposure allows simultaneous comparison of both hips, screens for SI disease, assesses leg-length discrepancy, and determines the position of the hips. Although these films are normal in the first 1 or 2 weeks, they form the basis for future comparison. Serial plain radiographs are an effective means of following the development of the fracture line, the osteoblastic repair, the loss of sphericity of the femoral head, and the secondary osteoarthritic changes.

SPECIAL TESTING Special testing is mandatory whenever the patient presents with the constellation of signs and symptoms described here. Changes on nuclear medicine bone scanning are too nonspecific to assist in the differential diagnosis (avascular necrosis characteristically shows an intense uptake of the radioactive tracer in the femoral head and in the joint, preventing a reliable discrimination between involvement of the joint from direct involvement of the femoral bone). MRI is the procedure of choice because it provides much more detailed changes. The localized osteopenia, effusion of the hip joint, subchondral bony edema, and, in later cases, evidence of early fracture line formation and loss of the normal sphericity of the femoral head identify the femur as the primary focus. In addition, MRI can identify benign and malignant changes in the bone.

DIAGNOSIS The diagnosis is based on acute and dramatic loss of hip function and the acute loss of hip rotation coupled with characteristic changes on MRI of the femur.

TREATMENT Nonweightbearing with crutches or a wheelchair is mandatory until the diagnosis is either made or excluded by special testing.

STEP 1 **Assess the general function of the hip, measure the patient's loss of internal and external rotation (normally 40 to 45 degrees in a 50-year-old person), and order a standing anteroposterior pelvis x-ray if weightbearing is tolerated or urgent MRI if pain is severe and weightbearing is not possible.**

Nonweightbearing with crutches is mandatory in hopes of preventing the collapse of the avascular segment.

Ice is applied over the upper outer thigh for 20 to 30 minutes three times a day.

Narcotics are prescribed to control the severe pain.

Laboratory testing is ordered to evaluate the general health of the patient and to assess the patient's underlying risk factors. Laboratory tests include complete blood count, erythrocyte sedimentation rate, glucose, liver function tests, serum protein electrophoresis, calcium, and alkaline phosphatase.

MRI is ordered to confirm the diagnosis and determine the bony integrity of the femur.

Consultation with an orthopedic surgeon is advised to assist in management. After confirming the diagnosis and assessing the medical stability of the patient, a decision when to intervene surgically is made.

Consider hyperbaric oxygen therapy for early presentations.

STEP 2 (AT 3 TO 4 WEEKS) **If surgery is not entertained, plain x-rays are repeated at 2- to 3-week intervals.**

Weightbearing must be avoided until rotation of the hip is no longer painful, and fracture healing has been shown radiographically.

Passive ROM stretching exercises are combined with active toning exercises of the hip flexors and extensors.

STEP 3 (6 TO 8 WEEKS FOR LONG-TERM FOLLOW-UP) **Patients are re-examined, and plain x-rays are repeated to determine the degree of arthritic change.**

Jogging, aerobic exercise, and other impact exercises are restricted.

Padded insoles are placed in every pair of shoes to reduce impact pressure (p. 262).

Passive hip-stretching exercises (p. 285) to preserve ROM are re-emphasized.

An NSAID (e.g., ibuprofen) is prescribed in full dose. Emphasize the need to take it regularly for at least 2 to 3 weeks for its anti-inflammatory effect.

A 3-week tapering dose of oral cortisone is prescribed as an alternative to NSAIDs.

Consultation with orthopedic surgeon for joint replacement is considered when pain becomes intractable, function is impaired, and ROM has gradually decreased.

SURGERY Core decompression with or without grafting and femoral neck osteotomy are used to obtain functional bone marrow studies and core biopsy for diagnosis. In addition, core decompression is used to reduce the pressure in the femoral head and theoretically to prevent the late segmental collapse of the femoral head (coxa plana) and secondary degenerative arthritis. For cases that progress to coxa plana and arthritis, hemiresurfacing, hemiarthroplasty, and total hip replacement are the procedures most commonly performed.

PROGNOSIS The outcome of avascular necrosis depends on making the diagnosis in a timely fashion, protecting the fracture segment from collapse by avoiding weightbearing, and choosing an appropriate surgical intervention. All patients must undergo plain radiography, MRI, and a full laboratory workup. The primary care provider should work with the surgical consultant in evaluating the patient.

SEVERE HIP PAIN (OCCULT FRACTURE OF THE HIP, SEPTIC ARTHRITIS, AND METASTATIC INVOLVEMENT OF THE FEMUR)

Occult fracture of the hip must be suspected if:

A fall has occurred in an elderly patient with known osteoporotic bones

Weightbearing is impossible because of moderate to severe hip pain

Internal and external rotation of the hip cause moderate to severe hip pain on examination

NOTE: Plain x-rays of the hip do not show a true fracture.

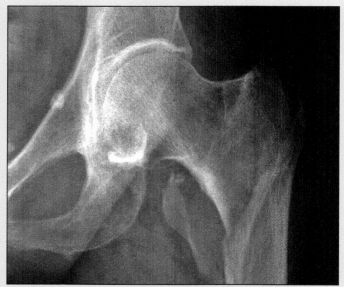

FIGURE 8–6. Occult fracture of the hip that progressed to complete fracture.

DESCRIPTION A patient with severe hip pain poses a unique clinical challenge. Most patients have a serious and potentially life-threatening process (occult fracture of the hip, pathologic fracture associated with benign or metastatic involvement of the femur, acute inflammatory arthritis, or septic arthritis) that requires emergent diagnostic studies and rapid therapeutic intervention. The clinician must be able to identify this group of patients and act rapidly to avoid catastrophic complications, such as complete fracture, avascular necrosis, or osteomyelitis.

SYMPTOMS The patient complains of acute and severe pain in the groin or upper thigh areas coupled with an acute change in the ability to bear weight.

"I've had this deep, achy pain in my thigh for weeks, but it suddenly got worse when I twisted my leg." (pathologic fracture in a patient with metastatic breast cancer)

"I fell out of bed in the nursing home and ever since I get this severe pain in my hip when the nursing assistant rolls me from side to side." (occult fracture in a elderly woman with osteoporosis)

"First I had biceps tendinitis. Then I had tendinitis along my instep. For the last several days I have had this severe pain in my hip and I can't put any weight on the leg or flex the hip." (track coach with migratory tenosynovitis and septic arthritis of the hip with gonorrhea)

"My hip hurts like hell and I can hardly put any weight on it." (pseudogout of the hip)

EXAM The exam assesses the patient's ability to bear weight and to walk and the ROM of the hip joint.

EXAM SUMMARY

1. Severely impaired function—inability to bear weight, the patient arrives using crutches or a wheelchair, or the patient is favoring one hip dramatically
2. Severely restricted internal and external rotation with severe end-point pain
3. Intolerant of the fabere maneuver (abnormal Patrick test)
4. Dramatic tenderness $1^1/_2$ inches below the inguinal ligament or severe pain with any type of torque applied to the femur

(1) Patients with an underlying fracture and patients with septic arthritis refuse to bear weight. Patients with inflammatory arthritis attempt walking, but display a dramatic antalgic gait and are unable to bear weight fully on the affected side. Most patients require assistance to move from chair to exam table. *(2)* The ROM of the hip is severely restricted. Rotation of the hip in internal or external rotation is extremely painful. Patients with septic arthritis tend to maintain the hip in partial flexion, relaxing the tension of the anterior joint capsule. *(3)* Whether because of acute hip joint effusion or underlying fracture,

most patients are intolerant of the fabere maneuver (also known as the Patrick test). (4) For patients with acute hip joint effusion, tenderness typically is located 1¹/₂ inches below the mid-portion of the inguinal ligament, close to the femoral artery. Tenderness over an underlying fracture depends on its exact location. Fracture line tenderness may be difficult to identify, however, in a patient with large overlying musculature or subcutaneous fat.

X-RAYS Specific x-rays (including anteroposterior, lateral, and frog-leg views of the hip) to evaluate the hip joint and the integrity of the femur are mandatory. An anteroposterior pelvis view also is obtained to compare both hips simultaneously and to evaluate the integrity of the bones of the pelvis. All of these films are performed in the lying position—to guard against aggravating the patient's pain or completing the underlying fracture.

SPECIAL TESTING Special testing is mandatory whenever a patient presents with the constellation of symptoms and signs. Bone scanning is performed in a patient with known metastatic disease. MRI is the test of choice for occult fracture. Fluoroscopy with aspiration of the hip joint is mandatory for a patient suspected to have septic or severe inflammatory arthritis.

TREATMENT The patient is kept nonweightbearing with crutches or in a wheelchair until the diagnosis is confirmed.

STEP 1 (ACUTE PERIOD) Assess the general function of the hip, measure the patient's loss of internal and external rotation (normally 40 to 45 degrees in a 50-year-old person), and order an anteroposterior pelvis x-ray or urgent MRI.

Nonweightbearing with crutches, a wheelchair, or bed rest is mandatory.

Urgent diagnostic studies are ordered, including complete blood count, erythrocyte sedimentation rate, calcium, alkaline phosphatase, plain films, MRI, and bone scan.

Consultation with an orthopedic surgeon is made urgently.

If diagnostic studies suggest either an inflammatory or a septic involvement of the hip joint, emergent consultation either with an orthopedic surgeon or interventional radiologist is mandatory to arrange for aspiration of the joint.

STEP 2 (RECOVERY PERIOD) The patient must be kept nonweightbearing through this interval.

ROM exercises are begun and combined with progressive ambulation after the patient has undergone definitive treatment and the acute pain has subsided.

Return to regular activities is gradual.

PHYSICAL THERAPY Physical therapy plays an adjunctive role in the recovery phase of these acute conditions affecting the hip.

PHYSICAL THERAPY SUMMARY

1. Stretching exercises of the adductors, rotators, and gluteus muscles and tendons, passively performed
2. Toning exercises of the iliopsoas and gluteus muscles, isometrically performed
3. Gradual return to regular activities

Acute Period, Recovery, and Rehabilitation
Passive stretching exercises are used to restore hip flexibility. Figure-of-four, Indian-style sitting, and knee-chest pulls are performed daily in sets of 20 to stretch the adductors, rotators, and gluteus muscles (p. 285). As flexibility returns, toning exercises of the iliopsoas and the gluteus muscles are added to the daily routine. Initially, straight-leg-raising is performed without weights in the supine and prone positions (p. 289). With improvement, 5- to 10-lb weights are added to the ankle to increase the tension. Regular activities must be postponed until flexibility and muscular tone is comparable to the unaffected side.

SURGERY The choice of surgery depends on the underlying diagnosis. Metastatic disease or benign tumors of the femur that are eroding through the cortex of the femur must be treated prophylactically with internal fixation with intramedullary rods. Patients with occult fracture of the femoral neck or head can be followed carefully over weeks for signs of healing (if the patient is a "poor" surgical candidate) or treated with hip pinning or total hip replacement. Patients with septic arthritis require repeated drainage and close observation for avascular necrosis from excessive intra-articular pressure.

DIFFERENTIAL DIAGNOSIS OF KNEE PAIN

Diagnoses	Confirmations
Patella (most common)	
Subluxation/dislocation	Exam; x-ray—sunrise view
Patellofemoral syndrome	Exam; x-ray—sunrise view
Dashboard knee (chondral fracture)	Arthroscopy (optional)
Patellofemoral osteoarthritis	X-ray—sunrise view
Patella alta	X-ray—lateral view of knee
Main joint	
Osteoarthritis: medial compartment, lateral compartment, or both	X-ray—bilateral standing anteroposterior knees
Inflammatory arthritis	Aspiration/synovial fluid analysis
Septic arthritis	Aspiration/synovial fluid analysis; culture
Hemarthrosis (anterior cruciate ligament [ACL] tear, medial collateral ligament [MCL] tear, meniscal tear, capsular tear, or tibial plateau fracture)	Aspiration/synovial fluid analysis; helical CT; MRI
Bursa	
Prepatellar ("housemaid's knee")	Aspiration/bursal fluid analysis
Anserine bursitis	Local anesthetic block
Baker's cyst	Aspiration or ultrasound
Infrapatellar (superficial or deep)	Local anesthetic block
Ligaments	
MCL injury—first, second, third	Exam; anesthetic block
Lateral collateral ligament injury—first, second, third	Exam; local anesthetic block
ACL injury	Exam; MRI
Posterior cruciate ligament injury	Exam; MRI
Iliotibial band syndrome	Exam; local anesthetic block
Snapping knee	Exam
Meniscal tear	
Traumatic or degenerative	MRI; arthroscopy
Referred pain	
Trochanteric bursitis	Exam; local anesthetic block
Hip joint	X-ray—standing anteroposterior pelvis
Femur	Bone scan
Lumbosacral spine radiculopathy	CT scan; MRI; electromyography

PATELLOFEMORAL SYNDROME

The patellofemoral family of conditions includes:

Patellofemoral syndrome
Patellofemoral subluxation
Patellofemoral arthritis
Patellar dislocation
Patella alta

These conditions all are characterized by abnormal tracking of the patella in the femoral groove. Intra-articular corticosteroid injection is indicated in patients with refractory symptoms and in rare patients with joint effusion.

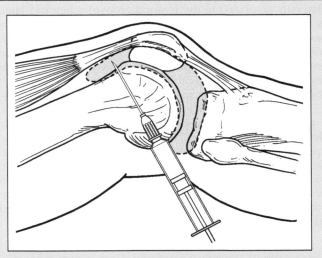

FIGURE 9–1. Injection of the knee for patellofemoral syndrome.

DESCRIPTION Patellofemoral syndrome represents a family of conditions that cause symptoms at the patellofemoral joint, including *patellofemoral syndrome* (formally *chondromalacia patellae*, the term describing the pathology), *patellar subluxation* (the mechanical term that describes the abnormal patellofemoral tracking), *patella alta* (excessive length of the patellar tendon), and *patellofemoral arthritis* (degenerative arthritis—the end result of years of symptoms). Although some cases are caused by direct trauma (dashboard knee), most cases result from the repetitive irritation of abnormal tracking of the patella in the femoral groove (patellar subluxation). An overdeveloped vastus lateralis muscle (a lack of balance with the weaker vastus medialis) and the Q angle formed by the tibial tubercle, the center of the patella, and the center of the quadriceps muscle contribute to the forces that cause lateral patellar subluxation. Arthroscopically the undersurface of the patella shows defects in the articular cartilage (pits and cracks). Over several decades, diffuse irregularities of the articular cartilage develop (e.g., osteoarthritis).

SYMPTOMS The patient complains of knee pain (in front of the knee), a "noisy" knee, and, occasionally, swelling. The patient often rubs the entire area around the patella or attempts to demonstrate the noise by actually flexing the knee when describing the condition.

"My knee caps ache after I run."

"I can't squat or kneel anymore."

"I have this grinding sound when I bend my knee."

"My knees have always had this grinding noise, but now they're swelling."

"I can't sit Indian-style anymore."

"Whenever I use the stair stepper or do aerobics, both my knees will ache that evening."

"Two years ago, I rammed my knees into the dashboard. Ever since then, my knees ache after skiing."

EXAM The patellofemoral articulation is examined for local irritation, alignment, and abnormal tracking, and the knee is examined for signs of effusion.

EXAM SUMMARY

1. Painful retropatellar crepitation (squatting, patellar compression, Insall maneuver)
2. Full range of motion (ROM) but with abnormal patellofemoral tracking
3. Clicking with passive flexion and extension
4. Negative apprehension sign for patellar dislocation
5. Knee effusion (uncommon)

(1) Painful retropatellar crepitation is best detected by passively moving the patella back and forth across the femoral groove. The leg is placed in the extended position, and the patient is asked to relax the quadriceps muscle. With the examiner's fingers on all four poles and with firm downward pressure, the patella is forced onto the lateral and medial femoral condyles and down into the inferior patellofemoral groove. Crepitation may be palpable only in the inferior portion of the groove, where the disease most often first develops. *(2)* Patellofemoral alignment

and tracking are assessed by inspection, by measurement of the Q angle, and by passive flexion and extension of the knee. Patellar subluxation may be obvious by visualization (laterally displaced in the femoral groove) when the knee is in the extended position. More often, subluxation is assessed by measuring the Q angle. The Q angle is determined at the intersection of the lines drawn from the anterior superior iliac spine, to the mid-patella, and from the mid-patella through the center of the tibial tubercle; the normal Q angle measures less than 20 degrees. (3) With the palm placed over the center of the patella, a patellar click may be palpable as the knee is passively flexed and extended. (4) The apprehension sign (pressure applied medially to laterally to reproduce patellar dislocation) should be absent. (5) Knee effusion is uncommon. Moderate to large effusion suggests severe exacerbation or advanced disease (p. •••). In the absence of a knee effusion, uncomplicated patellofemoral syndrome should have full ROM.

X-RAYS   Four views of the knee, including the sunrise (also referred to as the merchant view), standing postero-anterior, lateral, and tunnel views, are always recommended. Typical changes include lateral subluxation; a narrowing of the lateral patellofemoral articular cartilage; sclerosis of the lateral aspect of the patella (the reaction to the constant lateral pressure); and, in advanced cases, osteoarthritic changes, including osteophytes, severe sclerosis, and subchondral cyst formation of osteoarthritis. Early disease may show only subluxation.

DIAGNOSIS   The diagnosis of patellofemoral syndrome is based on clinical findings. Anterior knee pain associated with painful patellar crepitation and subluxation on x-rays is highly suggestive. Regional anesthetic block may be necessary to differentiate the articular pain arising from the patella from a complicating periarticular process, such as anserine bursitis. Arthroscopy to exclude osteochondritis dissecans, loose body, or meniscal tear is indicated when patellofemoral syndrome presents with a greater degree of mechanical symptoms or with a large knee effusion (1% to 2%).

TREATMENT   The goals of treatment are to improve patellofemoral tracking and alignment, to reduce pain and swelling, and to retard the development of patellofemoral arthritis. Restriction of repetitive flexion and isometrically performed quadriceps sets are the treatments of choice.

STEP 1   Evaluate the baseline quadriceps tone, perform a heel-to-buttock measurement to assess knee flexibility, measure or at least estimate the Q angle, and order x-rays of the knee.

   Apply ice, and elevate the knee, especially with effusion.

   Emphasize the absolute need to avoid squatting and kneeling.

Repetitive flexion must be restricted according to the severity of the condition (to 30 degrees for severe disease or to 60 degrees for moderate disease).

Recommend swimming, NordicTrack, and fast walking in place of jogging, bicycling, and stop-and-go sports that involve too much bending and impact.

Begin isometrically performed straight-leg raises with the leg externally rotated and in full extension to enhance the tone of the vastus medialis and improve patellofemoral tracking.

STEP 2 (4 TO 8 WEEKS FOR PERSISTENT CASES) Reinforce restrictions and exercises.

Prescribe a nonsteroidal anti-inflammatory drug (NSAID) (e.g., ibuprofen [Advil, Motrin]) at full dose for 3 weeks and with a taper at week 4.

Recommend a patellar strap (p. 256) or a Velcro patellar restraining brace (p. 257) to counter the deleterious effects of patellofemoral tracking, especially for patients active in sports.

STEP 3 (3 TO 4 MONTHS FOR PERSISTENT CASES) Perform a local corticosteroid injection with K40 or injection of hyaluronic acid for symptoms lasting longer than 6 to 8 weeks or for a patient with knee effusion.

Repeat the injection at 4 to 6 weeks if symptoms have not been reduced by 50%.

STEP 4 (4 TO 6 WEEKS FOR CHRONIC CASES) Re-emphasize the need to continue daily or thrice-weekly straight-leg-raising exercises.

Recommend long-term restrictions of squatting, kneeling, and bending for patients with chronic symptoms.

Consider orthopedic referral for persistent pain and dysfunction or in cases associated with patella alta, or Q angles greater than 20 degrees.

PHYSICAL THERAPY   Physical therapy exercises are the cornerstone of treatment for patellofemoral disorders.

PHYSICAL THERAPY SUMMARY

1. Ice
2. Isometrically performed quadriceps sets with the leg externally rotated and in full extension are used to increase the overall quadriceps tone and enhance the tone of the vastus medialis, counteracting the lateral forces applied to the patella.
3. Active exercises and apparatus that minimize impact and repetitive bending

Acute Period   Ice and elevation are used when symptoms are acute. *Ice* is an effective analgesic and may help to reduce swelling.

Recovery and Rehabilitation   Exercises are combined with activity restrictions to reduce patellofemoral irritation. *Muscle-toning exercises* help to stabilize the knee joint, reduce subluxation and dislocation, and improve patellofemoral tracking. Daily straight-leg-raising exercises in the supine and prone positions are performed in sets of 20 (p. 289). These exercises are performed initially without weights. With improvement, 5- to 10-lb weights are added at the ankle. *Active exercises,* especially on equipment, must be performed with caution. Stationary bicycle exercise, rowing machines, and universal gym requiring full-knee flexion must be avoided initially. Fast walking, swimming, and NordicTrack cross-country ski machines are preferable because of their low impact and the minimal bending required.

INJECTION   The indications for local corticosteroid injection are limited. Hyaluronic acid injection can be used for patients exhibiting chronic mechanical symptoms of pain, crepitation, and clicking. Patients with more inflammatory symptoms—intractable pain, persistent effusion, and poor responses to exercise and the NSAIDs—can be treated with corticosteroid injection. For the technique of intra-articular injection, see p. 150.

SURGICAL PROCEDURE   Lateral retinacular release, tibial tubercle transposition, and arthroscopic débridement are used in selected cases. All of these procedures attempt to reduce patellar irritation either directly (débridement) or indirectly by attempting to correct abnormal patellofemoral tracking (lateral retinacular release and tibial tubercle transposition). Surgery, similar to injection therapy, is not a substitute for regular quadriceps toning.

PROGNOSIS   The prognosis of patellofemoral syndrome—the most common diagnosis in young and middle-aged adults—is uniformly good. The condition is rarely disabling and rarely remains symptomatic beyond age 50. Symptoms can wax and wane over years, but the natural history of the condition for most is to fade gradually after age 50. Patients with frequently recurring or severe symptoms should undergo a thorough evaluation. Bilateral sunrise x-rays, synovial fluid analysis, or arthroscopy should be performed to evaluate for patellofemoral syndrome complicated by osteochondritis dissecans, inflammatory effusion, or focal, traumatic chondromalacia. Preventive exercises cannot be overemphasized. Improvement in quadriceps and hamstring tone and the use of oral glucosamine sulfate should retard the progression of the disease.

KNEE EFFUSION

Enter laterally between the lines formed by the underside of the patella and the middle of the iliotibial track; gently advance the needle to the mild resistance of the lateral retinaculum, angling just above the superior pole of the patella.

Needle: 1$\frac{1}{2}$- to 3$\frac{1}{2}$-inch spinal needle, 22- to 18-gauge
Depth: $\frac{1}{2}$ to 3 inches
Volume: 1 to 2 mL of anesthetic and 1 mL of K40

NOTE: The synovial cavity is $\frac{1}{2}$ to $\frac{5}{8}$ inch beyond the lateral retinaculum; aspirate with mild pressure as the needle is advanced to this depth.

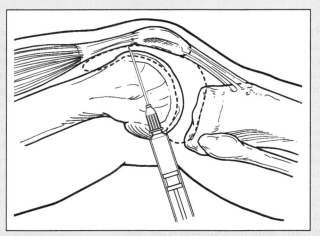

FIGURE 9–2. Intra-articular injection of the knee by the lateral approach entering the suprapatellar pouch.

DESCRIPTION   A knee effusion is an abnormal accumulation of synovial fluid. It is classified as noninflammatory, inflammatory, hemorrhagic, or septic depending on the cellular content (p. 300). Osteoarthritis, inflammatory arthritis, patellofemoral syndrome, hemarthrosis secondary to trauma, and infection (e.g., gonococcal, staphylococcal) are the most common causes. Increasing amounts of fluid interfere with the normal motion of the knee, restricting flexion first and eventually extension. The hydraulic pressure of repetitive bending forces the synovial fluid into the popliteal space, limiting flexion, causing the sensation of posterior knee tightness, and eventually leading to the formation of Baker's cyst (approximately 10% to 15% of cases). Large effusions stretch the supporting structures surrounding the knee, contributing to the instability of the knee.

SYMPTOMS   The patient complains of knee swelling, tightness in the knee, or restricted ROM. The patient often rubs over the front of the knee with both hands when describing the condition.

"My knee is swollen."

"I feel an egg behind my knee whenever I bend it back."

"My right knee seems to be so much bigger than the left."

"My whole knee feels achy and tight."

"At the end of the day the swelling is so great that I limp. It feels like it's going to burst."

"My knee is giving out. It feels like it won't hold my weight."

"I have a fever inside my knee."

"My knee has become so swollen that I can't bend it back or fully straighten it."

EXAM   Maneuvers to detect knee swelling are combined with an objective measurement of the ROM of the knee.

EXAM SUMMARY

1. General fullness and loss of the medial and lateral peripatellar dimples
2. Synovial milking sign
3. The patellar ballottement sign
4. Suprapatellar bulging
5. Needle aspiration of fluid
6. Loss of full knee flexion (the heel-to-buttock distance)

(1) With the knees in the extended position and the quadriceps muscle relaxed, the size and shape of both knees are compared, and the medial and lateral peripatellar dimples are inspected. Small effusions (5 to 10 mL) fill in these normal anatomic landmarks and create a general fullness to the knee. *(2)* For small effusions with high viscosity, the synovial milking sign may be positive. Pressure is held over the medial dimple (over the medial patellar retinaculum) to force the synovial fluid into the lateral compartment. When pressure is released, and a milking motion is applied to the lateral dimple (over the lateral patellar retinaculum), the fluid reappears medially. This test is practical only in asthenic patients with high-viscosity fluid. *(3)* The ballottement sign is positive with

10 to 15 mL of fluid. With the examiner using both hands, the synovial fluid is milked into the center of the knee from all four quadrants. With the index finger, the patella is forcibly snapped down against the femur. A moderate effusion is associated with a clicking or tapping sensation. (4) Large effusions (20 to 30 mL) fill the suprapatellar space. This area just above the superior pole of the patella is usually flat or slightly concave. Large effusions cause a convexity above the patella and a bulging under the distal vastus lateralis muscle and fascia. (5) Joint aspiration is the definitive test for knee effusion. This is especially true for an obese patient or for a patient with unusually large peripatellar fat pads. (6) A joint effusion always should be suspected if the affected knee is enlarged and lacks full flexion. Flexion can be compared between one side and the other or measured in degrees (0 degrees at full extension, 90 degrees with the knee bent at a right angle). A simple observation that provides an objective measurement of flexion is the heel-to-buttock distance. The knee is forced gently into full flexion, and the distance between the heel and the point on the buttock the heel ordinarily would come into contact with is measured. This measurement correlates well with the acute effusion. It also is abnormal with previous surgical treatment of the knee (e.g., total knee replacement, ACL repair) and with neuromuscular disorders that have affected the lower extremities. The measurement may not be abnormal in chronic effusion because chronic effusions gradually dilate all the supporting structures.

X-RAYS   X-rays of the knee (including weightbearing posteroanterior, lateral, sunrise, and tunnel views) always are recommended. The weightbearing view is used to determine the widths of the cartilage of the medial and lateral compartments and of the valgus carrying angle of the knee. The sunrise, or merchant, view is used to determine the degree of patellofemoral disease. The tunnel view is used to evaluate for osteochondritis dissecans and intra-articular loose bodies. The lateral view, with good soft-tissue technique, can provide clues to the presence of a large joint effusion, location of bony lesions, and soft-tissue calcifications.

SPECIAL TESTING   Synovial fluid analysis is an integral part of the evaluation of knee effusion.

DIAGNOSIS   A presumptive diagnosis of a knee effusion can be made on the basis of physical signs; however, a definitive diagnosis requires synovial fluid analysis obtained by aspiration. Joint aspiration is mandatory whenever infection is in the differential diagnosis (p. 300).

TREATMENT   The goals of treatment are to diagnose the underlying cause of the effusion, to reduce swelling and inflammation, and to restore the stability of the joint. Joint aspiration is the treatment of choice for tense hemarthrosis and tense effusions causing instability of the knee. Joint aspiration, synovial fluid analysis, and corticosteroid injection are the treatments of choice for large nonseptic effusions. Hospitalization and intravenous antibiotics are the treatments of choice for the septic effusion.

■ **STEP 1   Perform a heel-to-buttock measurement; aspirate the effusion for diagnostic studies (e.g., cell count and differential, crystals, glucose, Gram stain, and culture); and order standing posteroanterior, lateral, and sunrise views of the knees.**

Hospitalize and begin intravenous antibiotics empirically (covering for staphylococcal organisms) if infection is suspected.

Apply ice to reduce pain, and elevate the knee to reduce swelling.

Suggest crutches with touch-down weightbearing for severe cases.

Minimize squatting and kneeling.

Flexion of the knee must be restricted according to the degree of the problem (to 30 degrees for severe disease or 60 degrees for moderate disease).

Prescribe a patellar restraining brace if the knee is grossly unstable (giving out excessively).

Begin straight-leg-raising exercises without weights as soon as the acute symptoms resolve to restore muscle support, enhance stability, and reduce recurrent effusion.

■ **STEP 2 (DAYS TO 4 WEEKS FOR ACUTE FOLLOW-UP) Re-aspirate tense effusions.**

Re-emphasize the importance of straight-leg-raising exercises in restoring quadriceps support to the knee (with weights as tolerated).

Prescribe an NSAID (e.g., ibuprofen) for 4 weeks at full dose with a taper beginning at 3 weeks.

■ **STEP 3 (3 TO 6 WEEKS FOR PERSISTENT CASES)   Re-aspirate and inject the knee with K40.**

Repeat the injection at 4 to 6 weeks if symptoms are not reduced by 50%.

Re-emphasize the importance of weighted straight-leg raises.

■ **STEP 4 (2 TO 4 MONTHS FOR CHRONIC CASES)   Repeat plain x-rays or order MRI for cases that have failed to respond to treatment and especially for cases associated with symptoms of mechanical locking or severe giving-out.**

Consider orthopedic consultation, depending on the underlying cause (e.g., meniscal tear, loose body, advanced osteoarthritis).

The straight-leg-raising exercise combined with hamstring leg extensions completes the recovery.

PHYSICAL THERAPY   Physical therapy plays an essential role in the active treatment and prevention of knee effusion.

PHYSICAL THERAPY SUMMARY

1. Application of ice and elevation of the knee
2. Crutches with touch-down weightbearing
3. Straight-leg-raising exercises to restore support and stability, isometrically performed
4. Gradual resumption of active exercises, with caution

Acute Period   For the first few days, apply ice, elevate the knee, and restrict weightbearing. *Ice* and *elevation* always are recommended for acute knee effusions. An ice bag, a bag of frozen corn, or an iced towel from the freezer applied for 10 to 15 minutes is effective for swelling and analgesia. *Crutches,* a *walker,* or a *cane* may be necessary during the first few days.

Recovery and Rehabilitation   After the acute symptoms have subsided, toning exercises are begun and are combined with restricted use. *Straight-leg-raising* exercises always are recommended to restore muscular support to the knee (p. •••). Initially, they are performed without weights in sets of 20, with each held 5 seconds. With improvement in strength, a 5- to 10-lb weight is added to the ankle. These exercises are performed in the prone and supine positions to tone the quadriceps femoris and hamstring muscles. *Active exercises,* especially on apparatus, must be included with caution.

Exercise on a stationary bicycle, a rowing machine, or a universal gym may be irritating to an inflamed and recently distended joint. Fast walking, swimming, a NordicTrack-like glide machine, and other limited-impact exercise apparatus or exercises requiring much less flexion are preferred.

INJECTION   Aspiration of synovial fluid is performed to relieve the pressure of tense effusions and to obtain fluid for analysis. Injection of local anesthetic can be used to differentiate articular from periarticular conditions affecting the knee. Corticosteroid injection is used to treat nonseptic effusion, such as osteoarthritis, rheumatoid arthritis, and pseudogout.

Positioning   The patient is placed in the supine position with the leg fully extended. If the patient is uncomfortable and unable to relax the quadriceps muscle, a rolled-up towel is placed under the knee.

Surface Anatomy and Point of Entry   The midline of the iliotibial band, the lateral edge of the patella, and the superior pole of the patella are palpated and marked. Gently push the patella laterally to palpate its edge. The point of entry is along a line drawn halfway between the iliotibial band (the center of the femur) and the lateral edge of the patella and 1/2 inch below the superior pole of the patella. This point provides the safest and easiest access to the superolateral portion of the suprapatellar pouch.

Angle of Entry and Depth   The needle is angled up toward the superior pole of the patella. The lateral retinaculum (the first tissue plane) is 2 1/2 inches deep.

INTRA-ARTICULAR INJECTION OF THE KNEE

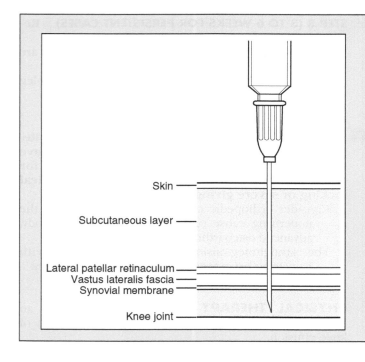

Skin
Subcutaneous layer
Lateral patellar retinaculum
Vastus lateralis fascia
Synovial membrane
Knee joint

Skin
Subcutaneous layer
Lateral patellar retinaculum
Vastus lateralis fascia
Synovial membrane
Knee joint

The superior pouch of the synovial cavity is always ¹/₂ to ⁵/₈ inch beyond the lateral retinaculum.

Anesthesia Ethyl chloride is sprayed on the skin. Local anesthetic is placed at the retinaculum (1 mL) and intra-articularly.

Technique A *lateral approach* to the suprapatellar pouch is most accessible, closer to the skin, and less likely to cause painful irritation. The needle is advanced at a 70-degree angle toward the superior pole of the patella (the suprapatellar pouch of the synovial cavity) until the resistance of the rubber-like tissue of the lateral retinaculum—the first tissue plane—is felt. Anesthetic (1 mL) is placed just outside the synovial lining. The needle is withdrawn. Next, an 18-gauge, 1¹/₂-inch needle attached to a 20-ml syringe is advanced down to the retinaculum and then into the joint (a giving-way sensation or pop is often felt, and the patient feels discomfort). To assist in aspirating fluid, gentle pressure against the medial retinaculum and joint line may shift the synovial fluid laterally. If the fluid is relatively clear (the examiner should be able to read newsprint through a low cell count fluid), 1 mL of K40 is injected through the same needle. If the first pass into the joint does not yield synovial fluid, the needle is withdrawn slowly with constant low suction. If fluid is not obtained with the slow withdrawal of the needle, the needle is redirected to just below the level of the superior pole of the patella. Aspiration is attempted at this site. If the second attempt is unsuccessful, a dry tap knee injection is recommended (p. 154).

INJECTION AFTERCARE

1. *Rest* for 3 days, avoiding all direct pressure, squatting, kneeling, and bending beyond 90 degrees.
2. Advise crutches with touch-down weightbearing for 3 to 7 days for severe cases.
3. Use *ice* (15 minutes every 4 to 6 hours) and *acetaminophen (Tylenol ES)* (1000 mg twice a day) for postinjection soreness.
4. *Protect* the knee for 3 to 4 weeks by limiting direct pressure, repetitive bending, prolonged standing, and unnecessary walking; continue to restrict squatting and kneeling.
5. Begin *straight-leg-raising exercises* for the quadriceps muscle on day 4 to enhance the support of the knee.
6. Recommend temporary bracing (3 to 4 weeks) with a patellar restraining brace or even a Velcro straight-leg brace for patients with poor quadriceps muscle tone or patients who have experienced frequent giving-out of the knee.

7. Repeat *injection* at 6 weeks with corticosteroid if swelling persists.
8. In chronic cases, order *plain x-rays* (standing posteroanterior, bilateral, and sunrise views) or *MRI* to identify advanced degenerative arthritis, high-degree subluxation of the patellofemoral joint, and degenerative or traumatic meniscal tear.
9. Advise long-term restrictions on bending of the knee (30 to 45 degrees) and the impact of weightbearing for the patient with advanced arthritis.
10. Request a *consultation* with an orthopedic surgeon for a second opinion if two consecutive injections fail to provide 4 to 6 months of improved function and decreased swelling.

SURGICAL PROCEDURE Surgical procedures vary according to the underlying pathology. Arthroscopic débridement can be considered for severe, protracted osteoarthritis flare. Meniscectomy is performed for a degenerative or traumatic meniscal tear (p. 175). Synovectomy is used for rheumatoid arthritis that has failed to respond to systemic therapy and intra-articular corticosteroids.

PROGNOSIS The response to aspiration and injection depends on the underlying cause. Mild to moderate inflammatory effusions (cell counts 1000 to 20,000) respond most dramatically, providing 6 to 18 months of relief. Further testing is usually unnecessary in patients with pseudogout, gout, and acute rheumatoid arthritis, who respond dramatically. Noninflammatory effusions (cell counts in the 100s) respond less predictably. Patients with osteoarthritis may respond gradually over several weeks. The response is often tempered, however, by an associated anserine bursitis, MCL strain, or degenerative meniscal tears; these complications must be addressed separately. Poor response to intra-articular steroids—either a low percentage improvement or short interval of time (≤4 to 6 weeks)—suggests either a noninflammatory process or a mechanical process, such as a meniscal tear, ACL insufficiency, severe varus or valgus deformity, loose body, or frayed or extremely injured articular cartilage. These patients require further workup, including repeat plain x-rays, MRI, or arthroscopy. A limited response to injection can be just as important as a successful response because it identifies patients needing further testing.

DRY TAP INJECTION OF THE KNEE

The same point of entry for aspiration of a knee effusion is used for this injection; direct the needle toward the undersurface of the patella.

Needle: 1^1/$_2$- to 3^1/$_2$-inch spinal needle, 22- to 18-gauge
Depth: ^{1}/$_2$ to 3 inches until the soft resistance of the patellar cartilage is felt
Volume: 1 to 2 mL of anesthetic and 1 mL of K40

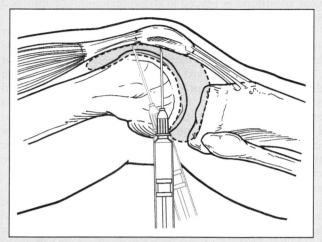

FIGURE 9–3. Dry tap intra-articular injection of the knee by the lateral approach to the patella.

DESCRIPTION When the lateral approach to the suprapatellar pouch does not yield synovial fluid, dry tap injection is an alternative injection technique to ensure an intra-articular placement of corticosteroid. If the tip of the needle is resting next to articular cartilage, an intra-articular injection is guaranteed. The symptoms, exam, plain x-rays, treatment protocol, and physical therapy are identical to information for knee effusion (p. 150).

INJECTION To ensure an intra-articular injection, an injection has to be placed immediately adjacent to articular cartilage. A *lateral approach* to the patella is preferred. It is less likely to damage articular cartilage than either a medial or a lateral joint line injection. The neurovascular structures are smaller over the lateral knee. The lateral patella is closer to the skin. The lateral approach avoids the obstacle of the contralateral leg.

Positioning The patient is placed in the supine position with the leg fully extended.

Surface Anatomy and Point of Entry The midline of the iliotibial band, the lateral edge of the patella, and the superior pole of the patella are palpated and marked. The patella should be moved gently laterally to palpate its lateral edge. The point of entry in the horizontal plane is halfway between the iliotibial band and the lateral edge of the patella and ^{1}/$_2$ inch caudal to the superior pole of the patella in the craniocaudal axis.

Angle of Entry and Depth The needle is angled up toward the undersurface of the patella. The lateral retinaculum (first tissue plane) ranges from ^{1}/$_2$ to 2^1/$_2$ inches deep. The articular cartilage of the patella is ^{1}/$_2$ to ^{3}/$_4$ inch beyond the firm tissue resistance of the retinaculum.

Anesthesia Ethyl chloride is sprayed on the skin. Local anesthetic is placed at the retinaculum (1 mL) and intra-articularly.

Technique A *lateral approach* is easiest and safest. The same point of entry used for knee aspiration (p. 152) is used to perform the dry tap injection. The needle is directed and advanced to the undersurface of the patella. Mild subluxation of the patella facilitates this injection. Firm pressure is necessary to "pop" into the joint. The bevel of the needle should be turned up so that the angle of the patella matches the bevel (less likely to damage the articular cartilage). The needle is advanced cautiously to the undersurface of the patella. The depth of injection is assessed by gently rocking the patella back and forth (pressure is applied from the medial edge of the patella). The medially applied pressure should be felt by the tip of the needle. At this exact point, 1 to 2 mL of anesthetic can be injected (diagnostic local anesthetic block for an intra-articular process) along with either 2 mL of hyaluronic acid or 1 mL of K40.

INJECTION AFTERCARE

1. *Rest* for 3 days, avoiding all direct pressure, squatting, kneeling, and bending beyond 90 degrees.
2. Advise *crutches* with touch-down weightbearing for 3 to 7 days for severe cases.
3. Use *ice* (15 minutes every 4 to 6 hours) and *acetaminophen* (1000 mg twice a day) for postinjection soreness.
4. *Protect* the knee for 3 to 4 weeks by limiting direct pressure, repetitive bending, prolonged standing, and unnecessary walking; continue to restrict squatting and kneeling.
5. Begin *straight-leg-raising exercises* for the quadriceps muscle on day 4 to enhance the support of the knee.
6. Recommend temporary *bracing* (3 to 4 weeks) with a patellar restraining brace or a Velcro straight-leg brace if quadriceps tone is poor, and the patient has

DRY TAP INJECTION OF THE KNEE

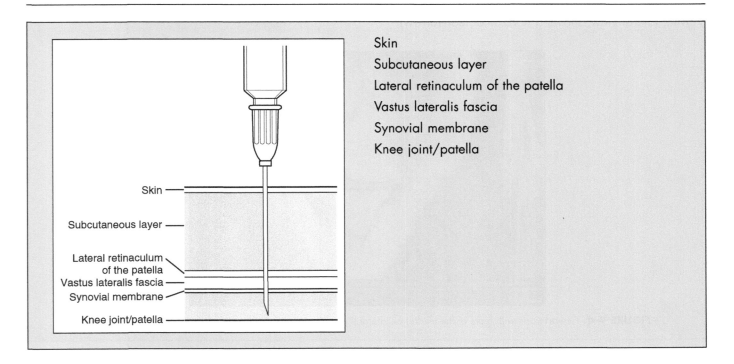

Skin
Subcutaneous layer
Lateral retinaculum of the patella
Vastus lateralis fascia
Synovial membrane
Knee joint/patella

Skin
Subcutaneous layer
Lateral retinaculum of the patella
Vastus lateralis fascia
Synovial membrane
Knee joint/patella

experienced repeated episodes in which the knee has given out.

7. Repeat *injection* at 6 weeks with corticosteroid if pain and swelling persist.

8. For persistent or chronic cases, obtain the following *plain x-rays* (standing posteroanterior and bilateral sunrise views) or CT or MRI to identify advanced degenerative arthritis, high-degree subluxation of the patellofemoral joint, and degenerative or traumatic meniscal tear.

9. Advise *long-term restrictions* on bending and the impact of weightbearing for a patient with advanced arthritis.

10. Request a *consultation* for a second opinion with an orthopedic surgeon if two consecutive injections fail to provide 4 to 6 months of improved function and decreased swelling.

PROGNOSIS The response and long-term outcome depend on the degree of inflammation, the stage of osteoarthritis (whether early or advanced), the degree of patellofemoral subluxation, and the association of mechanical dysfunction (e.g., poor quadriceps tone, ligamentous instability, malalignment from previous fracture, degenerative meniscal tear). Injection should provide 6 to 18 months of relief for knee effusion free of mechanical dysfunction.

HEMARTHROSIS

MRI, lateral view, shows a horizontal tear *(arrow)*.

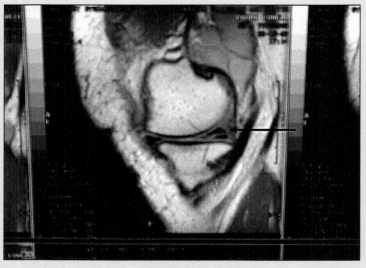

FIGURE 9–4. Hemarthrosis with tears of the medial collateral ligament, anterior cruciate ligament, and medial meniscus.

DESCRIPTION   The approach to a patient with an acute traumatic hemarthrosis is distinctly different than that to the typical patient presenting with a subacute or chronic effusion of the knee. Most patients presenting with a bloody effusion after trauma have underlying surgical pathology. ACL tears, meniscal tears, patellar tendon tears, and subcortical fractures constitute more than 90% of the underlying injuries. Less common causes include impingement of synovium, MCL avulsions, and coagulopathies (streptokinase and factor VII deficiencies). Aspirin and warfarin (Coumadin) are rare causes of hemarthrosis.

All tense effusions should be aspirated for diagnosis, to relieve pain, and to prevent an organized hematoma. Immediate surgical referral is necessary given the nearly universal presence of significant ligament, cartilage, or bony pathology. Exam, plain x-rays, treatment protocol, and physical therapy are identical to those for knee effusion.

SYMPTOMS   The patient complains of knee swelling, tightness and severe pain in the knee, inability to flex secondary to swelling and pain, and impaired weightbearing. The patient often rubs over the front of the knee with both hands when describing the condition.

"My knee is swollen."

"My knee twisted when I jumped off my skate board. I tried to walk, but after two steps I felt my knee shift." (ACL tear)

"I jumped off a rock, landed hard, my knee swelled immediately, and now I can't put any weight on it." (tibial plateau fracture)

"I went up for a lay up, and this guy came down on the side of my knee." (partial tear of the MCL and synovial membrane)

"I was tackled from the side, my knee immediately swelled, and now I can't bend it." (medial meniscus tear)

EXAM   Maneuvers to detect knee swelling are combined with an objective measurement of the ROM of the knee and carefully performed maneuvers to detect the underlying soft-tissue and bony injuries.

EXAM SUMMARY

1. General fullness and loss of the medial and lateral peripatellar dimples
2. Suprapatellar bulging often tense
3. Loss of full knee flexion (heel-to-buttock distance)
4. Abnormal anterior or posterior drawer signs
5. Abnormal varus and valgus stress testing
6. Tibial plateau bony tenderness
7. Needle aspiration of fluid

(1) With a significant injury, the knee rapidly fills with blood, causing a tense effusion, distending the suprapatellar space with 30 to 60 mL of blood. The fluid extends 3 to 4 inches above the superior pole of the patella, elevates the quadriceps tendon and muscle, and becomes

firm to hard to palpation. *(2)* Tense hemarthrosis inter-feres with flexion and extension of the joint. The patient may feel most comfortable with the knee in the partially flexed position, avoiding any attempt to extend the joint actively or passively. *(3)* Flexion is extremely compro-mised, often with less than 90 degrees of passive flexion. The heel-to-buttock distance remains a practical measure-ment of loss of full flexion (p. 151). *(4)* Varus and valgus stress testing of the integrity of the lateral collateral ligament and MCL are best performed after knee aspira-tion and placement of local anesthesia intra-articularly. *(5)* Similarly, the examiner should defer on testing the ACL and posterior cruciate ligament until after knee aspiration to avoid the difficulties in interpretation when patient cooperation, pain, and muscular guarding can interfere dramatically with these maneuvers. *(6)* Tibial plateau bony tenderness is located just below the joint lines at the level of the inferior pole of the plateau. *(7)* Lastly, joint aspiration is the definitive test for hemarthrosis. Removal of the blood effusion not only allows confirmation of the diagnosis, but also provides for pain relief; intra-articular anesthesia; and, after the bulk of the fluid is removed, a more reliable method of examining for the extent of injury to the supporting tissues.

X-RAYS   X-rays of the knee (including weightbearing posteroanterior, lateral, sunrise, and tunnel views) always are recommended. Weightbearing views are contra-indicated in the face of possible fracture. The sunrise, or merchant, view is used to determine the position and integrity of the patella. The tunnel view is used to evaluate for osteochondritis dissecans and intra-articular loose bodies. The lateral view, with good soft-tissue technique, can provide clues to the presence of a large joint effusion, the location of bony lesions, and the integrity of the patella.

SPECIAL TESTING   Because of the high degree of ligament and cartilage injury, all patients require MRI. Synovial fluid analysis is an integral part of the evaluation of knee effusion.

DIAGNOSIS   The diagnosis of hemarthrosis requires needle aspiration. A hematocrit and xanthochromia inspection performed on the synovial fluid determine whether the bleeding was recent or more remote.

TREATMENT   The goals of treatment are to confirm the diagnosis by simple needle aspiration, to relieve pain by removing most of the blood, and to determine the extent of the underlying soft-tissue and bony injuries by performing a full exam of the joint after anesthesia and MRI.

STEP 1   Aspirate the bulk of the blood; inject 2 mL of local anesthetic; perform a hematocrit on the aspirate; re-examine the joint for ligamentous instability; and order posteroanterior, lateral, tunnel, and sunrise views of the knees.

Apply ice to reduce pain, and elevate the knee to reduce swelling.

Strongly recommend crutches with touch-down weightbearing only.

Prescribe a Velcro straight-leg brace until the integrity of the bone and ligaments are determined.

Restrict flexion of the knee to 30 degrees even when sleeping.

Order urgent MRI of the knee.

Request a consultation with a knee arthroscopist for follow-up.

STEP 2 (DAYS TO 4 WEEKS FOR ACUTE FOLLOW-UP) If blood re-accumulates, re-aspirate for comfort.

Begin straight-leg-raising exercises without weights as soon as acute symptoms resolve.

Recovery is hastened if muscle support is maintained.

Re-emphasize the importance of straight-leg-raising exercises in restoring quadriceps support to the knee (with weights as tolerated).

Avoid aspirin and NSAIDs, which could aggravate bleeding.

STEP 3 (3 TO 6 WEEKS FOR PERSISTENT CASES) If a knee arthroscopist is unavailable, closely follow the patient at 2-week intervals with repeat exam of the effusion and the supporting ligaments.

Re-aspirate the effusion at 6 weeks, and consider corticosteroid injection with K40 if the bleeding has been replaced by an inflammatory effusion.

Minimize squatting, kneeling, and bending beyond 30 to 45 degrees.

STEP 4 (2 TO 4 MONTHS FOR CHRONIC CASES) Gradually resume activities of daily living and recreational activities.

Consider orthopedic consultation for definitive repair if instability persists, flexibility remains impaired, inflammatory effusion persists, and return to full function has not been achieved.

PHYSICAL THERAPY   Physical therapy plays an essential role in the active treatment and rehabilitation of hemarthrosis.

PHYSICAL THERAPY SUMMARY
1. Application of ice and elevation of the knee
2. Crutches with touch-down weightbearing
3. Straight-leg-raising exercises to restore support and stability, isometrically performed
4. Gradual resumption of active exercises, with caution

Acute Period For the first few days, apply ice, elevate the knee, and restrict weightbearing. *Ice and elevation* always are recommended for acute hemarthrosis. An ice bag, a bag of frozen corn, or an iced towel from the freezer applied for 10 to 15 minutes is effective for swelling and analgesia. The use of *crutches* is mandatory until the diagnosis is confirmed and thereafter when significant soft-tissue or bony injury has occurred.

Recovery and Rehabilitation After acute symptoms have subsided, toning exercises are begun and are combined with restricted use. *Straight-leg-raising* exercises always are recommended to restore muscular support to the knee (p. 289). Initially, exercises are performed without weights in sets of 20, with each held 5 seconds. With improvement in strength, a 5- to 10-lb weight is added to the ankle. These exercises are performed in the prone and supine positions to tone the quadriceps femoris and hamstring muscles. *Active exercises,* especially on apparatus, must be included with caution. Exercise on a stationary bicycle, a rowing machine, or a universal gym may be irritating to an inflamed and recently distended joint. Fast walking, swimming, a NordicTrack-like glide machine, and other limited-impact exercise apparatus or exercises requiring much less flexion are preferred.

INJECTION Because of the degree of swelling, the resulting discomfort, and the underlying soft-tissue and bony injuries, treatment for this unique cause of knee effusion is more aggressive than for bland or inflammatory effusions. Aspiration of synovial fluid is performed immediately to relieve the pressure of the tense effusion, to obtain fluid for hematocrit, and to begin the evaluation of the underlying injuries. Intra-articular injection of local anesthetic is used to relieve pain and allow a more thorough and reliable examination of the supporting structures. Corticosteroid injection has a limited role. It can be used for palliation if surgery is not considered because of poor medical risk. Corticosteroid injection occasionally is indicated when an inflammatory effusion persists after injury (p. 150).

SURGERY The appropriateness of surgery depends on the extent of tissue injury, the overall mechanics of the knee, the persistence of hemarthrosis or reactive inflammatory effusion, and the function of the patient. Ligament repair, ligament reconstruction, meniscal repair, partial or complete meniscectomy, and bone grafting are the procedures used most commonly.

PROGNOSIS Overall prognosis depends on the degree of underlying injury. Functional testing of the supporting ligaments and the meniscal cartilage must be combined with the findings of MRI and arthroscopy to determine which patients warrant close observation, partial repair, or reconstruction surgery. Partial ligament tears heal with a properly supervised rehabilitation program. The trend in meniscal surgery is to preserve as much tissue as possible, resorting to "partial meniscectomy" when severe, complex tears are encountered. Tibial plateau fracture management and the choice to repair osteochondral fractures require the input of a fracture specialist. Patients with significant injuries should be advised of the potential for arthritis later in life. Low-impact and limited flexing types of exercise and sports activities should be suggested. Emphasis is placed on maintaining high quadriceps muscle tone. Glucosamine sulfate should be used if cartilage damage has occurred.

OSTEOARTHRITIS OF THE KNEE

Medial joint narrowing (normally 6 to 8 mm)
Bone spur, squared-off tibial plateau
Tibial plateau sclerosis
Angulation of the tibia and femur (normally 8 to 10 degrees of valgus)

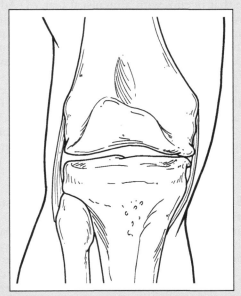

FIGURE 9–5. Wear-and-tear arthritis of the knee.

DESCRIPTION   Osteoarthritis of the knee is a wear-and-tear, mildly inflammatory arthritis that affects the three compartments of the joint—medial, lateral, and patellofemoral compartments. A family history, obesity, genu valgum and genu varum, previous meniscectomy, and previous fractures of the distal femur and tibia predispose to this condition. Pathologically, there is asymmetric wear of the articular cartilage, bony osteophyte formation, sclerosis of the subchondral bone, and subchondral cyst formation. Radiographically, a standing x-ray of the knee shows a narrowing of the articular cartilage between the tibia and the femur. Involvement of the medial compartment predominates owing to the fact that weight is carried medially, and the center of gravity is located adjacent to the medial compartment. Isolated involvement of the lateral compartment suggests previous injury, such as meniscal tear, articular cartilage injury, or tears to the supporting ligaments.

SYMPTOMS   The patient complains of knee pain, swelling, or deformity. The patient often rubs the inner aspect of the joint (along the medial compartment) when describing the condition.

"My knee gets stiff and painful at the end of the day."

"I can't do my 'folks walks' anymore ... my knees ache so bad."

"I'm too embarrassed to wear dresses anymore ... my knees look so bony."

"My knees make this awful sound every time I kneel down to pray in church."

"My knees have ached for a long time ... now they swell really badly and they give out all the time ... I'm afraid even to go to the store."

"I can't bend my knees anymore."

"When I was 22, I had the cartilage removed from my right knee. It swelled and popped a lot then. Now the whole thing just aches."

EXAM   Each patient is examined for local joint-line tenderness, loss of smooth mechanical function (crepitation), loss of ROM, and joint effusion.

EXAM SUMMARY

1. Joint-line tenderness (medial, lateral, or at the patella)
2. Loss of smooth mechanical motion (crepitation with passive or active motion)
3. Palpable bony osteophytes
4. Loss of full flexion or extension
5. Knee effusion

(1) Tenderness is present at the joint line, more commonly on the medial side. The joint lines are identified at the level of the lower third of the patella when the knee is in the extended position, and the quadriceps muscle is relaxed. *(2)* The hallmark of osteoarthritis is crepitation of the knee, palpable at the joint line when the knee is

passively flexed and extended. This is in contrast to the crepitation felt anteriorly that is seen with patellofemoral syndrome and the single popping sensation felt at the joint line that occurs with a meniscal tear. (3) Advanced cases have palpable bony osteophytes at the joint line. The enlargement is greatest at the medial tibial plateau. (4) As the condition progresses, the bony osteophytes and the damage to the articular cartilage interfere with full ROM. (5) Knee effusion commonly complicates osteoarthritis. Effusions that develop acutely and knee effusion greater than 20 to 25 mL interfere with full flexion. (6) Occasionally an acute change in the mechanical function of the knee occurs. Popping, locking, or other mechanical symptoms may suggest a degenerative meniscal tear.

X-RAYS X-rays of the knee (including standing posteroanterior, lateral, sunrise, and tunnel views) always are recommended. Standing weightbearing posteroanterior views are used to determine the widths of the cartilage of the medial and lateral compartments and the valgus carrying angle of the knee; the angle between the femur and the tibia normally measures 8 to 9 degrees. The distance between the medial tibial plateau and the medial femoral condyle is normally 6 to 8 mm. As the condition progresses, this space gradually narrows. Serial measurements can be used to predict when surgical consultation is necessary. The radiographic diagnosis of arthritis does *not* have to be accompanied by osteophytes, subchondral sclerosis, or subchondral cyst formation.

The sunrise, or merchant, view is used to determine the degree of patellofemoral arthritic involvement. The tunnel view is used to evaluate for osteochondritis dissecans and intra-articular loose bodies. The lateral view with good soft-tissue technique can provide clues to the presence of a large joint effusion, the location of bony lesions, and soft-tissue calcifications.

SPECIAL TESTING If mechanical symptoms dominate the clinical findings, MRI is ordered to evaluate for a degenerative meniscus tear or intra-articular loose body.

DIAGNOSIS A presumptive clinical diagnosis based on joint-line tenderness, crepitation, bony enlargement, and joint effusion should be confirmed by standing weightbearing x-rays. Occasionally a regional anesthetic block is used to differentiate the pain arising from the joint from the pain arising from the periarticular structures.

TREATMENT The goals of treatment are to relieve pain, to treat the accompanying effusion, to preserve function, and to evaluate the appropriateness of surgical referral. Restrictions of bending and impact combined with isometrically performed straight-leg-raising exercises are the treatments of choice for mild disease. Corticosteroid injection is the treatment of choice for osteoarthritis accompanied by a significant synovial effusion. Total knee replacement is the treatment of choice for advanced arthritis.

STEP 1 **Perform a heel-to-buttock measurement; aspirate the effusion for diagnostic studies (e.g., cell count and differential, crystals, glucose, Gram stain, and culture); and order standing posteroanterior, lateral, sunrise, and tunnel views of the knees.**

Suggest ice applications and elevation of the knee to reduce pain and swelling.

Recommend crutches with touch-down weightbearing for severe cases.

Minimize squatting and kneeling.

Restrict repetitive bending according to the severity of the condition (to 30 degrees for severe disease or to 60 degrees for moderate disease).

Advise on the importance of weight loss.

Recommend heat in the morning and ice for swelling after activities.

Prescribe a patellar restraining brace or Velcro straight-leg brace if the knee is grossly unstable (giving out frequently).

Begin straight-leg-raising exercises without weights as soon as the acute symptoms resolve, and advance to weighted exercises as tolerated.

Prescribe glucosamine sulfate, 1500 mg/day.

Prescribe an NSAID (e.g., ibuprofen) for 4 weeks at full dose with a taper beginning at 3 weeks.

STEP 2 (3 TO 6 WEEKS FOR PERSISTENT CASES) **If symptoms are persistent, prescribe a 3- to 4-week course of a second NSAID (from a different chemical class), or give a local corticosteroid injection for persistent effusion.**

Repeat the injection with corticosteroid or hyaluronic acid at 4 to 6 weeks if symptoms are not reduced by 50%.

Re-emphasize the importance of weighted straight-leg-raising exercises.

STEP 3 (2 TO 4 MONTHS FOR CHRONIC CASES) **Repeat plain films or order MRI for cases that have failed to respond to treatment and especially for cases associated with mechanical locking or severe giving-out.**

Consider orthopedic consultation for patients who do not have any medical contraindications for surgery and if (1) pain is intractable, (2) function is severely compromised, (3) 80% to 90% of the articular cartilage has worn away, or (4) progressive angulation of the lower extremity has occurred.

Order a Velcro patellar restraining brace, a walker, or a wheelchair for patients with advanced osteoarthritis who cannot undergo surgical replacement.

PHYSICAL THERAPY Physical therapy plays an essential role in the active treatment and prevention of osteoarthritis of the knee.

PHYSICAL THERAPY SUMMARY

1. Ice and elevation of the knee
2. Crutches with touch-down weightbearing
3. Straight-leg-raising exercises to restore support and stability, performed isometrically
4. Gradual resumption of active exercises, with caution

Acute Period   For the first few days apply ice, elevate the knee, and restrict weightbearing. *Ice* and elevation always are recommended for acute arthritic flares. An ice bag, a bag of frozen corn, or an iced towel from the freezer applied for 10 to 15 minutes is effective for swelling and analgesia. *Crutches,* a *walker,* or a *cane* may be necessary in the first few days.

Recovery and Rehabilitation   After acute symptoms subside, toning exercises are combined with restricted use. *Straight-leg-raising* exercises always are recommended to restore muscular support to the knee (p. 289). Initially, these exercises are performed without weights in sets of 20, with each held 5 seconds. With improvement in strength, a 5- to 10-lb weight is added to the ankle. These exercises are performed in the prone and supine positions to tone the quadriceps femoris and hamstring muscles. *Active exercises,* especially on apparatus, must be performed with caution. Exercise on a stationary bicycle, a rowing machine, or a universal gym may be irritating to an inflamed and recently distended joint. Fast walking, swimming, a NordicTrack-like glide machine, and other limited-impact exercise apparatus or exercises requiring much less flexion are preferred.

INJECTION   Local corticosteroid injection can provide dramatic short-term relief and is indicated when (1) NSAIDs are contraindicated, (2) NSAIDs are poorly tolerated, (3) inflammation and effusion fail to improve, (4) symptom palliation is necessary for a patient who has advanced disease and cannot undergo surgery, or (5) the patient prefers it. A lateral approach for aspiration and injection may not be suitable for all patients, especially patients with severe hypertrophic patellofemoral disease. In these cases, a medial approach can be performed that is analogous to the lateral approach. The point of entry is halfway between the medial edge of the patella and the midplane of the leg (the center of the femur).

SURGICAL PROCEDURE   Surgery is indicated for advanced disease. Arthroscopic débridement is indicated for degenerative meniscal tears and loose bodies. High tibial osteotomy is the procedure of choice for patients younger than age 62 to correct the loss of the normal 8- to 9-degree valgus angle and to shift the weightbearing pressure to the preserved lateral compartment articular cartilage. Total knee replacement is the procedure of choice for patients older than age 62.

PROGNOSIS   Osteoarthritis of the knee is a slowly progressive problem that is characterized by periodic flares of pain and swelling. Medication by mouth or by injection should be reserved for these exacerbations. Patients with osteoarthritis complicated solely by effusion respond predictably and completely to intra-articular injection. Patients with partial or very short-term responses to injection often have an associated anserine bursitis, MCL tear, ACL insufficiency, loose body, frayed or extremely injured articular cartilage, or meniscal tear. These patients require re-evaluation with a follow-up examination, repeat bilateral weightbearing x-rays, MRI, bone scan, or arthroscopy to exclude these complicating conditions. Patients with rapid arthritic progression as measured by dramatic changes in function, loss of ROM, or deterioration on serial weightbearing radiographs may have a degenerative meniscal tear, the poorly tolerated effects of increased angulation of the knee, developing underlying rheumatic disease, or the dramatic complication of septic arthritis.

PREPATELLAR BURSITIS

The bursa is entered at the base, paralleling the patella; the needle is passed into the center of the sac; alternatively the needle can be advanced to the lower third of the periosteum of the patella for injection of a small or chronically thickened bursa.

Needle: 1¹/₂-inch, 18- to 22-gauge
Depth: ¹/₄ to ³/₈ inch
Volume: 1 to 2 mL of anesthetic and 1 mL of K40

NOTE: Placement of the needle on the periosteum guarantees an intrabursal injection.

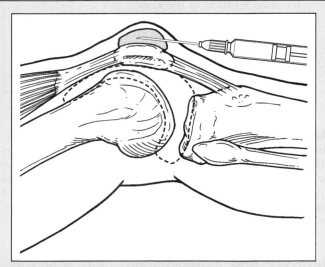

FIGURE 9–6. Aspiration and injection of the prepatellar bursa.

DESCRIPTION   Prepatellar bursitis is an inflammation of the bursal sac located between the patella and the overlying skin. The most common cause is trauma as a result of a fall or the direct pressure and friction of repetitive kneeling (90% "housemaid's knee"). It is one of two bursae in the body that can become infected (5% due to *Staphylococcus aureus*) or inflamed by urate crystals (5% due to acute gout). Normally the bursa is paper-thin, simply a fluid-filled potential space. With chronic bursal irritation and inflammation, the bursal walls dilate, thicken, and become fibrotic—the pathologic condition of chronic bursitis.

SYMPTOMS   The patient complains of knee swelling and knee pain just over the front of the knee. The patient often rubs over the bursa or points at the swelling when describing the condition.

"My knee is swollen."

"I bumped my knee against the kitchen cabinet, and within hours it had swelled up."

"It feels like a bunch of little marbles just under the skin." (chronic)

"I'm a housekeeper. I have to work on my knees a lot. Even though I am careful and wear knee pads, my right knee has begun to swell. Is this arthritis, doctor?"

"My knee is inflamed."

"I have a bump over my knee cap." (chronic)

EXAM   The exam includes degree of swelling and inflammation, the amount of bursal fluid, and the ROM of the knee.

EXAM SUMMARY

1. Swelling and inflammation directly over the inferior portion of the patella
2. Bursal sac tenderness versus bursal sac thickening (chronic)
3. Normal ROM of the knee (unless cellulitis accompanies)

(1) A cystic collection of fluid is palpable directly over the patella. Inflammatory signs vary, depending on the cause and the length of time symptoms have been present. *(2)* Tenderness is present over the entire sac in acute cases (i.e., gouty and septic bursitis). Tenderness may be minimal in chronically effused or thickened cases (10%). Chronic prepatellar bursitis has a characteristic cobblestone-like roughness or palpable thickening. This thickening is best appreciated by squeezing the bursa between two fingers and comparing the thickness with the contralateral side. *(3)* The ROM of the knee should be normal in an uncomplicated case of prepatellar bursitis that is unassociated with cellulitis or an underlying articular condition. This extra-articular accumulation of fluid does not interfere with motion, as opposed to the limitation of flexion commonly seen with acute knee effusion.

X-RAYS   Plain x-rays of the knee are unnecessary to make the diagnosis, and they rarely affect clinical management. The lateral view of the knee shows soft-tissue swelling above the patella. Calcification of the quadriceps tendon at the superior pole of the patella is not related to this condition. This calcification occurs commonly, but does not indicate disease of the quadriceps mechanism.

SPECIAL TESTING   Fluid analysis is the only special test indicated.

DIAGNOSIS   A clinical diagnosis of prepatellar bursitis is made easily by simple inspection and palpation of the anterior structures of the knee. Bursal fluid aspiration and analysis are necessary, however, to determine the cause of the condition.

TREATMENT   The goals of treatment are to identify the cause of the swelling, to reduce the swelling and inflammation, and to prevent chronic bursal thickening. Aspiration and drainage combined with padding and protection are the treatments of choice for acute prepatellar bursitis. Complete drainage of the distended bursa encourages the walls of the bursa to reapproximate, facilitates resolution, and reduces the chance of recurrent and chronic bursitis.

STEP 1   Aspirate the bursa for diagnostic studies: Gram stain and culture, crystals, and hematocrit.
> Apply a compression dressing for 24 to 36 hours after aspiration.
> Advise the patient to avoid direct pressure from kneeling and squatting and bending more than 90 degrees.
> Ice over the anterior knee is an effective analgesic and helps to reduce swelling.
> Recommend a neoprene pull-on knee brace (p. 256) or Velcro kneepads (p. 256).
> Prescribe an NSAID (e.g., ibuprofen).

STEP 2 (1 TO 2 DAYS AFTER FLUID ANALYSIS)   Immediately begin antibiotics for infection if infection is documented on Gram stain or is suspected clinically. Intravenous antibiotics are necessary if cellulitis accompanies septic bursitis. Evaluate and treat for gout if urate crystals are shown. Re-aspirate and inject with K40 if infection and gout have been excluded by fluid analysis.
> Advise patients whose occupations require constant kneeling or squatting of the possibility of recurrence, and strongly encourage them to wear protective knee padding.
> Educate the patient: *"Between 10% and 15% remain swollen or thickened regardless of treatment."*

STEP 3 (4 TO 6 WEEKS FOR PERSISTENT CASES)   Repeat the aspiration and injection of the bursa with K40 if symptoms have not been reduced by 50%.
> Limit squatting and kneeling.
> Straight-leg-raising exercises are combined with hamstring leg extensions for general conditioning of the knee if muscle tone has declined.

STEP 4 (MONTHS FOR CHRONIC CASES)   Consider an orthopedic consultation for definitive treatment of chronic bursal thickening.

PHYSICAL THERAPY   Physical therapy does not play a significant role in the treatment of prepatellar bursitis. General care of the knee is recommended with emphasis on toning the quadriceps and hamstring muscles by doing straight-leg-raising exercises.

INJECTION   Local corticosteroid injection is indicated for (1) recurrent nonseptic bursitis, (2) bursitis caused by gout when NSAIDs are contraindicated, (3) chronic bursal thickening (palpably thickened soft tissues above the patella—the "bursal pinch" sign), or (4) persistent post-infectious bursitis (with a negative postantibiotic culture).
  Positioning   The patient is placed in the supine position with the leg fully extended.
  Surface Anatomy and Point of Entry   The superior and inferior margins of the bursa are identified and marked. The point of entry is at the base of the inferior margin.
  Angle of Entry and Depth   The needle is inserted at the base of the bursa, paralleling the patella, and advanced to the center of the bursa. Alternatively the needle is entered above the bursa and advanced at a 45-degree angle down to the firm to hard resistance of the periosteum of the patella (for the chronically thickened bursa with little fluid).
  Anesthesia   Ethyl chloride is sprayed on the skin. Local anesthetic is placed at the base of the bursa in the subcutaneous tissue and dermis only.
  Technique   Complete aspiration combined with compression ensures the best outcome. After local anesthesia, an 18-gauge needle attached to a 10-mL syringe is passed into the center of the sac. The needle is rotated 180 degrees so that the bevel faces the patella. Aspiration with gentle suction combined with manual pressure from above and on the sides facilitates fluid removal. With the needle left in place, the syringe is replaced with the syringe containing the corticosteroid, and 1 mL of K40 is injected. The needle is withdrawn, and a gauze and Coban pressure dressing is applied.

INJECTION AFTERCARE
1. *Rest* for 3 days, avoiding all direct pressure, squatting, kneeling, and bending beyond 90 degrees.
2. Wear the compression dressing for 24 to 36 hours, then replace it with a neoprene pull-on knee sleeve.
3. Use *ice* (15 minutes every 4 to 6 hours) and *acetaminophen* (1000 mg twice a day) for soreness.
4. *Protect* the knee for 3 to 4 weeks by limiting pressure, repetitive bending, squatting, and kneeling.
5. Begin *straight-leg-raising exercises* for the quadriceps muscle on day 4 if muscle tone has declined.
6. Repeat the *aspiration and injection* at 6 weeks with corticosteroid if swelling recurs or persists.
7. Request a *consultation* with an orthopedic surgeon if two consecutive aspirations and injections fail to

PREPATELLAR BURSA INJECTION

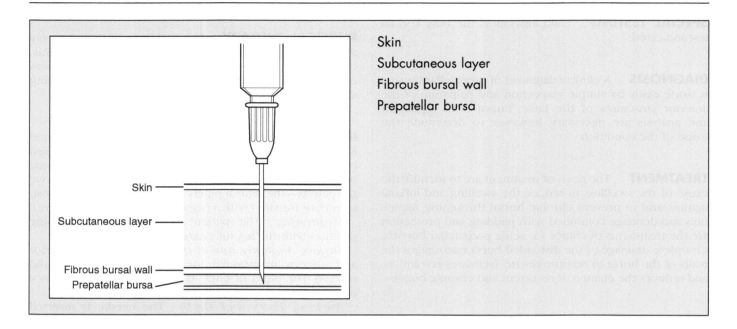

Skin
Subcutaneous layer
Fibrous bursal wall
Prepatellar bursa

Skin
Subcutaneous layer
Fibrous bursal wall
Prepatellar bursa

eliminate the swelling, and the patient still complains of pressure pain.

SURGICAL PROCEDURE Arthroscopic or open surgical bursectomy is reserved for patients with chronic, fibrotic bursitis (in 2% to 4% of cases).

PROGNOSIS About 50% to 60% of traumatic bursitis resolves spontaneously or responds to simple aspiration and protective padding. Approximately 30% to 40% of cases develop a persistent low-grade inflammatory reaction that requires one or two local injections of K40 to control swelling and pain. The remaining 5% to 10%

of cases fail to respond to these measures and progress to chronic bursitis—thickened fibrotic bursal walls caused by unremitting inflammation. The latter cases can be referred for definitive bursectomy. Patients with septic bursitis, especially staphylococcal, and patients who experience recurrent trauma have a greater risk of chronic bursitis (fibrosis, thickening, and recurrent effusion). Surgical treatment of these cases is individualized. This bursal sac does not interfere with the normal function of the knee. Persistent swelling or thickening of the bursal sac alone is not an indication for surgery. Patients troubled with persistent pain and irritation from repetitive kneeling (e.g., carpet layers, cement finishers) should be considered for surgery.

ANSERINE BURSITIS

Enter at the point of maximum tenderness, usually 1¹/₂ inches below the medial joint line or parallel to the tibial tubercle in the concavity of the tibial plateau.

Needle: 1- to 1¹/₂-inch, 22-gauge
Depth: ¹/₂ to 1¹/₂ inches exactly ¹/₈ inch above the periosteum of the tibia and outside the medial collateral ligament
Volume: 1 to 2 mL of anesthetic and 0.5 mL of D80

NOTE: Never inject under forced pressure. The flow of medication should require little pressure when the injection is placed properly between the medial collateral ligament and the conjoined tendon.

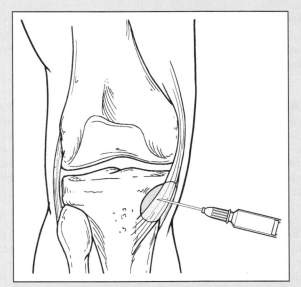

FIGURE 9–7. Anserine bursa injection.

DESCRIPTION Anserine bursitis is an inflammation of the bursal sac located between the attachment of the MCL at the medial tibial plateau and the conjoined tendon formed by the gracilis, sartorius, and semitendinosus tendons. Although it can result from direct trauma, it more commonly develops as a consequence of an abnormal gait. Any loss of the normal mechanical relationships between the knee, hip, and pelvis causes an abnormal pull at the insertion point of the three tendons (the gracilis originates at the pubis, the sartorius at the ilium, and the semitendinosus at the ischium). The increased friction and pressure resulting from this gait disturbance cause anserine bursitis. It frequently accompanies osteoarthritis of the knee, chronic knee effusion, or any other intrinsic knee condition.

SYMPTOMS The patient complains of knee pain that is often localized to a well-defined area of the inner knee. The patient often points to the area with one finger when describing the local irritation.

"I have a very sharp knee pain right here (pointing to the inner aspect of the knee)."

"I can't sleep on my side. When my knees touch, I get this really sharp pain on the inside of my knee."

"I don't know what happened. I didn't have an injury. I slowly developed this sharp pain inside my knee."

"The inside of my knee looks a little swollen and is very tender to the touch."

"I sleep with a pillow between my legs because my knee is tender."

"I was hit with a line drive when I was playing baseball. The ball hit me in the inside of my knee. The pain was so sharp I couldn't walk for several days."

EXAM The exam comprises an assessment of tenderness at the medial tibial plateau, a thorough exam of the knee, and an analysis of the patient's gait.

EXAM SUMMARY

1. Local tenderness in the concavity of the medial tibial plateau at the level of the tibial tubercle
2. Painless valgus stress testing of the MCL
3. Associated intrinsic knee joint abnormalities or abnormal gait
4. Successful anesthetic block at the bursa

(1) Local tenderness is present 1 to 1¹/₄ inches below the medial joint line at the level parallel the tibial tubercle. The quarter-sized area is located in the midline in the concavity of the medial tibial plateau. *(2)* Valgus stress testing of the MCL does not aggravate the pain; that is, the signs of an MCL strain are absent. *(3)* The knee and lower extremities are examined for any primary musculoskeletal process that would affect the gait.

X-RAYS X-rays of the knee are unnecessary for the diagnosis. No specific changes are seen either in the soft tissues or along the medial tibial plateau. X-rays of the knee are strongly recommended, however, to assess the degree of associated osteoarthritis or rheumatoid arthritis (the most common causes of knee effusions).

SPECIAL TESTING
Special testing is not required to confirm an uncomplicated case of anserine bursitis. Plain x-rays, arthrocentesis, or MRI is necessary when bursitis is the result of an underlying gait disturbance.

DIAGNOSIS
The diagnosis is based on localized medial tibial plateau tenderness, the absence of signs indicating an MCL strain, and pain relief with local anesthetic. Regional anesthesic block placed within the bursal sac is used to differentiate the symptoms of bursitis from symptoms of medial compartment osteoarthritis, patellofemoral syndrome, and medial meniscus tear.

TREATMENT
The goals of treatment are to reduce the pain and swelling in the bursa and to identify and treat any underlying cause of abnormal gait. Restrictions of bending, protection from direct pressure, and ice are the treatments of choice for acute bursitis. When symptoms and signs of bursitis persist, corticosteroid injection is the preferred initial treatment. When bursitis complicates one of the articular disorders of the knee, hip, or ankle, treatment must be directed at both.

STEP 1   Obtain plain x-rays of the knee, including the sunrise view; assess quadriceps tone; and evaluate the gait. Direct treatment of the underlying gait disturbance (e.g., knee effusion, osteoarthritis of the knee, leg-length discrepancy, muscle imbalance from stroke) is indicated if symptoms arising from the primary condition outweigh the symptoms arising from the bursa.

Perform local anesthetic block of the bursa, have the patient walk and determine the degree of pain relief, and assess the contribution of the bursa to the patient's current symptoms.

Recommend elimination of squatting and repetitive bending.

Avoid all direct pressure and recommend using a pillow between the knees at night.

Suggest a pull-on neoprene sleeve to provide protection against direct pressure during the day.

Advise the patient to avoid crossing the legs.

Limit repetitive bending.

Suggest ice applications for acute symptoms.

Prescribe an NSAID (e.g., ibuprofen). *Note:* An oral medication may not concentrate sufficiently in this relatively isolated structure.

STEP 2 (6 TO 8 WEEKS FOR PERSISTENT CASES)   Perform an injection of D80.

If the first injection does not reduce symptoms and signs by 50%, then the injection of D80 is repeated at 4 to 6 weeks.

Continue to investigate for a primary cause.

STEP 3 (8 TO 10 WEEKS AFTER IMPROVEMENT) Begin straight-leg-raising exercises with weights (p. 289). Suggest cautious squatting, kneeling, and repetitive knee flexion until symptoms have been controlled.

PHYSICAL THERAPY
Physical therapy does not play a direct role in the treatment of anserine bursitis. General toning exercises of the quadriceps and hamstring muscles are used in the recovery period. *Ice* over the bursa effectively controls pain and some of the swelling. *Phonophoresis* with a hydrocortisone gel may provide temporary relief in asthenic individuals. *General care of the knee* is recommended, with emphasis on toning the quadriceps femoris and the hamstring muscles through straight-leg-raising exercises.

PHYSICAL THERAPY SUMMARY

1. Ice applied to the medial tibial plateau
2. Phonophoresis with a hydrocortisone gel in asthenic individuals
3. General care of the knee (p. 288)

INJECTION
Local injection is used (1) to confirm the diagnosis, (2) to treat primary bursitis, and (3) to treat bursitis that persists after the primary gait disturbance has been addressed.

Positioning   The patient is placed in the supine position with the leg extended and externally rotated.

Surface Anatomy and Point of Entry   The tibial tubercle, medial joint line, and the midline of the medial lower leg are identified and marked. The point of entry is in the midline directly across from the tibial tubercle or approximately $1^1/_2$ inches below the medial joint line.

Angle of Entry and Depth   The needle is inserted perpendicularly to the skin and is directed slightly upward toward the concavity of the medial tibial plateau. The injection depth is always $^1/_8$ inch above the periosteum of the tibia or $^1/_2$ to $1^1/_2$ inches deep.

Anesthesia   Ethyl chloride is sprayed on the skin. Local anesthetic is placed at the tissue plane of the tendon and $^1/_8$ inch above the periosteum of the tibia (0.5 mL in both places).

Technique   A 22-gauge needle is passed through the subcutaneous fat until the subtle resistance of the conjoined tendon is felt. Anesthetic can be injected here for comfort. Then the needle is gently passed an additional $^3/_8$ inch to the firm periosteum of the tibia and immediately withdrawn $^1/_8$ inch to avoid injection into the MCL. The bursa is located between the MCL and the tendon, and anesthetic and corticosteroid are injected here. Injection should be free flowing, with little resistance. Pressure on injection usually suggests improper position (too deep).

ANSERINE BURSA INJECTION

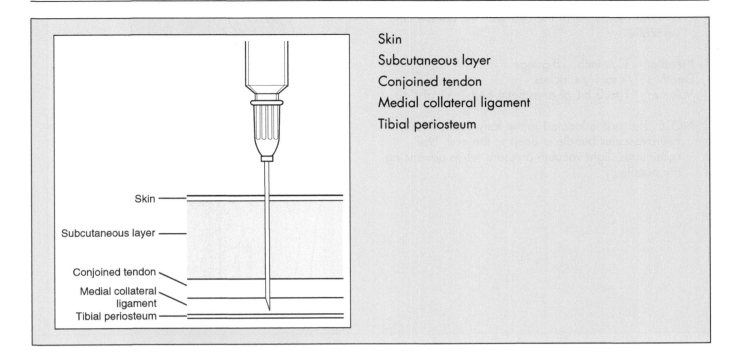

Skin
Subcutaneous layer
Conjoined tendon
Medial collateral ligament
Tibial periosteum

Skin
Subcutaneous layer
Conjoined tendon
Medial collateral ligament
Tibial periosteum

INJECTION AFTERCARE

1. *Rest* for 3 days, avoiding all direct pressure, squatting, kneeling, repetitive bending beyond 90 degrees, and unnecessary standing and walking.
2. Recommend *crutches* with touch-down weightbearing for 3 to 7 days only if the underlying gait disturbance is severe.
3. Use *ice* (15 minutes every 4 to 6 hours) and *acetaminophen* (1000 mg twice a day) for postinjection soreness.
4. *Protect* the knee for 3 to 4 weeks by limiting repetitive bending, squatting, and kneeling and unnecessary walking.
5. Begin *straight-leg-raising exercises* for the quadriceps muscle on day 4 to enhance the support of the knee.
6. Recommend *temporary bracing* (3 to 4 weeks) with a patellar restraining brace or a Velcro straight-leg brace for patients with poor quadriceps muscle tone or with frequent giving-out of the knee.
7. Repeat *injection* at 6 weeks with corticosteroid if pain recurs or persists.
8. Perform repeat *plain x-rays* (standing posteroanterior and bilateral sunrise views) or obtain *MRI* if the initial treatment response is unsatisfactory (e.g., to identify underlying advanced degenerative arthritis, high degree of subluxation of the patellofemoral joint, degenerative or traumatic meniscal tear).
9. Advise on long-term restrictions of bending (30 to 45 degrees) and the impact of weightbearing for patients with chronic symptoms.
10. Request a *consultation* with an orthopedic surgeon if two consecutive aspirations and injections fail to eliminate the swelling, and the patient still complains of pain on weightbearing.

SURGICAL PROCEDURE Bursectomy is rarely required (<1% of cases).

PROGNOSIS Primary involvement of the bursa and secondary anserine bursitis—associated with an underlying gait disturbance—respond dramatically to corticosteroid injection. Primary bursitis typically resolves completely with a properly placed injection. Further workup is unnecessary in these cases. The injection response may be short-lived, however, with secondary bursitis if the underlying knee effusion, arthritis, short leg, or other gait disturbance is not treated concurrently. Any patient with persistent anserine bursitis must undergo a thorough evaluation of the gait, knee, hip, and ankle by physical exam and radiographically.

BAKER'S CYST

Enter over the center of the cyst with the needle held vertically.

Needle: 1 1/2-inch, 18-gauge
Depth: 3/4 to 1 1/4 inches
Volume: 1 to 2 mL of anesthetic and 1 mL of K40

NOTE: The cyst is located in the fatty layer. The neurovascular bundle is deep to the cyst. Use continuous, light vacuum pressure while advancing the needle.

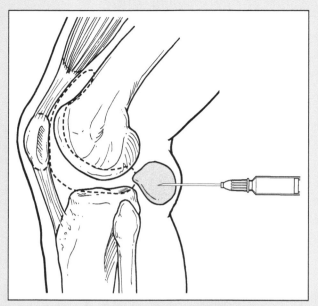

FIGURE 9–8. Baker's cyst aspiration and injection.

DESCRIPTION   Baker's cyst is an abnormal collection of synovial fluid in the fatty layers of the popliteal fossa. Fluid that escapes from the normal confines of the synovial lining causes a fibrotic reaction in the subcutaneous tissue and cyst formation. It must be distinguished from the more common dilated semimembranosus bursa—an evagination of the synovial lining of the knee, which gradually enlarges as a result of the hydraulic pressure of repetitive flexing of the knee. Both are located on the medial side of the popliteal fossa, and both become enlarged as a result of an overproduction of synovial fluid. Only Baker's cyst is a separate anatomic structure, however.

Small cysts should be observed. Large Baker's cysts that interfere with flexion of the knee can be aspirated and injected with corticosteroids. Dilated semimembranosus bursae are not aspirated and injected directly. The treatment for a dilated bursa is directed at the underlying cause (e.g., osteoarthritis, rheumatoid arthritis, meniscal tear).

SYMPTOMS   The patient complains of tightness behind the knee or pain down the back of the leg (the latter symptom suggests cyst rupture). The patient often rubs the back of the knee when describing the condition.

"My doctor did an ultrasound of my leg and told me that I have a cyst behind my knee."

"I felt a lump behind my knee."

"When I bend my knee back, it feels like an egg is behind my knee."

"My knee seems swollen and tight."

"My regular doctor told me I have bad circulation. The doctor in the emergency department thought I had a blood clot in my leg. I'm really confused. I've had all these tests, and I still don't know why I have this pain in my leg."

EXAM   The patient is examined for a palpable, cystic mass in the medial aspect of the popliteal fossa, and a thorough exam of the knee is done to determine the cause of synovial fluid overproduction.

EXAM SUMMARY

1. Cystic mass in the popliteal fossa
2. Impaired knee flexion when the cyst is large
3. Evidence of a current or past chronic knee effusion
4. No evidence of peripheral vascular insufficiency or deep venous thrombosis

(1) With the patient in the prone position and the leg fully extended, an oblong cystic mass is palpable and visible in the medial popliteal fossa. *(2)* Large cysts may impair knee flexion by 10 to 15 degrees. *(3)* Signs of a knee effusion may be present. *(4)* Signs of vascular insufficiency (suggesting popliteal aneurysm) and signs of deep venous thrombosis of the popliteal veins (pain in the posterior calf) are absent.

X-RAYS X-rays of the knee are unnecessary for this specific diagnosis. Plain films of the popliteal fossa are normal. X-rays of the knee are recommended, however, to assess the degree of osteoarthritis or rheumatoid arthritis (more common causes of knee effusions).

SPECIAL TESTING Diagnostic ultrasound can be used to define the size and extent of the cyst. This test is of questionable utility, however, if the cyst is not obviously palpable (small cysts discovered by ultrasound rarely interfere with knee function). Arthrography may reveal the sinus tract originating from the synovial cavity. This test may be helpful in planning the correct surgical exposure.

DIAGNOSIS A tentative diagnosis is based on the presence of a palpable, popliteal mass or on the demonstration of a fluid-filled cyst on ultrasound. A definitive diagnosis requires, however, aspiration of the characteristic clear, nonbloody, highly tenacious fluid.

TREATMENT Whether the cyst is a Baker's cyst or simply a dilated bursa, few need to be treated directly. In general, small cysts should be observed. The treatment approach for large cysts that interfere with full function of the knee is to aspirate the abnormal accumulation of fluid, to reduce the size of the cyst by corticosteroid injection, to identify any underlying cause of chronic knee effusion, and to determine the need for surgery.

STEP 1 **Evaluate and treat any underlying cause of chronic knee effusion (e.g., rheumatoid arthritis, osteoarthritis), assess the strength of the quadriceps, and measure the ROM of the knee.**

Aspirate the bursa to confirm the diagnosis (typical high-viscosity fluid), and treat large cysts that interfere with full knee flexion with corticosteroid injection with K40.

Educate the patient: *"The Baker cyst can resolve on its own over time."*

Advise the patient to restrict squatting, kneeling, repetitive bending (flexion limited to 30 to 45 degrees), and unnecessary walking and standing.

Encourage straight-leg-raising exercises with weights (p. 289).

Consider a neoprene pull-on knee brace to provide warmth and nominal support (p. 256).

STEP 2 (4 TO 6 WEEKS FOR FOLLOW-UP TREATMENT) **Repeat the aspiration (remove as much fluid as possible).**

Continue the use of the neoprene brace (p. 256).

Educate the patient: *"These types of cysts frequently recur regardless of which treatment is used."*

STEP 3 (8 TO 10 WEEKS FOR PERSISTENT CASES) **Re-aspirate and inject with K40.**

Repeat the injection in 4 to 6 weeks if the size of the cyst has not decreased by 50%.

STEP 4 (3 TO 6 MONTHS FOR CHRONIC CASES) **If improved, perform straight-leg-raising exercises with weights (p. 289).**

Advise patients with recurrent or chronic symptoms to avoid repetitive flexion and squatting.

Consider surgical removal if the patient is a surgical candidate, if all causes of excessive fluid production have been treated optimally, and if the cyst is interfering with the normal function of the knee.

PHYSICAL THERAPY Physical therapy plays a minor role in the treatment of Baker's cyst. General care of the knee is recommended, with emphasis on toning the quadriceps femoris and hamstring muscles by doing straight-leg-raising exercises.

INJECTION Local injection is used to confirm the diagnosis (simple aspiration showing typical high-viscosity fluid), and corticosteroid injection with K40 is used to treat large cysts that compromise full flexion of the knee.

Positioning The patient is placed in the prone position with the leg fully extended.

Surface Anatomy and Point of Entry The outline of the cyst is marked; it is typically an oblong structure located medially in the popliteal fossa and extending inferiorly. The point of entry is directly over the center of the cyst.

Angle of Entry and Depth The needle is inserted perpendicular to the skin and is advanced through the subcutaneous tissue to the subtle tissue resistance of the cyst wall ($3/4$ to $1^1/4$ inches below the skin surface).

Anesthesia Ethyl chloride is sprayed on the skin. Using a 22-gauge needle, local anesthetic is placed intradermally, subcutaneously, and just outside the cyst wall (0.5 mL).

Technique An 18-gauge needle attached to a 20-mL syringe is held vertically and passed down to the subtle resistance of the cyst wall. *Note:* The neurovascular bundle is deep to the cyst; only skin and subcutaneous tissue overlie the cyst cavity. Continuous negative pressure is used while advancing. The outer wall is often thick, and a giving-way or popping sensation is often felt as the cyst is entered. After the cyst is punctured, the needle is advanced until the subtle tissue resistance of the back wall is felt or fluid no longer can be aspirated easily. At this point, the needle is withdrawn $1/8$ to $3/8$ inch. This needle position ensures optimal aspiration of the fluid as the cyst collapses. Manual pressure is applied to either side of the needle to assist in fluid recovery. With the needle left in place, 1 mL of K40 is injected into the cyst.

INJECTION AFTERCARE

1. *Rest* for 3 days, avoiding all direct pressure, squatting, kneeling, and repetitive bending beyond 90 degrees.
2. Use of crutches with touch-down weightbearing for 3 to 7 days is necessary only if the underlying condition affecting the knee is severe.

BAKER'S CYST INJECTION

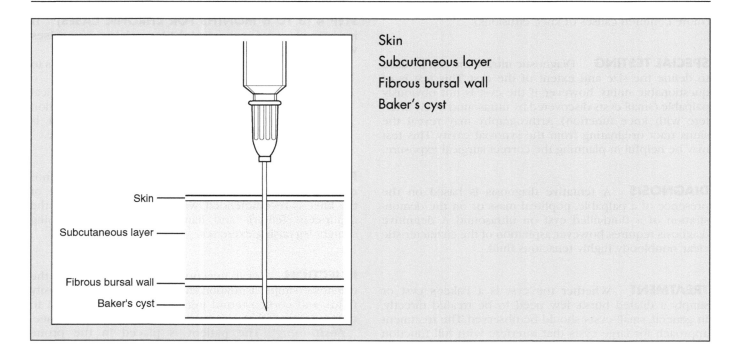

Skin
Subcutaneous layer
Fibrous bursal wall
Baker's cyst

Skin
Subcutaneous layer
Fibrous bursal wall
Baker's cyst

3. Use *ice* (15 minutes every 4 to 6 hours) and *acetaminophen* (1000 mg twice a day) for postinjection soreness.
4. *Protect* the knee for 3 to 4 weeks by limiting direct pressure, repetitive bending, squatting, kneeling, impact, and prolonged standing.
5. Maximize the treatment of the associated conditions affecting the knee (e.g., osteoarthritis, rheumatoid arthritis).
6. Begin *straight-leg-raising exercises* for the quadriceps muscle on day 4 to enhance the support of the knee.
7. Repeat the *aspiration and injection* with corticosteroid at 6 weeks if pain recurs or persists (at the cyst or intra-articularly).
8. Request a *consultation* with an orthopedic surgeon if two consecutive aspirations and injections fail to eliminate the swelling, and the patient still complains of pressure and swelling in the popliteal fossa.

SURGICAL PROCEDURE Bursectomy is indicated when full flexion of the knee is interfered with, and two consecutive injections fail to reduce the overall size of the cyst.

PROGNOSIS In the short-term, the optimal treatment of Baker's cyst depends on the complete aspiration of its contents and the accurate placement of the corticosteroid. Aspiration and injection with corticosteroids can provide symptomatic relief for months. The long-term prognosis always depends, however, on the underlying process affecting the knee. This explains why a Baker cyst, similar to ganglion cysts at the wrist and ankle, recurs frequently. If the underlying cause of the overproduction of synovial fluid is not addressed, the cyst is likely to reform. Recurrent Baker's cysts that interfere with the function of the knee can be referred for surgical removal. As with medical therapy, Baker's cyst recurs frequently despite surgical excision if the underlying cause is not adequately addressed.

MEDIAL COLLATERAL LIGAMENT SPRAIN

Enter in the midline over the tibial plateau just below the joint line.

Needle: ⁵/₈-inch, 25-gauge or 1¹/₂-inch, 22-gauge
Depth: varies according to the thickness of the dermis, averaging ¹/₂ to ³/₄ inch; alternatively, ¹/₈ inch above the periosteum of the tibia
Volume: 1 to 2 mL of anesthetic and 1 mL of D80

NOTE: Never inject between the medial collateral ligament and the bone, and always brace after injection.

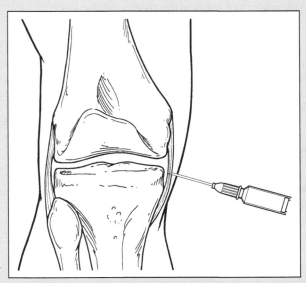

FIGURE 9–9. Medial collateral ligament injection.

DESCRIPTION An MCL strain is an irritation, inflammation, or partial separation of the inner "hinge" ligament of the knee. Strains are classified as first, second, or third degree on the basis of the amount of motion on valgus stress testing. Dramatic twisting of the knee or falls that place the knee in a valgus position are the types on injuries that are common to all degrees of sprain. Ligaments that are irritated and inflamed but otherwise intact are classified as first-degree strains. Ligaments that are partially torn are classified as second-degree separations. Ligaments that are completely disrupted with gross instability of the knee are classified as third-degree separations. Patients with third-degree separations must be evaluated for coexisting injuries to the ACL, medial meniscus, or both.

SYMPTOMS The patient complains of knee pain along the inner aspect of the knee joint and has difficulty walking, pivoting, and twisting. The patient often points to or rubs along the joint line down to the tibial plateau insertion site when describing the condition.

"I was playing football, and I was tackled from the right side, causing immediate pain along the inner part of my knee."

"I was getting out of the bathtub when my leg caught, my body twisted, and my leg was wrenched. Ever since, I have had pain and sensitivity along the inside of my knee."

"I sprained my knee when I tripped on the rug."

"Every time I twist my leg, I get this sharp pain along the side of my knee."

"I can't even turn over in bed. My leg gets snagged up in the sheets, and any amount of twisting just kills me."

"My knee has been swollen for months, but now it feels different. It feels loose and sloppy."

EXAM The patient is examined for the degree of irritation, inflammation, and laxity of the MCL, and overall knee stability is assessed.

EXAM SUMMARY

1. A 1-inch-long band of local tenderness located between the medial joint line and the insertion on the tibia
2. Pain aggravated by valgus stress testing
3. Laxity of the MCL (with higher degrees of rupture)
4. Associated knee effusion, ACL tear, or medial meniscal tear

(1) Tenderness is located from the medial joint line down the insertion of the MCL on the tibial plateau. The tenderness is usually about 1 inch long and parallels the length of the ligament. *(2)* Valgus stress testing, applied with the leg in the extended position and at 30 degrees of flexion, causes acute pain. *(3)* Valgus stress testing also may show laxity. In addition, medial knee pain may be aggravated by forcibly externally rotating the tibia on the femur with the knee bent at 90 degrees. *(4)* The remaining

exam of the knee may show effusion, laxity, or disruption of the ACL or a medial meniscal tear. Trauma severe enough to cause a third-degree separation is often enough to disrupt other supporting tissues of the knee.

X-RAYS X-rays of the knee are unnecessary for the diagnosis. Routine views are usually normal. Avulsion fractures are unusual. Calcification of the ligament can occur months to years later. A 1- to $1^1/4$-inch, crescent-shaped calcification along the medial joint line is referred to as *Pellegrini-Stieda syndrome*. This radiographic finding is unique, but does not correlate directly with clinical findings.

SPECIAL TESTING MRI is indicated when other injuries are suspected. Tears of the joint capsule, the ACL, the meniscal cartilage, or the articular cartilage (osteochondritis dissecans) are more likely with second-degree or third-degree MCL tears.

DIAGNOSIS The diagnosis is based on a history of a line of pain crossing the medial joint line and an exam showing local tenderness along the medial knee that is consistently aggravated by valgus stress testing. A regional anesthetic block is rarely used to differentiate this local periarticular process from an intra-articular condition.

TREATMENT The goals of treatment are to allow the ligament to reattach to its bony origins, to strengthen the muscular support to the knee, and to avoid activities that would reinjure the ligament. The initial treatment of choice comprises immobilization with a Velcro straight-leg immobilizer or a patellar restraining brace combined with crutches and physical therapy exercises.

STEP 1 Determine the stage of the condition, assess for secondary injuries, estimate the quadriceps strength, and establish a baseline level of function (e.g., can walk, can limp, cannot bear weight).

Advise walking with crutches for the first 7 days of the acute injury.

Prescribe a Velcro straight-leg knee immobilizer (p. 257) with metal stays for second-degree and third-degree injuries and a patellar restraining brace for first-degree sprains to be worn continuously during the day.

Recommend ice applications at the joint line to reduce pain and swelling.

Avoid bending, twisting, and pivoting even when in bed.

Prescribe an NSAID (e.g., ibuprofen) to control the pain.

Advise sleeping with the leg straight and with loose covers.

Restrict activities of daily living for the first 2 to 4 weeks; advise no sports.

STEP 2 (2 TO 4 WEEKS FOR PERSISTENT CASES) Recommend straight-leg-raising exercises without weights (as soon as acute pain subsides).

Advise continuing use of the brace during activities.

Educate the patient: *"This ligament injury can take months to heal."*

STEP 3 (6 TO 8 WEEKS FOR PERSISTENT CASES) Perform a local injection of D80 coupled with continuous bracing for the next 3 to 4 weeks.

Gradually transition out of the brace, using it only for longer walks or more vigorous activities.

Advise on a graduated return to normal activities and a graduated exercise program.

Perform straight-leg-raising exercises with weights (p. 289).

Strongly encourage the use of a brace during sports and the avoidance of pivoting and twisting.

Recommend orthopedic consultation for third-degree sprains with associated injuries and for lesser sprains that have failed to improve after 2 to 3 months.

PHYSICAL THERAPY Physical therapy plays a minor role in the active treatment of MCL strain, but a major role in rehabilitation.

PHYSICAL THERAPY SUMMARY
1. Ice for acute pain and swelling
2. Straight-leg-raising exercises without weights (while in the brace), isometrically performed
3. Straight-leg-raising exercises with weights in the recovery and rehabilitation phase
4. Cautious return to sports and use of exercise equipment

Acute Period Ice, elevation, crutches, and limited activities are advised during the first 7 to 14 days. Application of *ice* over the medial tibial plateau is an effective local analgesic. Activity restrictions are necessary to allow the injured ligament to reattach to the bone.

Recovery After 7 to 10 days, exercises are begun to strengthen the supporting structures of the knee. While continuing with the knee brace, *straight-leg-raising exercises* (p. 289) are performed daily. The leg is kept perfectly straight to avoid placing stress on the ligament.

Rehabilitation As the ligament strengthens, *weighted straight-leg-raising exercises* can be started to enhance the tone of the quadriceps and hamstring muscles (p. 289). *Sports and active exercising,* especially on equipment, must be delayed until the quadriceps muscle tone is restored to the strength and tone of the contralateral muscle. A knee brace should be worn during the first several weeks of retraining. Exercises and equipment that place torque through the knee must be avoided. Fast walking, swimming (kicking with the knees held straight), and NordicTrack-like equipment are preferred.

INJECTION Immobilization combined with physical therapy strengthening exercises is the treatment of choice. The use of local corticosteroid injection is adjunctive at best and is appropriate only for first-degree and second-degree separations that fail to improve with immobilization, quadriceps-toning exercise, and several weeks of restricted use.

Positioning The patient is placed in the prone position with the leg extended and externally rotated.

Surface Anatomy and Point of Entry The MCL is located in the midplane, originating at the medial femoral condyle and inserting on the medial tibial plateau. The point of entry is just below the medial joint line on the tibia (the joint line is located parallel to the lower third of the patella when the leg is in the extended position).

Angle of Entry and Depth The needle is inserted in the midplane on the tibial side of the medial joint line perpendicular to the skin. The depth is $1/8$ inch above the periosteum of the tibia, approximately $1/2$ to $3/4$ inch from the skin.

Anesthesia Ethyl chloride is sprayed on the skin. Local anesthetic is placed subcutaneously and $1/8$ inch above the tibial periosteum (0.5 mL in both places).

Technique The tibial plateau is identified, just below the medial joint line. A 25-gauge needle is inserted, held perpendicular to the skin, and advanced down to the firm resistance of the periosteum of the tibia. When the bone has been encountered, the needle is withdrawn $1/8$ inch to ensure that the injection is above the MCL attachment (err on the superficial side rather than going too deep; deep injections may detach a portion of the ligament). The injection is stopped if firm or hard pressure is encountered. After local anesthesia, local tenderness is retested, and valgus stress testing is performed. If these signs are significantly reduced and pain is significantly improved, the same area is injected with 0.5 mL of D80. The medication is massaged in for 5 minutes.

INJECTION AFTERCARE

1. *Rest* for 3 days, avoiding direct pressure, twisting, squatting, kneeling, and repetitive bending.
2. Strongly suggest the use of *crutches* with touch-down weightbearing for the first 3 to 7 days.
3. Wear the *Velcro straight-leg immobilizer* (p. 257) continuously during the day for mild to moderate injuries and 24 hours for severe injuries.
4. Use *ice* (15 minutes every 4 to 6 hours) and *acetaminophen* (1000 mg twice a day) for postinjection soreness.
5. *Protect* the knee for 3 to 4 weeks by limiting direct pressure, twisting, pivoting, bending, squatting, and kneeling.
6. Begin *straight-leg-raising exercises* (p. 289) for the quadriceps muscle on day 4 (perform these in the brace for the first 1 or 2 weeks).
7. Repeat the *injection* with corticosteroid at 6 weeks if pain recurs or persists.

MEDIAL COLLATERAL LIGAMENT INJECTION

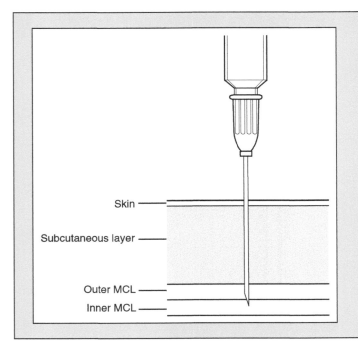

Skin

Subcutaneous layer

Outer medial collateral ligament

Inner medial collateral ligament

8. Request a *consultation* with an orthopedic surgeon if two consecutive injections fail, and the patient still complains of pain with pivoting and twisting (possibly internal derangement).

SURGICAL PROCEDURE The decision to proceed with surgery with higher grade ligament injuries must be made early. A choice between primary repair or delayed reconstruction for third-degree tears is based on the degree of instability and coexistent injuries.

PROGNOSIS Most MCL sprains occur as a result of trauma. The sprain is either an isolated process (minor twisting injuries or simple falls—better prognosis) or associated with tears to the meniscal cartilage or ACL (major trauma—guarded prognosis). MCL injury also may develop as a complication of an underlying effusion or arthritis.

The ligament has a greater vulnerability to injury in the presence of a large chronic effusion (stretching of the supporting structures) and the arthritic narrowing of the medial cartilage (laxity of the ligament secondary to narrowing of the joint). In either case, depending on the severity of the injury, MRI, arthroscopy, or both are necessary to define the extent of the injury. Immobilization, physical therapy, and rest are the mainstays of early treatment for first-degree and second-degree sprains, and surgical intervention is the treatment of choice for third-degree sprains. Ultimately the outcome depends on the degree of injury, associated injuries, and underlying knee pathology. First-degree sprains heal completely 90% of the time. Healing may take several months in some cases, however. Second-degree tears with greater tissue disruption heal less predictably. The primary physician rarely encounters third-degree tears. These injuries often are triaged from the emergency department directly to the orthopedic surgeon.

MENISCAL TEAR

Tears are classified by size as partial or complete; by location as anterior, lateral, or posterior; by cause as traumatic or degenerative; or by description as horizontal, vertical, radial, parrot-beak, or bucket-handle.

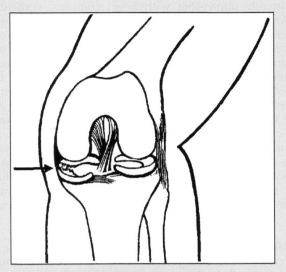

FIGURE 9–10. Medial meniscal tear.

DESCRIPTION   A torn meniscus is a disruption of the unique fibrocartilage pads located between the femoral condyles and the tibial plateaus. Tears are classified as partial or complex; anterior, lateral, or posterior; traumatic or degenerative; and horizontal, vertical, radial, parrot-beak, or bucket-handle. Because of the strategic location and inherent shock-absorbing properties of the meniscus, significant tears can lead to loss of smooth motion of the knee, variable degrees of the classic locking phenomenon, knee effusion, and premature osteoarthritis. Patients suspected to have a torn meniscus must undergo either MRI or arthroscopy to confirm the diagnosis. Small tears that do not extend to the articular cartilage of the femur or tibia can be observed; these have the least potential for further joint damage. Moderate to large tears that extend to the articular cartilage are more significant, tending to cause greater degrees of knee swelling and loss of normal mechanical function of the knee, and as such are more likely to require surgery.

SYMPTOMS   The patient complains of an ill-defined loss of smooth motion, inexplicable or unpredictable giving-out, or, less commonly, popping or locking. Athletic patients attempt to demonstrate the catching or locking phenomenon when describing their symptoms.

"My knee locks up whenever I get it in certain bent positions."

"My knee catches."

"My knee locks up on me when I bend down. When I stand up, it won't straighten right away. When it pops, I feel a bunch of pain and then it releases. It's always right here (pointing to the inner knee)."

"I can't squat anymore."

"If I twist a certain way, I get this real sharp pain."

"I was getting out of the car. My leg was twisted. I tried to shift my weight when I felt this loud pop and immediate sharp pain inside my knee."

"I can't put my finger on it, but whenever I try to shift my weight, the pain inside my knee practically kills me."

EXAM   The patient is examined for loss of smooth motion, for the presence of a joint effusion, and for specific meniscal signs.

EXAM SUMMARY

1. Loss of smooth motion of the knee, passively performed
2. Inability to squat or kneel
3. Palpable popping on the joint line (McMurray maneuver)
4. Joint effusion

(1) Patients with certain types of meniscal tears can have a completely normal knee exam. Partial tears, horizontal tears, and anterior tears may not produce abnormal knee signs because of their size and anatomic location. These types of tears are less likely to interfere with the normal mechanics of the knee and are less likely to compromise function or cause mechanical locking. (2) Screening tests for significant meniscal tears should start with an

assessment of general knee function. The knee can be assessed by observing gait, passive and active flexion and extension, squatting, and duck waddling. The latter is virtually impossible with large, complex, vertical, or bucket-handle tears. *(3)* The McMurray test and the Apley grinding test are relatively specific for meniscal tears; however, their sensitivity is poor. These tests have a false-negative rate of 20% to 25%. The McMurray maneuver should be performed several times. The knee is fully flexed. The tibia is internally rotated (relative to the femur) to trap the lateral meniscus and externally rotated to trap the medial meniscus. A popping sensation under the examiner's fingers held firmly along the joint line is considered abnormal. *(4)* Large or complex tears and tears associated with degenerative arthritis often have an associated joint effusion. Signs of underlying osteoarthritis may be present, either as a cause of the degenerative meniscus or as a result of a long-standing meniscal tear.

X-RAYS   X-rays of the knee (including sunrise, tunnel, posteroanterior, and lateral views) are recommended. Plain films of the knee may show degenerative change, calcification of the meniscus, or calcified loose bodies. The tunnel view shows the intercondylar notch and may show a sequestered loose body.

SPECIAL TESTING   MRI defines the extent and type of meniscal tear, but must be interpreted cautiously. The images obtained from MRI provide information that may or may not be clinically relevant or useful. Mucinoid degenerative change (increased signal arising from the center of the meniscus) is a common finding; this is a normal part of the aging process of the meniscus and should not be misinterpreted as a traumatic meniscal tear. Arthroscopy is the definitive diagnostic and therapeutic test.

DIAGNOSIS   A tentative diagnosis is based on a history of mechanical catching or locking along with corroborative signs on exam. The diagnosis is confirmed by MRI or, preferably, by arthroscopy. The decision to proceed to MRI or arthroscopy should be based on the patient's age, the patient's operative candidacy, and the need to proceed with surgery. The surgical decision should be based on frequency of symptoms (daily), the general function of the knee (e.g., unable to squat, unstable knee), the type of tear (complex tear extending to the articular surfaces), the location (correlating with the patient's symptoms), and the likelihood that leaving it in place might lead to further articular cartilage damage.

TREATMENT   The goals of treatment are to define the type and extent of the tear, to strengthen the muscular support of the knee, and to determine the need for surgery. Meniscal tears that are small, cause infrequent symptoms, and do not interfere with the general function of the knee should be observed. Large, complex tears

associated with persistent knee effusion should be referred for surgical repair or removal.

STEP 1   Assess the general function of the knee, determine the frequency of locking, and order plain x-rays.

Aspirate and drain "tense" hemorrhagic effusions to reduce pain, allow greater involvement in recovery exercises, and decrease the chance of further cartilage damage.

Recommend applications of ice with leg elevation.

Strongly encourage the use of crutches for acute and severe cases.

Prescribe a patellar restraining brace (p. 257) if quadriceps tone is poor and giving-out is frequent.

Restrict activities and all sports.

Begin straight-leg-raising exercises without weights as the pain begins to wane (p. 289).

STEP 2 (2 TO 4 WEEKS FOR PERSISTENT CASES) Aspirate persistent knee effusions for diagnostic studies and to relieve pain.

Order MRI if mechanical symptoms and effusion persist.

All twisting and pivoting must be absolutely avoided, and impact and repetitive bending need to be limited.

Observe a patient with a small meniscal tear unassociated with persistent effusion or mechanical dysfunction because it will gradually or spontaneously resolve over time.

STEP 3 (4 TO 6 WEEKS FOR PERSISTENT CASES) Consider consultation with an orthopedic surgeon experienced in arthroscopy for persistent effusion, frequent locking, and disabling symptoms.

Educate the patient: *"Arthritis can result if severely damaged cartilage remains in the joint. However, removal of a large part of the 'shock-absorber' cartilage may lead to premature arthritis."*

Straight-leg-raising exercises (p. 289) combined with hamstring leg extensions complete the recovery.

PHYSICAL THERAPY   Physical therapy does not play a significant role in the active treatment of a surgical meniscal tear but is important in the preoperative preparation and the postoperative rehabilitation process. *General care of the knee* is always recommended, with particular emphasis on strengthening the quadriceps and hamstring muscles that have been weakened by disuse (p. 289). For nonsurgical meniscal tears, even greater emphasis is placed on toning the thigh muscles. *Quadriceps and hamstring toning exercises* provide greater stability to the knee, allow the joint surfaces to approximate better, and increase the knee's endurance. In addition, these treatments combine to reduce the knee's susceptibility to future injury.

PHYSICAL THERAPY SUMMARY

1. Ice and elevation for acute symptoms
2. Straight-leg-raising exercises, performed isometrically
3. Quadriceps and hamstring toning on apparatus (initially, only to 30 to 45 degrees)
4. Gradual resumption of activities

INJECTION For large meniscal tears that interfere with the normal smooth motion of the knee, arthroscopy with débridement is the treatment of choice. Aspiration of the knee can be used as an interim treatment, however, and is recommended to reduce rapidly the pressure symptoms of the acute, tense, bloody effusion. In addition, local corticosteroid injection is recommended in the select group of patients with osteoarthritis complicated by a degenerative meniscal tear (p. 150).

SURGICAL PROCEDURE Partial meniscectomy is the preferred surgical procedure because it attempts to preserve as much of the normal shock-absorbing properties of the meniscus as possible.

PROGNOSIS Meniscal tear is a classic mechanical problem affecting the knee. Surgical evaluation and treatment rather than anti-inflammatory treatment is relied on to restore the normal function of the knee. Unless the meniscal tear occurs in the setting of a primary arthritis (with a component of active inflammation), corticosteroid injection provides minimal relief. Short-lived responses (days) to a properly placed intra-articular injection of corticosteroid often suggests mechanical issues are the dominant process.

The management of meniscal tears depends on the type of tear (e.g., intrasubstance, horizontal, or vertical), the presence of significant mechanical symptoms, and the presence of persistent knee effusion. Intrasubstance and horizontal tears can be managed medically with rest, restriction, exercises, and aspiration. Vertical tears (in contact with articular cartilage); tears associated with large, persistent effusions; and tears with frequently disabling symptoms should be evaluated by arthroscopy. Repair of the tear, partial meniscectomy, or complete removal of the meniscus is determined at the time of operation. Size, location, vascularity of the tissue, and the patient's age and general health are the major variables determining repair or removal.

DIFFERENTIAL DIAGNOSIS OF ANKLE AND LOWER LEG PAIN

Diagnoses	Confirmations
Ligaments (most common)	
Ankle sprain (first, second, third degree)	Exam; x-ray (if indicated)
Ankle sprain with fibular avulsion	Exam; x-ray—ankle series
Ankle sprain with peroneus tendon avulsion fracture	Exam; x-ray—ankle series
Ankle sprain with osteochondritis dissecans or chondral fracture	Exam; x-ray; MRI
Ankle sprain with interosseous membrane disruption	Exam; x-ray—stress views
Ankle sprain with instability	Exam; x-ray—stress views
Tendons	
Achilles tendinitis	Exam; MRI
Achilles tendon rupture	Exam; MRI
Peroneus tenosynovitis	Local anesthetic block
Posterior tibialis tenosynovitis	Local anesthetic block
Bursa	
Pre-Achilles bursitis	Local anesthetic block
Retrocalcaneal bursitis	Local anesthetic block
Joint	
Osteoarthritis, post-traumatic	X-ray—ankle series
Inflammatory or septic arthritis	Aspiration/synovial fluid analysis
Heel	
Heel pad syndrome	Exam
Plantar fasciitis	Local anesthetic block
Sever's disease (<18 years old)	X-ray—ankle series
Calcaneal stress fracture	X-ray; bone scan
Os trigonum syndrome	Bone scan
Tarsal tunnel syndrome	Nerve conduction velocity testing
Referred pain	
Lumbosacral spine radiculopathy	CT; MRI; electromyography
Compartment syndrome/shin splints	Calf exam
Baker's cyst	Knee exam; ultrasound

ANKLE SPRAIN

Enter $^1/_2$ inch anterior to the lateral malleolus for the anterior talofibular ligament and $^1/_2$ inch below the tip of the lateral malleolus for the fibulocalcaneal ligament.

Needle: $^5/_8$-inch, 25-gauge
Depth: $^1/_2$ to $^5/_8$ inch
Volume: 1 to 2 mL of anesthetic and 0.5 mL of D80

NOTE: Confirm the placement with local anesthetic first; immobilize for 1 to 4 weeks after corticosteroid injection, depending on the severity.

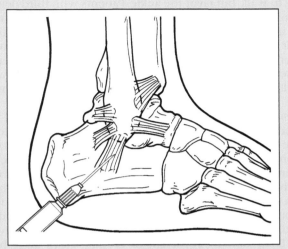

FIGURE 10–1. Fibulocalcaneal ligament injection just below the inferior tip of the lateral malleolus.

DESCRIPTION   An ankle sprain is an injury of the supporting ligaments of the ankle joint. The tissue injury ranges from ligament microtears to complete tears through the body of the ligament or its bony attachments (avulsion of the ligament). The anterior talofibular ligament is injured most commonly, followed closely by the fibulocalcaneal; the most common type of injury is ankle inversion, which places abnormal force across these ligaments. Sprains are classified as first, second, or third degree corresponding to the extent of the tissue disruption—microtears, partial tears, and full-thickness tears. Sprains also are classified as acute, recurrent, or chronic. Ligaments that do not reapproximate their torn filaments or do not reattach to their bony origins and insertions can cause significant ankle instability, which can lead to recurrent ankle sprain, osteochondritis dissecans, or late-developing osteoarthritis.

SYMPTOMS   The patient with an acute injury complains of ankle pain, ankle swelling, bruising, and difficulty with weightbearing. In a recurrent or chronic case, the patient may have additional complaints of instability of the ankle (e.g., giving-out, loss of smooth motion).

"I stepped off a high curb, higher than I thought, and came down on the side of my foot. My ankle immediately swelled, and I couldn't put any weight on it."

"I tried to turn a corner while running, and my ankle suddenly gave out."

"I jumped up and landed on the side of my foot. Ever since, I have had sharp pain along the outside."

"I injured my ankle years ago, and it has been weak ever since."

"Four weeks ago I sprained my ankle. I had this huge black-and-blue spot that went away. My ankle still feels weak."

"Every time I try to play basketball my ankle gives out. I wear high-top shoes, but I still can't run or jump very well."

"Ever since I injured my ankle, I can't trust it when I'm climbing my ladder. In certain positions, it seems as if it is going to give out."

EXAM   The exam begins with assessment of general ankle alignment and function (weightbearing and walking). The patient is examined for irritation, inflammation, and laxity of the individual lateral ankle ligaments.

EXAM SUMMARY

1. Exam begins by assessing the patient's ability to bear weight and walk
2. Tenderness, swelling, or bruising anterior and inferior to the lateral malleolus
3. Pain aggravated by forced inversion, plantar flexion, or both
4. No pain with resisted plantar flexion and eversion, isometrically performed
5. Full range of motion (ROM) of the ankle (in nonacute cases)
6. Ankle instability (positive drawer sign or talar knock sign) documented in the recovery phase

(1) The exam of the patient with an ankle sprain always begins with an assessment of the patient's ability to stand, bear weight, and walk. Patients with minor injuries are able to walk, but favor the ankle. Patients with third-degree sprains and patients with accompanying fibular fractures are unwilling to bear weight and refuse to demonstrate their impaired walking. (2) Minor ankle sprains are tender anterior and inferior to the lateral malleolus. Moderate to severe ankle sprains have tenderness combined with swelling and bruising. The severe sprain may be so intensely sore that the remaining portions of the exam are not possible. (3) Passive inversion and plantar flexion of the ankle aggravates the pain, depending on which ligaments have been injured. This passive stretching sign should improve gradually as the condition resolves. (4) Isometric testing of the peroneus tendons may show pain inferior to the lateral malleolus (active tendinitis) or may show pain and tenderness at the insertion at the base of the fifth metatarsal (avulsion fracture). (5) The ROM of the ankle should be normal after the acute symptoms have resolved. (6) Long-standing recurrent or chronic cases may show instability of the ankle. An anterior or posterior drawer sign may be present. In addition, rocking the ankle back and forth passively may produce a knocking (the talar knock sign). The latter usually indicates a separation of the interosseous membrane between the tibia and the fibula. Lastly, long-standing ankle instability may lead to signs of limited ROM, crepitation, and pain at the extremes of motion (i.e., osteoarthritis of the ankle).

X-RAYS   X-rays of the ankle (including routine postero-anterior, mortise, and lateral views) are ordered to evaluate the ankle joint, the subtalar joint, and the malleoli. In addition, the special posteroanterior oblique and subtalar views are used to assess further the integrity of the tibiotalar and subtalar joints and to exclude an avulsion fracture at the lateral malleolus at the base of the fifth metatarsal—the attachment of the peroneus tendon. Most routine x-rays are normal. Special stress views of the ankle are ordered occasionally in patients with persistent symptoms in the recovery phase and in patients with recurrent ankle sprains. Widening of the tibiotalar joint space when inversion stress is applied to the ankle provides strong evidence of joint instability.

SPECIAL TESTING   Patients with persistent localized findings despite immobilization, recovery-oriented physical therapy exercises, and time may benefit from MRI. Osteo-chondritis dissecans of the talar dome or early arthritic changes may be seen.

DIAGNOSIS   The diagnosis is based on the history of inversion injury coupled with the obvious physical findings. Plain x-rays are used to exclude avulsion or complete fracture of the lateral malleolus or the base of the fifth metatarsal. Rarely, regional anesthetic block is indicated to differentiate the symptoms and signs of ankle sprain from peroneus tenosynovitis and subtalar arthritis.

TREATMENT   The goals of treatment are to allow the lateral ligaments of the ankle to reattach to their bony insertions, to strengthen the tendons that cross the ankle, and to prevent recurrent ankle sprains. Limited weight-bearing and immobilization of the ankle, lower leg, or both (high-top shoes, overlap taping, an air cast, or a short-leg walking cast) are the treatments of choice for acute ankle sprain.

STEP 1   Examine the patient, assess the severity of the injury using the Ottawa criteria (ability to bear weight and walk, bony tenderness, tissue swelling and bruising, and severity of the injury), and obtain plain x-rays of the ankle if two of the four criteria are met.

Strongly advise on limited weightbearing using crutches.

Advise on the use of ice and elevation to reduce swelling and pain.

Restrict walking, standing, impact, and repetitive bending.

Prescribe immobilization with an Ace wrap and crutches, overlap taping, an air cast, an Unna boot, or a short-leg walking cast, depending on the severity of the injury. Because 10% to 20% of patients are at risk for recurrent ankle sprain (nonanatomically or poorly healing ligaments), emphasis should be placed on immobilization that prevents inversion and eversion.

STEP 2 (1- TO 3-WEEK FOLLOW-UP EVALUATION) Perform gentle stretching exercises beginning with dorsiflexion and plantar flexion.

Begin isometric toning exercises of eversion when flexibility has improved significantly.

Advise the patient to wear high-top shoes or a Velcro ankle brace (p. 259).

Recommend limiting stop-and-go sports, basketball, running, and impact aerobics.

Educate the patient: *"Healing is measured in months rather than weeks."*

Complete the rehabilitation process by gradually returning to exercise and sports activities.

STEP 3 (6 TO 8 WEEKS FOR PERSISTENT CASES)   Perform a local injection of D80, and combine it with a short-leg walking cast.

Repeat the injection in 4 to 6 weeks if symptoms have not been reduced by 50%.

Re-emphasize the need to perform daily stretching and toning exercises.

Order MRI of the ankle for persistent swelling, intractable pain, or instability.

Consider referral to an orthopedic surgeon if symptoms and instability persist.

PHYSICAL THERAPY   Physical therapy plays an essential role in the active treatment and rehabilitation of ankle sprain.

PHYSICAL THERAPY SUMMARY

1. Ice and elevation for acute pain and swelling
2. Heating and ankle stretching for postimmobilization rehabilitation
3. Toning exercises in eversion, isometrically performed

Acute Period　Ice and elevation are used in the first few days to reduce the acute pain and swelling effectively. Treatments lasting 15 to 20 minutes several times a day reduce tissue distortion resulting from bleeding and swelling.

Recovery Rehabilitation　After acute pain and swelling have subsided, exercises are performed to restore normal ROM and to strengthen the ankle joint. *Stretching exercises* (p. 292) of the ankle joint are performed after immobilization, especially with fixed casting. Dorsiflexion and plantar flexion stretching is performed initially, followed by gentle inversion and eversion. The ankle is heated before stretching. Sets of 20 passive stretches in each direction are performed daily. *Isometric exercises* (p. 293) are used to strengthen and stabilize the ankle joint and are the most effective means of preventing further injuries. Toning exercises are necessary to overcome the weakness of a tear or of severe separation of the ligaments. Both types of recovery exercises are necessary before resumption of normal activities.

INJECTION　The treatment of choice comprises immobilization combined with physical therapy (strengthening exercises). Local corticosteroid injection is performed uncommonly, being reserved for patients with persistent inflammation despite immobilization (first-degree sprains only).

Positioning　The patient is placed in the supine position. The ankle is kept in a neutral position.

Surface Anatomy and Point of Entry　The tip of the lateral malleolus and the point of maximum tenderness are identified and marked. The point of entry is $1/2$ inch anterior or inferior to the lateral malleolus depending on which ligament has been injured (talofibular and fibulocalcaneal ligaments).

Angle of Entry and Depth　The needle is inserted directly over the point of maximum tenderness, perpendicular to the skin. The depth is $1/2$ to $5/8$ inch beneath the skin.

Anesthesia　Ethyl chloride is sprayed on the skin. Local anesthetic (0.5 mL) is placed subcutaneously and at the firm resistance of the lateral ligament $1/4$ to $1/2$ inch from the skin.

Technique　All medication injections should be placed atop the ligament—between the subcutaneous tissue and the ligament. This tissue plane can be identified easily by

FIBULOCALCANEAL LIGAMENT INJECTION

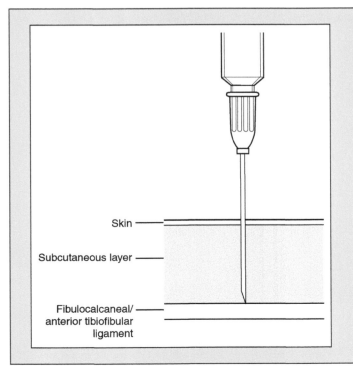

Skin

Subcutaneous layer

Fibulocalcaneal ligament

Anterior tibiofibular ligament

advancing the needle gradually until the firm resistance of the ligament is appreciated or until the tip of the needle stays in place when skin traction is applied (if the needle is above the ligament, the needle will move with the skin and subcutaneous tissue when traction is applied). After local anesthesia, the ankle is re-examined for instability and pain relief. If local tenderness and passive inversion are no longer painful and the anterior drawer and talar knock signs are negative (no sign of gross instability), 0.5 mL of D80 is injected.

INJECTION AFTERCARE

1. *Rest* for 3 days, avoiding all unnecessary weightbearing (*"It takes 3 days for the medication to set up."*).
2. Use *crutches* with touch-down weightbearing for the first few days in severe cases.
3. Recommend *immobilization* with lace-up high-top shoes, an air cast, or a short-leg walking cast for 1 to 4 weeks, depending on the severity of the original injury.
4. Use *ice* (15 minutes every 4 to 6 hours) and *acetaminophen (Tylenol ES)* (1000 mg twice a day) for postinjection soreness.
5. *Protect* the ankle for 3 to 4 weeks by avoiding all twisting and pivoting and limiting unnecessary walking and standing.
6. Begin *isometric toning exercises* (p. 293) of ankle eversion and inversion at 3 to 4 weeks.
7. Repeat the *injection* at 6 weeks with corticosteroid if pain recurs or persists.
8. Order *MRI* for persistent instability or intractable pain, or consider aspirating the ankle joint if joint swelling develops.
9. Request a *consultation* with an orthopedic surgeon if two consecutive injections fail, and the patient still complains of giving-out (instability), pain and swelling (osteochondritis dissecans, chondral fracture), or pain when pivoting and twisting (fracture of the talus, peroneus tendinitis).

SURGICAL PROCEDURE   Advanced third-degree tears can be repaired primarily or undergo delayed reconstruction if the ankle remains unstable.

PROGNOSIS   Most sprained ankles respond to rest and immobilization and heal without residual effects. Severe ankle sprains (unable to bear weight, goose egg–sized swelling, intolerance of passive ROM testing in inversion, and bony tenderness) must be managed carefully to avoid the 25% to 30% chance of persistent ankle instability and recurrent ankle sprain. Inadequate activity restriction, immobilization, or physical therapy rehabilitation exercises can lead to nonanatomic healing, weakness of the supporting ligaments, recurrent ankle sprains, and, ultimately, osteoarthritis of the joint in later years. To avoid the consequences of incomplete healing (recurrent ankle sprain and instability), treatment should emphasize strict immobilization, physical therapy toning exercises, and gradual resumption of activity. This management strategy ensures optimal protection for patients who are at the greatest risk for postrecovery instability.

Persistent pain and swelling suggest poor healing of the original ligament injury or possible unrecognized injury to the adjacent bones, tendons, or ankle cartilage. Patients who fail to resolve their injury in 4 to 6 weeks should undergo stress views of the ankle for instability, MRI for osteochondritis dissecans, nuclear medicine bone scanning for occult bony fracture, and synovial fluid analysis for injury to the ankle or subtalar joint.

ARTHROCENTESIS OF THE ANKLE

The ankle can be entered anteromedially just medial to the extensor hallucis longus or anterolaterally just lateral to the extensor digiti minimi

Needle: 1¹/₂-inch, 22-gauge
Depth: 1 to 1¹/₄ inch through either the tibionavicular ligament medially or the fibulonavicular ligament laterally
Volume: 2 to 3 mL of anesthetic and 0.5 mL of K40

NOTE: If bone is encountered, withdraw back through the ligament, redirect with skin traction either toward the midline or inferiorly, and advance again.

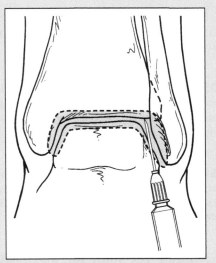

FIGURE 10–2. Arthrocentesis and injection of the ankle.

DESCRIPTION   Effusion of the ankle is an uncommon problem. Swelling at the ankle is more often due to edema (fluid retention, congestive heart failure, varicosities, deep venous thrombosis), ankle sprain, or fracture. True ankle effusion presents as a bandlike swelling that forms over the anterior ankle joint, obliterates the malleolar prominences, and impairs dorsiflexion and plantar flexion of the joint. Aspiration and synovial fluid analysis of the tibiotalar joint are necessary to distinguish among the variety of causes of ankle effusion, which include traumatic bloody effusions, noninflammatory effusions secondary to osteoarthritis, inflammatory effusions secondary to rheumatoid disease, and the rare case of septic arthritis.

SYMPTOMS   The patient complains of swelling in front of or along the sides of the ankle and stiffness or pain in the ankle. Patients often gaze at the ankle and ask the provider if the ankle appears swollen while they are describing the condition.

"I think my ankle is swollen."

"At the end of my shift—I have to stand all day at the cash register—my ankle feels tight inside."

"My ankle feels loose. If I get in a certain position, my ankle gives out."

"I can't find a pair of shoes that fit."

"I didn't fall, but my ankle feels like it did when I broke it years ago."

EXAM   The patient is examined for joint effusion, local joint-line tenderness, and ROM of the tibiotalar joint.

EXAM SUMMARY

1. Anterior swelling or general fullness to the ankle
2. Anterior joint-line tenderness
3. Loss of or painful plantar flexion or dorsiflexion
4. Characteristic aspirate or confirmation with local anesthetic block

(1) The detection of an effusion of the ankle joint can be elusive. Small effusions cause mild general fullness of the anterior ankle (which is difficult to differentiate from lower extremity edema). Moderate to large effusions should be ballotable. With finger pressure placed behind both malleoli (all four fingers hooked around the malleoli to compress the soft tissues anteriorly), the synovial fluid should be palpable as a softness or spongelike quality when alternating pressure is applied on either side of the extensor tendons with the thumbs. *(2)* Tenderness is present along the anterior joint line (a line drawn between the two points, ¹/₂ inch above the tip of the medial malleolus and ³/₄ inch above the tip of the lateral malleolus). *(3)* Acute synovitis causes end-point stiffness, end-point pain, or absolute loss of plantar flexion or dorsiflexion. *(4)* Aspiration of joint fluid or a beneficial response to intra-articular injection is necessary to confirm the involvement of the joint.

X-RAYS   Plain x-rays of the ankle (posteroanterior, lateral, and oblique views) are strongly recommended. Osteoarthritic narrowing between the tibia and the talus with accompanying medial or lateral osteophytes is best appreciated on the lateral and posteroanterior projections. The width of the articular cartilage averages 2 to 3 mm.

SPECIAL TESTING   Synovial fluid analysis should be performed. MRI is indicated to exclude osteochondritis of the talar dome or loose body.

DIAGNOSIS   The diagnosis is suggested by general fullness and ballotable fluid anteriorly. The diagnosis and determination of specific cause require arthrocentesis and synovial fluid analysis.

TREATMENT   Diagnostic aspiration and synovial fluid analysis are the procedures of choice for acute effusion. Ice, elevation, limited weightbearing, and ROM exercises are the treatments of choice.

STEP 1   **Aspirate the joint for diagnostic studies (Gram stain and culture, uric acid crystal analysis, and cell count and differential); order plain x-rays of the ankle; and measure the baseline ROM of the ankle, especially dorsiflexion.**
>   Ice and elevation are effective in reducing pain and swelling.
>   Strongly advise on limited weightbearing.
>   Prescribe immobilization with an Ace wrap, high-top shoes (mild disease), Velcro ankle brace, an air cast, an Unna boot (moderate disease), or a short-leg walking cast (severe disease), and combine with touch-down weightbearing with crutches.
>   Restrict walking, standing, impact, and repetitive bending until the swelling and pain are well controlled.
>   A 2- to 3-week trial of a nonsteroidal anti-inflammatory drug (NSAID) is effective for mild involvement.
>   Prescribe glucosamine sulfate, 1500 mg/day.

STEP 2 (1 TO 3 DAYS AFTER LABORATORY ANALYSIS)   **Evaluate and treat for gout, repeat drainage of hemarthrosis, or perform an intra-articular injection of K40 for an osteoarthritic or inflammatory arthritic flare.**
>   Perform passive ROM stretching exercises beginning with dorsiflexion and plantar flexion after immobilizing the ankle for 3 weeks (p. 292).
>   Begin isometric toning exercises of eversion after flexibility has improved significantly (p. 293).
>   Advise the wearing of high-top shoes or a Velcro ankle brace (p. 259).
>   Recommend limiting stop-and-go sports, basketball, running, and impact aerobics.

STEP 3 (3 TO 4 WEEKS FOR PERSISTENT CASES)   **Repeat local injection of K40, and couple this with limited weightbearing or joint immobilization.**
>   Re-emphasize the need to perform daily Achilles tendon–stretching exercises and peroneus tendon

toning exercises to maintain joint flexibility and support.

STEP 4 (8 TO 10 WEEKS FOR CHRONIC CASES)   **Consider surgical referral for advanced disease characterized by greater than 50% loss of ROM and for persistent symptoms that interfere with activities of daily living.**

PHYSICAL THERAPY   Physical therapy plays an important role in the rehabilitation of ankle effusion. During the acute period, ice and elevation are used in the first few days to reduce acute pain and swelling effectively.

PHYSICAL THERAPY SUMMARY

1. Ice and elevation for acute pain and swelling
2. Heat before ROM exercises, passively performed
3. Toning exercises in eversion to enhance ankle support, isometrically performed

---

Recovery and Rehabilitation   After acute pain and swelling have subsided, exercises are performed to restore normal ROM and to strengthen the ankle joint. *Stretching exercises* (p. 292) of the ankle joint are performed after heating the joint for 15 to 20 minutes. Emphasis is placed on restoring dorsiflexion and plantar flexion first. Eversion and inversion often are restored naturally after the return to regular activities. Sets of 20 passive stretches in each direction are performed daily. *Eversion and inversion toning exercises* (p. 293), *isometrically performed,* are used to strengthen and stabilize the ankle joint. Emphasis is placed on enhancing the tone of the everter tendons, the peroneus longus in particular. Sets of 20 ankle eversions and inversions, each held 5 seconds, are performed daily. Recovery of eversion and inversion strength is necessary before resuming normal activities.

INJECTION   Ice, elevation, and limited weightbearing are the mainstays of treatment for recurrent arthritic flares. Diagnostic aspiration is mandatory if septic arthritis is suspected. Local corticosteroid injection is indicated for large or persistent nonseptic effusions.
Position   The patient is placed in the supine position, and the ankle is held in 15 to 20 degrees of plantar flexion (this tightens the anterior capsule).
Surface Anatomy and Point of Entry   A horizontal line is drawn $^1/_2$ inch above the medial malleolar tip and $^3/_4$ inch above the lateral malleolar tip. The point of entry is at the intersection of these lines and just lateral to the extensor digit minimi (*anterolateral approach*) or, alternatively, just medial to extensor hallucis longus (*anteromedially*).
Angle of Entry and Depth   The needle is inserted perpendicular to the skin and angled toward the center of the joint. The depth is 1 to $1^1/_4$ inches from the skin.

ANKLE JOINT INJECTION

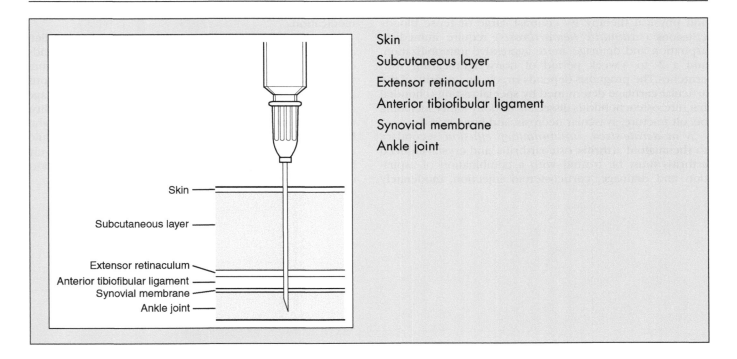

Skin
Subcutaneous layer
Extensor retinaculum
Anterior tibiofibular ligament
Synovial membrane
Ankle joint

Skin
Subcutaneous layer
Extensor retinaculum
Anterior tibiofibular ligament
Synovial membrane
Ankle joint

Anesthesia Ethyl chloride is sprayed on the skin. Local anesthetic (0.5 mL) is placed subcutaneously, at the firm resistance of the extensor retinaculum, and intra-articularly.

Technique The *anterolateral* approach is preferred because the lateral synovial cavity is larger, and there are fewer obstructing structures. After anesthetic placement in the superficial tissues, the 22-gauge needle is advanced slowly to the firm resistance of the extensor retinaculum and superficial ligaments. If bone is encountered at a superficial level (^{1}/$_2$ inch), the needle is redirected more inferiorly or medially with the aid of skin traction. If the needle is centered over the joint, the passage of the needle to a depth of 1 to 1^1/$_4$ inches should be smooth and unobstructed. *Note:* The joint cannot be entered if the needle is more than 15 to 20 degrees from perpendicular. If active infection is excluded by fluid inspection or subsequent synovial fluid laboratory analysis, 0.5 mL of K40 is injected intra-articularly.

INJECTION AFTERCARE

1. *Rest* for 3 days, avoiding all unnecessary weightbearing.
2. Use *crutches* with touch-down weightbearing for the first few days in severe cases.
3. Recommend *immobilization* with lace-up high-top shoes, an air cast, or a short-leg walking cast for 1 to 4 weeks, depending on the severity of the arthritis and swelling.
4. Use *ice* (15 minutes every 4 to 6 hours) and *acetaminophen* (1000 mg twice a day) for postinjection soreness.

5. *Protect* the ankle for 3 to 4 weeks by avoiding twisting and pivoting and limiting unnecessary walking and standing.
6. Begin *passive stretching* of the ankle in flexion and extension after the pain and swelling have improved significantly. Follow this with drawing out the alphabet with the foot to restore full ROM.
7. Begin *isometric toning exercises* of ankle eversion and inversion at 3 to 4 weeks to enhance support of the ankle (always maintaining the ankle in neutral position).
8. Repeat *injection* at 6 weeks with corticosteroid if swelling recurs or persists.
9. Request MRI and a *consultation* with an orthopedic surgeon if two consecutive injections fail, and the patient still complains of weightbearing pain (e.g., loose bodies, osteochondritis dissecans of the talar dome).

SURGICAL PROCEDURE Patients with moderate involvement can be considered for arthroscopic débridement, particularly patients with loose bodies, osteochondritis dissecans, and advanced arthritis. Patients with advanced wear and tear of the joint, intractable pain, and poor function are candidates for arthrodesis.

PROGNOSIS In general, the long-term prognosis depends on the underlying presenting diagnosis (e.g., traumatic osteochondritis dissecans, rheumatoid arthritis), the integrity and thickness of the articular cartilage, and the ability of the patient to perform physical therapy recovery exercises to restore joint flexibility and muscular support. *Small ankle effusions* (ROM restrictions <20%) secondary to minor trauma can be managed effectively with ice, elevation, high-top shoes, reduced activities, and physical therapy. By contrast, large or tense bloody effusions (*traumatic hemarthrosis*) require immediate aspiration and drainage, more aggressive immobilization, and a 2- to 4-week period of nonweightbearing with crutches. The prognosis depends largely on integrity of the articular cartilage determined by special testing (chondral fracture; osteochondritis dissecans; or bony injury, including occult fracture, avascular necrosis, and bony cysts).

A *moderate-sized, inflammatory effusion* secondary to rheumatoid arthritis, osteoarthritis, and crystal-induced arthritis must be treated with a combination of aspiration and drainage, corticosteroid injection, moderately restrictive immobilization, and limited weightbearing. The prognosis depends on the intensity of the inflammatory flare, the integrity of the articular cartilage, and the ability to control the underlying process with systemic medication.

Patients with *septic arthritis* have the most unpredictable prognosis. The outcome in these patients depends on the infective pathogen, the interval of time from presentation to the institution of effective intravenous antibiotics, and the degree of articular cartilage damage caused by the infection. Because of the unpredictability, these patients must be hospitalized, be kept nonweightbearing, have repeated aspiration and drainage (if fluid continues to reaccumulate), and be treated aggressively by a physical therapist with ROM and muscular support exercises.

ACHILLES TENDINITIS

This is a peritendinous injection; enter along the outer edge of the tendon, approximately $1^1/2$ inches above the calcaneus.

Needle: $1^1/2$-inch, 22-gauge
Depth: superficial—$^3/8$ to $^1/2$ inch
Volume: 2 to 3 mL of anesthetic and 1 mL of D80 (0.5 mL injected on either side of the tendon)

NOTE: Do not enter the tendon; minimal pressure is needed when injecting; immobilize with an air cast or short-leg walking cast for 3 to 4 weeks.

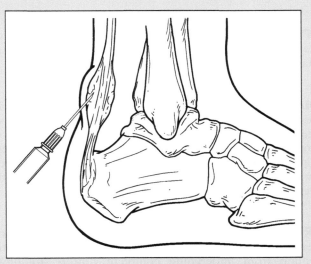

FIGURE 10–3. Peritendinous injection for Achilles tendinitis.

DESCRIPTION   Achilles tendinitis is an inflammation of the musculotendinous junction of the Achilles tendon, located approximately $1^1/2$ inches above the calcaneal insertion. Repetitive jumping, pivoting, and impact lead to microtearing of the tendon and secondary inflammation. These pathologic changes weaken the tendon and can lead to complete tendon rupture in 10% of cases. Runners, patients with short tight Achilles tendons, and patients with Reiter's syndrome are at particular risk. Dramatic changes in the level of activity, incomplete warm-ups before physical activity, and inadequate stretching of the tendon predispose to tendinitis.

SYMPTOMS   The patient complains of pain behind the ankle with walking, standing, or weightbearing sports activities. The patient often points to the back of the heel when describing the condition.

"I have to stop running after 2 miles because the back of my ankle begins to hurt."

"I get sharp pain through my ankle and up the back of my leg whenever I jump."

"My shoes feel like they're rubbing against the bone."

"I've had to shorten my jogging stride because my cords hurt."

"My Achilles tendon is larger on the right side."

"If I try to do my leg stretches, I get a sharp pain up the back of my leg."

"I was playing basketball when I got this sudden shock of pain right behind my ankle. I looked back to see who might have kicked me, but no one was there. Every step I take now causes pain behind my ankle."

EXAM   The patient is examined for Achilles tendon irritation, paratendinous thickening at the musculotendinous junction, and signs of tendon rupture.

EXAM SUMMARY

1. Tenderness and "cobblestone" thickening $1^1/2$ inches above the calcaneus
2. Pain aggravated by resisting plantar flexion, isometrically performed
3. Pain aggravated by stretching in dorsiflexion, passively performed
4. ROM of the ankle that is otherwise normal
5. Strength and tendon integrity intact

(1) The Achilles tendon is enlarged at the musculotendinous junction. The thickening is 1 to $1^1/2$ inches above the calcaneal insertion, fusiform in shape, and cobblestone-like to the touch. The entire area is sensitive to pressure, especially when compressing the tendon from side to side. *(2)* The pain is aggravated by resisting active plantar flexion isometrically. *(3)* Passive stretching in dorsiflexion also aggravates the pain. Passive stretching is definitely much more sensitive in the average case. *(4)* The ROM of the ankle is preserved, although pain may limit the ability to measure dorsiflexion accurately. *(5)* Palpation of the length of the tendon shows that it is free of defects. The strength of the calf muscles is preserved, attenuated only by the patient's acute pain.

X-RAYS   Plain x-rays of the ankle and lower extremity bony structures are normal. Calcification does not occur at the musculotendinous junction. Incidental calcification of the calcaneal insertion of the tendon commonly occurs, but it does not correlate with signs of tendinitis.

SPECIAL TESTING   MRI often is used for preoperative staging. Peritendinous swelling, degenerative change, and macrotears of the tendon can be shown.

DIAGNOSIS   The diagnosis is based on the abnormalities found on physical exam. MRI is used to distinguish the tendon with a microtear with inflammatory reaction from the tendon with partial-thickness or full-thickness rupture. Alternatively, regional anesthetic block followed by careful palpation and stress testing may disclose subtle weakness or difficult-to-feel tendon separations.

TREATMENT   The goals of treatment are to reduce peritendinous swelling and thickening, to protect the tendon from undergoing complete rupture, to allow the tendon with a microtear to heal, and to stretch out the muscle and tendon gradually to prevent recurrent tendinitis. Treatment must be individualized. Passive stretching and limited weightbearing are the treatments of choice for mild tendinitis. Immobilization with an air cast or a short-leg walking cast is the treatment of choice for moderate to severe involvement.

STEP 1   Measure the extent of the process (side-to-side width and the length of the swelling superior to inferior), measure the ROM of the ankle in flexion and extension, and order MRI if partial tendon rupture is suspected.

 Mildly symptomatic Achilles tendinitis should respond to the following recommendations:

 Educate the patient on the importance of rest and reduced weightbearing.

 Strongly recommend the use of crutches for 7 to 10 days if symptoms are hyperacute.

 Recommend ice for acute swelling and pain.

 Advise on shortening the walking stride.

 Prescribe padded heel cups or a heel lift (p. 261).

 Recommend New-Skin, moleskin, or double socks to reduce friction over the tendon thickening (p. 259).

 Recommend v-notched tennis shoes.

STEP 2 (3 TO 6 WEEKS FOR PERSISTENT CASES)   Prescribe an NSAID (e.g., ibuprofen [Advil, Motrin]) at full dosage for 3 to 4 weeks and discuss its partial effectiveness owing to poor penetration into these avascular tissues.

 Prescribe a Velcro ankle brace or an air cast (p. 259).

STEP 3 (6 TO 8 WEEKS FOR PERSISTENT CASES)   Moderate to severe cases should be treated with more aggressive fixed immobilization for 3 to 4 weeks.

 If immobilization fails to control symptoms, order MRI to rule out a partial or complete tear of the tendon.

 If MRI is negative for tear, perform a local injection of D80, and combine it with an air cast or a short-leg walking cast (in "equinous" position).

STEP 4 (10 TO 12 WEEKS FOR CHRONIC CASES) **Prescribe daily Achilles tendon–stretching exercises (p. 292).**

 Recommend following stretching exercises with toning exercises (p. 293).

 Recommend high-top tennis shoes.

 Restrict running, jumping, and repetitive bending until all signs of irritation have resolved, full flexibility has been restored, and strength has been recovered.

 Advise on resuming activities gradually (e.g., increasing time or distance by 10% each week, alternating running days with weight training).

 Recommend continued reduction of friction over the back of the heel.

 Limit high-impact sports, jumping, and long-distance running.

 Consider a surgical consultation for persistent pain and swelling despite adequate immobilization and local injection.

PHYSICAL THERAPY   Physical therapy plays an important role in the treatment and rehabilitation of Achilles tendinitis.

PHYSICAL THERAPY SUMMARY

1. Ice for acute swelling and pain
2. Phonophoresis with a hydrocortisone gel
3. Stretching exercises in dorsiflexion, passively performed
4. Active stretching exercises in dorsiflexion
5. Toning exercises in plantar flexion, isometrically performed

Acute Period   Ice and phonophoresis are used in the first few weeks to reduce the acute pain and swelling. *Ice* and *phonophoresis* applied directly to the musculotendinous junction provide short-term relief of pain and swelling. *Gentle passive stretching* in dorsiflexion always is recommended after acute symptoms abate. A foreshortened, inflexible tendon is susceptible to continued irritation. Stretching applied with hand pressure or very gentle wall stretches should be performed daily (p. 292). Mild discomfort in the calf is normal, but acute or sharp pain in the tendon area must be avoided. This stretching is performed after heating.

Recovery and Rehabilitation Complete healing requires continued daily stretching of the tendon. Prevention of recurrent tendinitis requires stretching and toning exercises. *Passive stretching exercises* are continued in the recovery period. Vigorous stretching exercises to achieve 30 degrees of dorsiflexion without experiencing pain are started 3 to 4 weeks after the acute symptoms have resolved. When full dorsiflexion has been obtained, *isometric toning exercises* are begun. These exercises should be performed daily using a TheraBand, oversized rubber bands, or a bungee cord. Sets of 20 are performed with the ankle kept in a neutral position. As strength and tone increase, weightbearing active toning exercises can be performed (p. 293). With increasing strength, full weightbearing activities can be resumed.

INJECTION The role of local injection is controversial. Local corticosteroid injection can reduce the chronic peritendinous inflammation and thickening effectively. The benefits of injection must be balanced, however, against the risk of tendon rupture. To reduce this risk, it is strongly advised that injection be combined with rigid immobilization.

Position The patient is placed in the prone position with the foot hanging over the end of the exam table. The ankle is kept in a neutral position.

Surface Anatomy and Point of Entry The peritendinous thickening surrounding the tendon is identified. The two points of entry are on either side of the thickening.

Angle of Entry and Depth The needle is inserted alongside the tendon in the peritendinous thickening, at an angle paralleling the tendon. The depth is $^3/_8$ to $^1/_2$ inch from the surface.

Anesthesia Ethyl chloride is sprayed on the skin. Local anesthetic is placed subcutaneously (0.5 mL) and within the peritendinous thickening (0.5 mL on each side).

Technique A *peritendinous injection* is performed; the anesthetic and the corticosteroid are injected in a 1-inch-long linear track within the peritendinous thickening. *Note: Never* inject into the body of the tendon. The optimal injection is accomplished by entering at the most inferior portion of the peritendinous thickening, advancing the needle to the most superior point of the thickening, and slowly withdrawing the needle inferiorly, leaving a track of medication parallel to the tendon. If local tenderness is significantly relieved and dorsiflexion strength is unquestionably normal, 0.5 mL of D80 is injected similarly. The procedure is repeated on the opposite side of the tendon. Although the peritendinous thickening affects the medial aspect of the tendon more often, injection is still performed in equal amounts on either side of the tendon.

INJECTION AFTERCARE

1. Strongly recommend *immobilization* in a short-leg walking cast or air cast for 3 to 4 weeks: *"A cast is necessary to protect the tendon from rupture after injection."*

ACHILLES TENDINITIS INJECTION

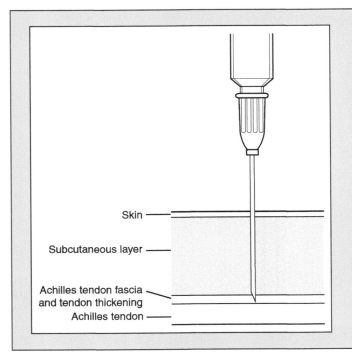

Skin

Subcutaneous layer

Achilles tendon fascia and tendon thickening

Achilles tendon

2. Recommend the use of *crutches* with touch-down weightbearing for the first few days if an air cast has been chosen.
3. Use *acetaminophen* (1000 mg twice a day) for soreness.
4. Begin *passive stretching* of the ankle in flexion and extension after the cast is removed, first by hand and then with gentle wall stretches.
5. Restrict jumping, twisting, and impact during the recovery phase.
6. Keep the stride short while in the recovery phase.
7. Use high-top shoes with padding over the tendon (double socks, felt ring, or mole foam).
8. Begin *isometric toning exercises* of ankle eversion and inversion after flexibility has been partially restored followed by isometric toning of the ankle in plantar flexion.
9. Request *MRI* and a *consultation* with an orthopedic surgeon if injection and immobilization fail.

SURGICAL PROCEDURE   Operative intervention for chronic Achilles tendinitis involves close inspection for subtle tendon tears followed by stripping away the peritendinous fibrosis. Primary repair of the tendon is the procedure of choice when the tendon has been torn.

PROGNOSIS   Achilles tendinitis can be dishearteningly persistent or recurrent, probably owing to the variability in tendon disruption (microtears to full-thickness tears), the degrees of inflammation, and the patient's ability to perform ankle-stretching exercises to increase ankle dorsiflexion. Treatment must be individualized based on the degree of thickening, the length of time symptoms have been present, the risk of tear, and the acceptance of treatment by the patient. Patients who have had mild symptoms for 2 to 3 months respond favorably to rest, immobilization, and stretching exercises. Patients with moderate to severe symptoms lasting 4 to 6 months, patients with tendon thickening more than two to three times normal in width, and patients with a history of trauma require strict immobilization for at least 3 to 4 weeks, require more intense physical therapy recovery exercises, and have a greater risk of partial tendon tear. Despite the inconvenience of casting and the risk of corticosteroid use, the decision to treat with rigid immobilization or local injection should not be postponed for moderate to severe disease. Chronic inflammation around and through the tendon contributes in a major way to spontaneous tendon rupture. Significant degrees of tendon inflammation must be treated in a timely fashion. Local injection should be strongly considered at 2 to 3 months if tendon thickening is dramatic. Lastly, all spontaneous tendon ruptures and most cases of persistent tendinitis should be evaluated by an orthopedic surgeon. Primary tendon repair can be combined with surgical stripping of the peritendinous tissue or sharp dissection of the mucinoid degeneration.

PRE-ACHILLES BURSITIS

Enter over the posterior-superior aspect of the calcaneus, directly in the midline.

Needle: $^5/_8$-inch, 25-gauge
Depth: $^1/_4$ to $^3/_8$ inch
Volume: 0.5 to 1 mL of anesthetic and 0.5 mL of D80

NOTE: The injection should be superficial to the tendon; high pressure when injecting suggests an intratendinous position.

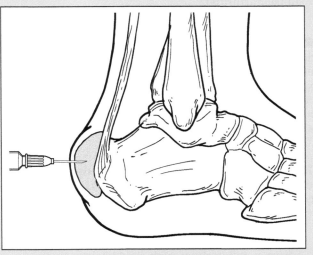

FIGURE 10–4. Pre-Achilles bursa injection.

DESCRIPTION Pre-Achilles bursitis (also called the "pump bump") is an inflammation of the bursal sac located between the calcaneal insertion of the Achilles tendon and the overlying skin. Its function is to reduce the friction between the skin and the tendon caused by poorly fitted or tight shoes. Although frequently misdiagnosed as Achilles tendinitis, it is distinctly different in pathology, location, and response to treatment. The tenderness and inflammation of pre-Achilles bursitis are located directly over the calcaneus. By contrast, the tenderness and tendon thickening of Achilles tendinitis are located 1½ inches above the calcaneus. Chronic irritation of the bursa can lead to calcification just posterior to the calcaneus (Haglund's deformity). Pre-Achilles bursitis is rarely disabling and does not contribute directly to tendon rupture.

SYMPTOMS The patient has pain and localized swelling behind the heel. The patient attempts to rotate the foot to show the swelling or rubs along the posterior heel when describing the condition.

"I can't find a comfortable pair of shoes. I can't stand any pressure over the back of my heel."

"There's a lump over the back of my heel."

"My doctor tells me that I have a calcium deposit over the back of my heel. He referred me to you because he didn't know how to treat it."

"The back of my heel hurts."

EXAM The exam assesses local bursal tenderness and swelling.

EXAM SUMMARY

1. Local tenderness and swelling directly over the posterior calcaneus
2. Minimal pain with stretching of the ankle in dorsiflexion, passively performed
3. Painless resisted plantar flexion of the ankle, performed isometrically
4. Normal ROM of the ankle

(1) Local tenderness and swelling are present directly over the posterior calcaneus. The quarter-sized area of inflammation is 1 inch superior to the heel pad, in the midline. *(2)* Signs of Achilles tendinitis are absent. Passive stretching of the tendon in dorsiflexion is minimally aggravating. *(3)* Actively resisted plantar flexion also is minimally aggravating. *(4)* The ROM of the ankle is normal.

X-RAYS Plain x-rays of the ankle are often ordered, but are unnecessary for the diagnosis. The lateral view may show calcification arising at the posterior calcaneus. In most cases, the presence of the calcification does *not* influence either the clinical decision making or the long-term outcome. Calcific deposits approaching 1 cm in length are large enough to cause pressure and affect walking, however.

SPECIAL TESTING No special testing is indicated.

DIAGNOSIS The diagnosis is based on the findings of swelling and tenderness on physical exam. A regional anesthetic block is rarely necessary to distinguish superficial involvement of the bursa from any involvement of the underlying calcaneus (stress fracture, epiphysitis, or subtalar arthritis).

TREATMENT The goals of treatment are to reduce the friction over the heel, to reduce the bursal inflammation, and to prevent recurrent bursitis by means of stretching exercises. The treatment of choice involves measures to reduce friction over the back of the heel (a large felt ring, moleskin, New-Skin, v-notched tennis shoes, or padded heel cups).

STEP 1 Prescribe padded heel cups, moleskin, double socks, or adhesive New-Skin (p. 259) to reduce heel friction.

Suggest the use of a large felt ring (p. 263).

Recommend the wearing of fleece heel pads while lying in bed.

Advise avoiding shoes with rigid backs.

Recommend v-notched tennis shoes.

Advise on shortening the walking and running stride.

Recommend passive Achilles tendon stretching exercises (p. 292) after acute swelling and inflammation have resolved.

STEP 2 (3 TO 6 WEEKS FOR PERSISTENT CASES) Perform a local injection of D80.

Re-emphasize the recommendations of Step 1.

STEP 3 (8 TO 10 WEEKS FOR PERSISTENT CASES) Repeat the injection at 4 to 6 weeks if symptoms are not relieved by at least 50%.

Encourage the patient to combine the second injection with a walking cast.

STEP 4 (2 TO 3 MONTHS FOR CHRONIC CASES) Consider an orthopedic consultation for large calcifications or chronic inflammation.

Delay full activities until all signs of irritation have resolved, and full flexibility is restored.

PHYSICAL THERAPY Physical therapy plays a minor role compared with measures to reduce friction, local injection, and immobilization. Ice is an effective analgesic because the bursa is located in the superficial tissues, $1/2$ to $3/8$ inch below the skin surface. Stretching exercises of the Achilles tendon are generally helpful (p. 292).

INJECTION Local injection with anesthetic is often used to confirm the diagnosis and can be combined with corticosteroid to arrest the local inflammation effectively. Injection and fixed immobilization (air or walking cast) can be combined to improve the outcome in severe or recurrent cases.

Position The patient is placed in the prone position with the foot over the edge of the table. The ankle is kept in neutral position.

Surface Anatomy and Point of Entry The insertion of the Achilles tendon on the calcaneus is identified. The point of entry is in the midline, directly over the superior portion of the tendon attachment.

Angle of Entry and Depth The angle of entry is perpendicular to the skin. The depth is located at the interface of the dermis and the firm to hard resistance of the tendon insertion, approximately $1/4$ to $3/8$ inch from skin.

Anesthesia Ethyl chloride is sprayed on the skin. Local anesthetic is placed just under the skin in the subcutaneous tissue (0.25 mL) and just posterior to the tendon (0.25 to 0.5 mL).

Technique A *special pressure technique* is used to identify the bursal sac accurately. The skin is puckered in the midline to facilitate entry of the needle. The needle is advanced down to the firm to hard tissue resistance of the tendon (felt with the needle tip as increased tissue resistance or as increased pressure when attempting to inject anesthetic). With a constant, moderate injection pressure, the needle is withdrawn very slowly until the anesthetic flows easily. The proper placement should create a visible bulge the size of a dime. *Note:* The bursa accepts only a small volume. The least possible amount of anesthetic should be used to confirm the diagnosis. The patient is then re-examined. If the local tenderness is significantly relieved, 0.5 mL of D80 is injected. *Caution:* Firm to hard pressure on injection suggests an intratendinous injection.

INJECTION AFTERCARE

1. *Rest* for 3 days, avoiding all unnecessary weightbearing.
2. Recommend lace-up high-top shoes with generous heel padding (double socks, felt ring, or mole-foam) to protect the heel from direct pressure.
3. Use *ice* (15 minutes every 4 to 6 hours) and *acetaminophen* (1000 mg twice a day) for postinjection soreness.
4. *Protect* the ankle for 3 to 4 weeks by avoiding all unnecessary walking and standing.
5. Recommend shortening the stride: *"Take extra time when walking to and from work."*
6. Begin *passive stretching* of the ankle in flexion and extension after the pain and swelling have resolved.
7. Repeat *injection* at 6 weeks with corticosteroid if swelling recurs or persists.
8. Request *plain x-rays* and a *consultation* with an orthopedic surgeon or podiatrist if two consecutive injections fail, and the patient still complains of posterior heel pain.

SURGICAL PROCEDURE Surgical removal of large calcaneal calcification is necessary when chronic irritation of the bursa accompanies calcification greater than 1 cm in length.

PROGNOSIS This lower extremity bursa is sensitive to pressure and friction from shoes and may be difficult

PRE-ACHILLES BURSA INJECTION

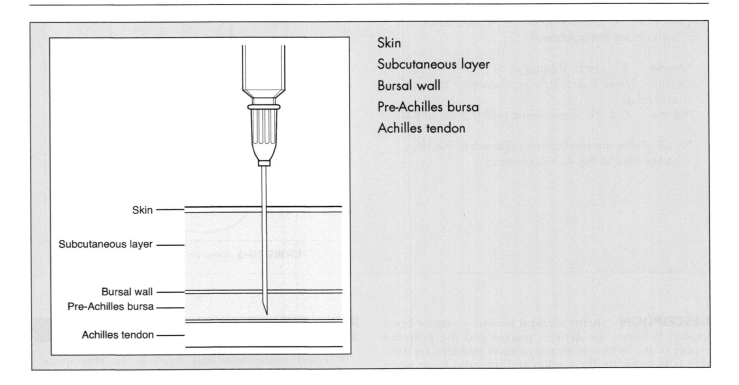

Skin
Subcutaneous layer
Bursal wall
Pre-Achilles bursa
Achilles tendon

Skin ——
Subcutaneous layer ——
Bursal wall ——
Pre-Achilles bursa ——
Achilles tendon ——

to heal. Re-treatment is not unusual. Mildly symptomatic bursitis responds to ice, shortening of the stride, measures to reduce friction over the tendon (double socks, molefoam, New-Skin, heel cups, or adhesive pads), and gradual tendon stretching, Moderate to severe cases usually require corticosteroid injection (D80) combined with an air cast or a short-leg walking cast for 3 weeks (p. 260).

Patients who fail to experience long-term relief from local injection should have plain x-rays of the ankle to evaluate the integrity of the calcaneus and to determine the presence of Achilles tendon calcification. Patients with calcaneal spurs greater than 1 cm have a guarded prognosis; they are more likely to require surgery.

RETROCALCANEAL BURSITIS

Enter from the lateral side of the Achilles tendon, 1 inch above the calcaneus.

Needle: 1 1/2-inch, 22-gauge
Depth: 3/4 to 1 inch (1/2 inch posterior to the tibia and talus)
Volume: 0.5 mL of anesthetic and 0.5 mL of K40

NOTE: Place the medication adjacent to the talus rather than to the Achilles tendon.

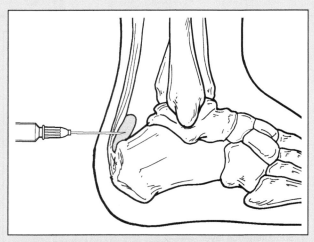

FIGURE 10–5. Retrocalcaneal bursa injection.

DESCRIPTION   Retrocalcaneal bursitis—a minor bursa located between the Achilles tendon and the posterior aspect of the ankle—is an uncommon problem. Its function is to lubricate the tendon and the talus bone when the foot is in extreme plantar flexion. Symptoms consist of a vague posterior heel pain aggravated by extreme plantar flexion. The diagnosis is suggested by fullness in the space behind the ankle and local tenderness in the soft-tissue space between the Achilles tendon and the ankle and is confirmed by a regional anesthetic block placed in the bursa. The differential diagnosis includes calcaneal stress fracture, arthritis of the ankle, and tarsal tunnel syndrome.

SYMPTOMS   The patient has ankle pain behind the ankle and painful walking. The patient often takes two fingers and rubs along either side of the Achilles tendon.

"The back of my ankle hurts whenever I go upstairs too fast."

"I've lost my ankle bones ... the back of my foot is all swollen."

"No one seems to know what's wrong with me. My x-rays are normal. My blood tests don't show gout or anything. Even my MRI is okay. The back of my ankle still hurts."

"My knee has been swollen, and I've been limping. Now I have a pain in the back of my ankle."

"I can't see any swelling. My ankle still moves okay, but I'm having this pain behind my ankle."

EXAM   The patient is examined for local tenderness and swelling in the soft tissues behind the ankle, and Achilles tendon flexibility is evaluated.

EXAM SUMMARY

1. Local tenderness and swelling in the space between the Achilles tendon and the ankle
2. Pain aggravated by ankle plantar flexion, passively performed
3. Painless resisted ankle eversion, inversion, and plantar flexion, isometrically performed
4. Normal ROM of the ankle

(1) Local tenderness and swelling are present in the soft-tissue space between the Achilles tendon and the posterior ankle. Pressure applied to the soft tissues just posterior to the talus is painful. Severe cases may swell dramatically, filling in the space between the talus and the Achilles tendon and obscuring the posterior aspects of the medial and lateral malleoli. *(2)* The pain is aggravated by forcing the ankle into extreme plantar flexion, compressing the bursa. *(3)* The bursa is unaffected by isometric testing of the tendons that cross the ankle. Resisted ankle dorsiflexion, plantar flexion, inversion, and eversion are painless. *(4)* The ROM of the ankle is normal.

X-RAYS   X-rays of the ankle are unnecessary for the diagnosis. Calcification does not occur. Ankle films or a radionuclide bone scan may be necessary in a long-distance runner to exclude a stress fracture of the calcaneus.

SPECIAL TESTING   No special testing is indicated.

DIAGNOSIS   A presumptive diagnosis is based on the characteristic findings on physical exam. The diagnosis is confirmed by a regional anesthetic block placed in the bursa adjacent to the talus.

TREATMENT   The goals of treatment are to reduce the swelling and inflammation in the bursa and to prevent a recurrence by recommending Achilles tendon–stretching exercises. The treatment of choice comprises restrictions placed at the ankle and local corticosteroid injection.

STEP 1   Define the extent of the swelling, measure the ROM of the ankle, and perform local anesthetic block to distinguish involvement of the bursa as opposed to the adjacent bone or ankle joint.

Advise restriction of repetitive ankle motion (e.g., limit stair climbing, walk on flat surfaces, no jumping or jogging).

Advise the patient to avoid high heels.

Suggest shortening the stride when walking.

Prescribe padded heel cups (p. 261) to reduce the effects of impact.

STEP 2 (3 TO 6 WEEKS FOR PERSISTENT CASES)   Prescribe an NSAID (e.g., ibuprofen), and note that it may have limited benefit because of poor tissue penetration.

Perform a local injection of K40 if NSAIDs are ineffective or contraindicated.

Suggest high-top shoes or apply a Velcro ankle brace (p. 259).

STEP 3 (8 TO 10 WEEKS FOR PERSISTENT CASES)   Repeat the injection in 4 to 6 weeks if symptoms have not decreased by 50%.

STEP 4 (12 TO 14 WEEKS)   Recommend stretching exercises for the Achilles tendon (p. 292) if ankle flexibility has been diminished.

PHYSICAL THERAPY   Physical therapy plays a minor role in the treatment of retrocalcaneal bursitis. Ice and elevation always are recommended for pain and swelling. Recommendations are made for the general care of the ankle. There are no other specific treatments for this isolated bursitis.

INJECTION   Local injection with anesthetic is used to confirm the diagnosis and to differentiate this soft-tissue condition from ankle arthritis, calcaneal bony lesions, and tarsal tunnel. Local corticosteroid injection is the preferred anti-inflammatory treatment.

Position   The patient is placed in the prone position with the foot hanging over the end of the exam table. The ankle is kept in neutral position.

RETROCALCANEAL BURSA INJECTION

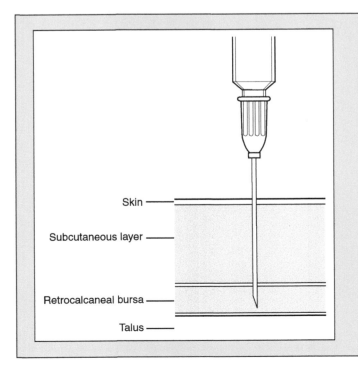

Skin
Subcutaneous layer
Retrocalcaneal bursa
Talus

Surface Anatomy and Point of Entry The Achilles tendon, the superior portion of the calcaneus, and the posterior aspect of the ankle are identified and marked. The point of entry is lateral to the Achilles tendon, 1 inch above the calcaneus.

Angle of Entry and Depth The needle is angled from the lateral aspect of the Achilles tendon toward the center and midline of the talus. The depth is approximately 1 inch.

Anesthesia Ethyl chloride is sprayed on the skin. Local anesthetic is placed in the subcutaneous tissue (0.5 mL) and just posterior to the talus (0.5 mL).

Technique A *lateral approach* is used to avoid the neurovascular bundle of the foot and the posterior tibialis artery and nerve. The needle is advanced down to the hard resistance of the talus. Local anesthetic is injected just posterior to the talus, and the patient is re-examined. If local tenderness and pain with forced plantar flexion are relieved, 0.5 mL of K40 is injected.

INJECTION AFTERCARE

1. *Rest* for 3 days, avoiding all unnecessary weightbearing.
2. Recommend *lace-up high-top shoes with generous heel padding* (double socks, felt ring, or mole-foam) to protect the heel from direct pressure.
3. Use *ice* (15 minutes every 4 to 6 hours) and *acetaminophen* (1000 mg twice a day) for postinjection soreness.

4. *Protect* the ankle for 3 to 4 weeks by avoiding all unnecessary walking and standing.
5. Recommend shortening the stride: *"Take extra time when walking to and from work."*
6. Begin *passive stretching* of the ankle in flexion and extension at 3 to 4 weeks after the pain and swelling have resolved.
7. Repeat the *injection* at 6 weeks with corticosteroid if pain recurs or persists.
8. Request *plain x-rays* of the ankle (look for subtle changes in the tibiotalar joint) and a *consultation* with an orthopedic surgeon or podiatrist if two consecutive injections fail, and the patient still complains of posterior heel pain.

SURGICAL PROCEDURE No surgical procedure is indicated.

PROGNOSIS Retrocalcaneal bursitis is an uncommon condition. Local corticosteroid injection is an effective treatment. Stretching and strengthening exercises of the Achilles tendon decrease the likelihood of a recurrence. If symptoms and signs persist, subtle abnormalities of the ankle joint (pronation, arthritis, tarsal coalition), the talus (subtalar arthritis, talar dome osteochondritis dissecans), or the calcaneus (bony lesions) need to be excluded. Bursectomy is not performed.

POSTERIOR TIBIALIS TENOSYNOVITIS

Enter just below the posterior edge of the medial malleolus.

Needle: ⁵/₈-inch, 25-gauge
Depth: ³/₈ to ¹/₂ inch
Volume: 1 to 2 mL of anesthetic and 0.5 mL of D80

NOTE: Keep the bevel of the needle parallel to the tendon.

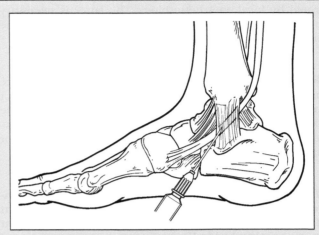

FIGURE 10–6. Posterior tibialis tendon injection.

DESCRIPTION Tenosynovitis of the posterior tibialis, an inverter of the foot, is an inflammation of the tendon as it courses around the medial malleolus. It is covered by a tenosynovial sheath that provides lubrication and reduces friction as it curves under the bone. The patient complains of medial ankle pain. The exam reveals local tenderness and swelling just under the medial malleolus, pain aggravated by resisted inversion and plantar flexion, and pain aggravated by passively stretching the ankle in eversion. Ankle pronation, pes planus, ankle arthritis, and excessive body weight are predisposing factors to active tenosynovitis. In cases of severe pronation, tenosynovitis may be accompanied by the entrapment of the posterior tibial nerve (tarsal tunnel syndrome).

SYMPTOMS The patient complains of pain and swelling on the inner aspect of the ankle and painful walking. The patient points to the area of irritation when describing the symptoms.

"I have this sharp pain around the inside of my ankle whenever I step."

"There's swelling around the back of my ankle (pointing to the inner aspect of the ankle)."

"Tight shoes have rubbed the inside of my ankle raw .... It must be inside because the skin looks normal."

EXAM The patient is examined for inflammation and swelling of the tendon sheath, and ankle ROM and alignment are assessed.

EXAM SUMMARY

1. Local tenderness and swelling just inferior and posterior to the medial malleolus
2. Pain aggravated by resisting ankle inversion and plantar flexion, isometrically performed
3. Pain aggravated by stretching in eversion, passively performed (variably present)
4. Normal ROM of the ankle
5. Associated conditions, including ankle pronation, pes planus, or pes cavus

(1) Local tenderness and swelling are located in a crescent-shaped area inferior and posterior to the medial malleolus. The swelling may be so dramatic as to fill in the space below the inferior tip of the malleolus. *(2)* The pain consistently is aggravated by resisting the action of the tendon isometrically. Inversion is usually more painful than resisting plantar flexion. *(3)* The pain is aggravated less predictably by forced eversion of the ankle, passively performed. *(4)* The ROM of the ankle is normal in an uncomplicated case. *(5)* Pes planus, pes cavus, or ankle pronation may be present.

X-RAYS X-rays are unnecessary for the diagnosis. Calcification does not occur. Ankle views are normal, unless there is a concomitant arthritic process.

SPECIAL TESTING No special testing is indicated.

DIAGNOSIS A presumptive diagnosis is based on a history of medial ankle pain and an exam showing local tenosynovial tenderness and isometric pain that is confirmed by local anesthetic block. The latter is necessary to distinguish tenosynovitis from the pain arising from the ankle joint or tarsal tunnel.

TREATMENT The goals of treatment are to reduce the inflammation in the tendon sheath and to correct any underlying abnormalities of the ankle joint or ankle alignment. The initial treatment of choice involves correction of ankle pronation, pes planus, or pes cavus or management of ankle arthritis.

STEP 1 **Perform a local anesthetic injection to confirm the diagnosis and to distinguish involvement of the tendon from involvement of the ankle joint or supporting ankle ligaments.**

Evaluate and correct ankle pronation (high-top shoes, arch supports, or a medial wedge), pes planus (arch supports), or metatarsalgia (padded insoles).

Advise the patient to limit direct pressure or impact and unnecessary standing and walking.

Suggest shortening the walking stride to reduce the tension across the tendon.

Recommend ice applications to reduce pain and swelling.

Prescribe a Velcro pull-on ankle brace (p. 259).

Prescribe an NSAID (e.g., ibuprofen) for 4 weeks at full dosage.

STEP 2 (6 TO 8 WEEKS FOR PERSISTENT CASES) **Perform a local injection of D80, and combine it with immobilization (e.g., short-leg walking cast, air cast).**

Repeat the injection of D80 if symptoms have not improved by 50%.

Strongly suggest combining the second injection with rigid immobilization if this was not recommended with the first injection.

STEP 3 (8 TO 10 WEEKS FOR RECOVERY) **Advise gentle performance of passive stretching exercises of the ankle in all four directions.**

Recommend isometric toning of ankle inversion and eversion (p. 293) when symptoms have nearly resolved.

Consider a referral to a podiatrist for custom-made, plaster-molded, rigid orthotics.

PHYSICAL THERAPY Physical therapy is important in the rehabilitation of posterior tibialis tenosynovitis in the postcast recovery period. Gradual stretching exercises of the ankle (emphasizing dorsiflexion and eversion) are performed daily (p. 292). These exercises are performed in sets of 20 after heating the ankle. They are begun immediately after casting or approximately 4 weeks after local injection.

INJECTION Local injection with anesthetic can be used to confirm the diagnosis and to differentiate this soft-tissue condition from subtalar arthritis. Local corticosteroid is indicated for persistent symptoms that fail to respond to correction of ankle alignment, arch abnormalities, and ankle immobilization.

Position The patient is placed in the supine position. The leg is kept straight, and the lower leg is externally rotated.

Surface Anatomy and Point of Entry The tip of the medial malleolus is identified. The needle is inserted just behind the posterior edge of the bone.

Angle of Entry and Depth The needle is inserted perpendicular to the skin and is advanced to the firm resistance of the tendon ($^3/_8$ inch) or the hard resistance of the bone ($^1/_2$ inch).

Anesthesia Ethyl chloride is sprayed on the skin. Local anesthetic is placed in the subcutaneous tissue (0.5 mL) and at the firm resistance of the tendon (0.5 mL).

Technique An *intratenosynovial* injection is the aim of this technique. It can be performed in two ways. If the rubbery-firm resistance of the tendon is identified easily as the needle is advanced, the injection can be placed at this more superficial site. If the tendon is not readily identified, however, the needle is advanced down to the hard resistance of the bone. The injection is placed just off the bone by withdrawing $^1/_8$ inch. *Note:* The bevel must be kept parallel to the course of the tendon fibers. Always note the position of the bevel relative to the printing along the side of the syringe before entering the skin. In either case, the pressure of injection is minimal if the needle is in the tenosynovial sheath. Finally, if the local tenderness and isometric pain with resisted ankle inversion are improved, 0.5 mL of D80 is injected.

INJECTION AFTERCARE

1. *Rest* for 3 days, avoiding all unnecessary weight-bearing.
2. Recommend *lace-up high-top shoes, an air cast, or a short-leg walking cast,* depending on the severity of the symptoms and signs and the associated conditions (e.g., pronation, arthritis).
3. Use *ice* (15 minutes every 4 to 6 hours) and *acetaminophen* (1000 mg twice a day) for postinjection soreness.
4. *Protect* the ankle for 3 to 4 weeks by avoiding all unnecessary walking and standing.
5. Recommend *shortening the stride* to reduce the stress on the tendon.
6. Begin *passive stretching* of the ankle in flexion and extension at 3 to 4 weeks.
7. Begin *isometric toning exercises* of ankle inversion and eversion after flexibility has been partially restored.
8. Repeat *injection* at 6 weeks with corticosteroid if pain recurs or persists.
9. Request *plain x-rays* of the ankle (look for subtle changes in the tibiotalar joint) and a *consultation* with an orthopedic surgeon or podiatrist if two consecutive injections fail, and the patient still complains of medial ankle pain and swelling.

POSTERIOR TIBIALIS TENDON INJECTION

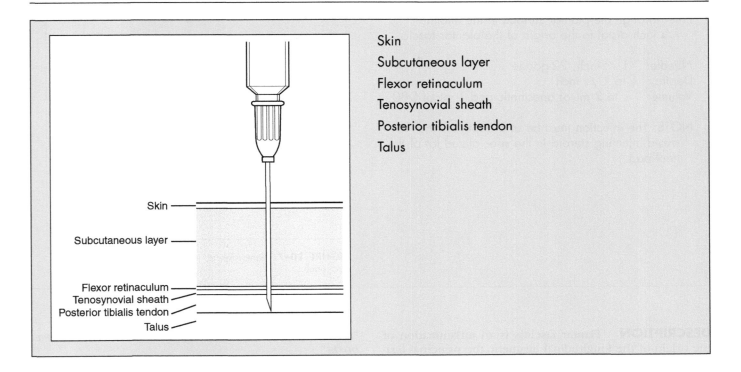

Skin
Subcutaneous layer
Flexor retinaculum
Tenosynovial sheath
Posterior tibialis tendon
Talus

Skin ———
Subcutaneous layer ———
Flexor retinaculum ———
Tenosynovial sheath ———
Posterior tibialis tendon ———
Talus ———

SURGICAL PROCEDURE   No surgical procedure is indicated.

PROGNOSIS   An injection combined with immobilization is usually successful in uncomplicated cases (e.g., no pronation or pes planus). Recurrent tenosynovitis is often a result of the biomechanical stresses of difficult-to-manage ankle instability, ankle deformity, obesity, or old trauma. Long-term success depends on the correction of these associated conditions. Surgery usually is reserved for tendon rupture, a rare event.

PLANTAR FASCIITIS

Enter through the plantar surface in the midline
  ³/₄ inch distal to the origin of the plantar fascia.

Needle: 1¹/₂-inch, 22-gauge
Depth: 1 to 1¹/₂ inch
Volume: 1 to 2 mL of anesthetic and 1 mL of D80

NOTE: The injection must be at a depth >1 inch to
  avoid injecting steroid in the specialized fat of the
  heel pad.

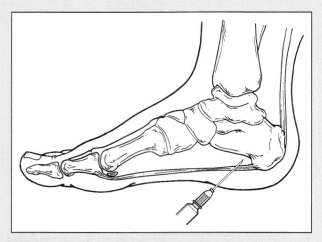

FIGURE 10–7. Plantar fascial injection from the plantar approach.

DESCRIPTION   Plantar fasciitis is an inflammation of the origin of the longitudinal ligament, the principal ligament that forms the arch of the foot. Flat feet (pes planus), high arches (pes cavus), turned-in ankles (ankle pronation), and short Achilles tendons predispose to this condition. Obesity, working on concrete, poorly fitted shoes, and prolonged daily standing aggravate the condition. A few cases are purely inflammatory in nature and are associated with Reiter's syndrome.

Patients with plantar fasciitis complain of localized tenderness at or just medial to the origin of the fascia with minimal pain when compressing the calcaneus. By contrast, patients diagnosed with heel pad syndrome complain of diffuse heel pain and exhibit diffuse heel tenderness. Patients with calcaneal fracture, calcaneal stress fracture, or Sever's epiphysitis complain of diffuse heel pain that can be reproduced by side-to-side compression of the calcaneus on exam.

SYMPTOMS   The patient complains of heel pain aggravated by walking and standing. The patient grabs the bottom of the heel and rubs it back and forth when describing the condition.

"Whenever I put pressure down on my heel, I get a severe, sharp pain under my heel."

"The pressure over my heel is so bad that I have started to walk on my tiptoes."

"My flat feet never bothered me until I took this job where I have to stand on concrete all day long."

"I can't wear these kinds of shoes (flats) because my heel will really start to hurt."

"It's like the bottom of my heel is bruised."

"I can't wear high heels any more because my heel hurts."

"I can't do my aerobics any more because of my heel."

EXAM   The patient is examined for local irritation and inflammation of the origin of the plantar fascia, and ankle alignment, Achilles tendon flexibility, and the configuration of the arch of the foot are evaluated.

EXAM SUMMARY

1. Local tenderness at the calcaneal origin of the plantar fascia
2. Pain with calcaneal compression
3. Achilles tendon inflexibility
4. Associated conditions include ankle pronation, pes planus, and pes cavus
5. Anesthetic block at the origin of the plantar fascia

(1) Local tenderness is present in the midline or slightly medial of midline at the origin of the longitudinal arch of the foot. The dime-sized area of tenderness is located 1¹/₄ to 1¹/₂ inches from the posterior heel. Firm pressure may be needed. *(2)* Medial to lateral compression of the calcaneus may be mildly painful, but rarely more painful than the local tenderness. If the calcaneal compression sign is more painful than the local tenderness, studies should be obtained to exclude a calcaneal stress fracture. *(3)* Achilles tendon flexibility may be limited, especially in cases with a duration of 2 to 3 months. The tendon often

shortens as a result of a shortened stride or favoring the foot. Normally the ankle should dorsiflex 25 to 30 degrees. *(4)* Ankle pronation, pes planus, and pes cavus may be associated findings. Ankle alignment and arch configuration must be examined in the standing position.

X-RAYS Plain x-rays of the ankle are unnecessary to make the diagnosis. X-rays are indicated for long-distance runners to exclude a stress fracture of the calcaneus, for patients with calcaneal injuries to exclude a routine fracture, and for patients with chronic symptoms to exclude a large (>1 cm), pressure-aggravated heel spur. Small calcaneal calcifications at the origin of the fascia are exceedingly common (10% of the population—much greater than the incidence of fasciitis); they are a reflection of the chronic inflammatory response. These small heel spurs, protected by the shelf of the calcaneus, are not an indication for surgery.

SPECIAL TESTING Nuclear medicine bone scanning is used to exclude a stress fracture in a long-distance runner. A bone scan should be obtained when the calcaneal compression sign is more painful than the local heel tenderness.

DIAGNOSIS The diagnosis is based on the history and the characteristic findings on physical exam. A regional anesthetic block at the origin of the plantar fascia can be used to differentiate heel pad syndrome (self-limited irritation to the specialized fat of the heel), calcaneal stress fracture (seen nearly exclusively in runners), and subtalar arthritis.

TREATMENT The goals of treatment are to reduce the inflammation in the longitudinal arch and to improve the mechanics of the heel and ankle. Treatment always should start with padded arch supports, correction of ankle pronation, and reduced weightbearing.

STEP 1 **Examine the heel, evaluate the configuration of the arch with the patient standing, and confirm the diagnosis with local anesthesia in selected cases.**

　Recommend cushioning for the heel with heel cups, foam to stand on at work, and padded insoles for mild disease (p. 262).

　Recommend padded arch supports (e.g., Spenco, Sorbothane) to be worn continuously in well-fitted shoes (p. 262).

　Advise the patient to avoid tiptoeing or pressure across the ball of the feet (e.g., stairs, pedals, exercise equipment) and to limit standing and walking.

　Recommend application of ice to the heel.

　Recommend Achilles tendon–stretching exercises performed by hand pressure initially, followed by wall stretches as flexibility is regained (p. 292).

　Suggest massage over the heel with a rubber ball.

STEP 2 (3 TO 4 WEEKS FOR PERSISTENT CASES) **Prescribe an NSAID (e.g., ibuprofen), and note that the response may be limited because of poor penetration.**

　Offer taping of the ankle and the arch to support the arch.

　Re-emphasize the use of padding.

STEP 3 (6 TO 8 WEEKS FOR PERSISTENT CASES) **Obtain x-rays of the foot (including posteroanterior, posteroanterior oblique, and lateral views).**

　Perform a local injection of D80, and combine with immobilization using high-top shoes with soft arch supports in place.

　Repeat the injection in 4 to 6 weeks if symptoms have not decreased by 50%, and combine with immobilization using either an air cast or a short-leg walking cast for greater protection.

　Recommend custom-made arch supports for patients with dramatic degrees of pes planus or pes cavus.

STEP 4 (3 TO 4 MONTHS FOR CHRONIC CASES) **Consider a referral to a podiatrist for surgical débridement.**

PHYSICAL THERAPY Physical therapy plays a significant role in the active treatment of plantar fasciitis and in its prevention.

PHYSICAL THERAPY SUMMARY

1. Ice for acute pain
2. Heat and massage of the heel
3. Achilles tendon stretching, passively performed

Acute Period Ice, massage, and padding are used in the first several weeks to reduce pain and swelling. *Ice* placed over the center of the heel provides effective analgesia and may help to reduce swelling. Cold must be applied for 10 to 15 minutes to penetrate $^3/_4$ to 1 inch down to the origin of the fascia. For other patients, *heating and massage* provide more effective analgesia and may help to disperse swelling. Massage can be accomplished by rolling a tennis ball under the heel or using a vibrating foot massage unit.

Recovery and Rehabilitation After the acute symptoms have decreased significantly, stretching exercises are begun. The most important treatment for plantar fasciitis is *Achilles tendon–stretching exercises* (p. 292). Increasing Achilles tendon flexibility lessens the tension over the plantar fascia. The fascia, calcaneus, and Achilles tendon must share the workload of ankle motion. Stiffness in one area increases the tension and stress in other areas. Passive and active stretching exercises should be performed daily. The combined use of padded insoles, arch supports, and shoes with good support makes plantar fasciitis less likely to recur.

INJECTION   Treatment focuses on padding the heel (heel cups, heel cushions, padded insoles), supporting the arch (padded arch supports, shoes with good support), and doing Achilles tendon–stretching exercises. Local injection with corticosteroids is indicated for persistent symptoms. Difficult cases may require two injections and rigid immobilization.

Position   The patient is placed in the prone position with the foot hanging just off the edge of the exam table.

Surface Anatomy and Point of Entry   The inferior surface of the calcaneus and the origin of the plantar fascia (approximately 1 to 1½ inches from the back of the heel) are identified. The point of entry is ¾ inch *distal* to the origin of the fascia in the midline.

Angle of Entry and Depth   The needle is inserted at a 45-degree angle and is advanced to the firm resistance of the fascia (1 inch) and then to the hard resistance of the bone (1½ inches).

Anesthesia   Ethyl chloride is sprayed on the skin. Local anesthetic is placed in the subcutaneous tissue (0.5 mL), intradermally (0.25 mL), at the firm resistance of the fascia (0.5 mL), and in between the fascia and the calcaneus (0.5 mL).

Technique   To inject accurately between the plantar fascia and the calcaneus and avoid injecting into the specialized fat of the heel pad, a *plantar approach* is strongly suggested. Generous anesthesia is given at the plantar surface. The needle is advanced through the low-resistance fat to the subtle to firm resistance of the fascia. A popping or giving-way often is felt when passing through the fascia. *Caution:* The patient may experience pain as the periosteum is touched. If the local tenderness is significantly relieved, 1 mL of D80 is injected slowly. *Caution:* The space is small; a rapid injection of medication can be painful.

INJECTION AFTERCARE

1. *Rest* for 3 days, avoiding all unnecessary weightbearing.
2. Recommend *immobilization* with lace-up high-top shoes, an air cast, or a short-leg walking cast, depending on the severity and associated pronation or arthritis.
3. Use *ice* (15 minutes every 4 to 6 hours) and *acetaminophen* (1000 mg twice a day) for postinjection soreness.
4. *Protect* the ankle for 3 to 4 weeks by limiting all unnecessary walking and standing.
5. Recommend *shortening the stride* to reduce the stress on the fascia.
6. Begin *passive stretching* of the Achilles tendon at 3 to 4 weeks after pain and swelling have resolved.
7. Repeat *injection* at 6 weeks if pain recurs or persists, and combine with immobilization.
8. Request a *consultation* with an orthopedic surgeon or podiatrist if two consecutive injections and fixed immobilization fail.

PLANTAR FASCIITIS INJECTION

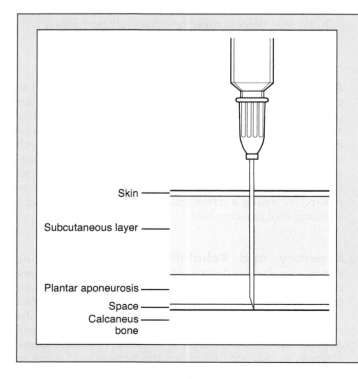

Skin
Subcutaneous layer
Plantar aponeurosis
Space
Calcaneus

Skin
Subcutaneous layer
Plantar aponeurosis
Space
Calcaneus
bone

SURGICAL PROCEDURE   Surgical procedures include fascial débridement and calcaneal spur removal.

PROGNOSIS   Corticosteroid injection combined with padded arch supports and limited weightbearing is successful in approximately 60% of cases. Because plantar fasciitis results from the biomechanical stresses caused by tight Achilles tendons, ankle pronation, and abnormalities of the arch, the response to treatment can be enhanced by combining the injection with 3 to 4 weeks of rigid immobilization (a short-leg walking cast). Persistent or recurrent fasciitis (approximately 10% of cases) is seen most often in patients with obesity, with abnormal arch and ankle conditions, with calcaneal spurs greater than $1/2$ to $3/4$ inch in length, or with jobs demanding prolonged standing or walking on concrete surfaces. Surgical débridement of the devitalized tissue or resection of the accompanying bone spur (>1 cm) can be considered in these cases.

HEEL PAD SYNDROME

Treatment of choice is padded heel cups.

Calcaneus
Specialized
Fat of the heel
Plantar fascia

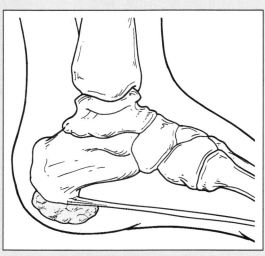

FIGURE 10-8. Heel pad syndrome.

DESCRIPTION Traumatic irritation of the specialized fat that covers and protects the calcaneus is referred to as *heel pad syndrome*. The diagnosis is suggested by a history of trauma, diffuse tenderness over the entire heel, pain aggravated by squeezing the fat pad from either side, and an absence of focal bony tenderness (calcaneal fracture or plantar fasciitis). Radiographic studies are normal. The goal of treatment is to reduce the direct pressure over the fat pad, allowing the tissues to heal and to return to normal.

SYMPTOMS The patient complains of diffuse heel pain aggravated by walking and standing. The symptoms are nearly identical to the symptoms of plantar fasciitis.

"It's like the bottom of my heel is bruised."

"I came down hard on my heel when I jumped off the lowest rung of my ladder. Ever since I can't put my full weight down on my heel."

"I have a stone bruise on my heel. I was hiking in the gorge and I came down too hard on a rock."

"I'm walking on the side of my foot because the bottom of my heel hurts too much."

EXAM The patient is examined for sensitivity over the entire bottom of the heel compared with the focal tenderness of the origin of the plantar fascia and the focal bony tenderness characteristic of stress fracture of the calcaneus.

EXAM SUMMARY

1. The entire heel is tender
2. Side-to-side compression of the heel pad is painful
3. Calcaneal compression is nontender
4. Tenderness is present at the origin of the plantar fascia, but it is not more tender than the rest of the heel
5. ROM of the ankle is normal

(1) The entire bottom of the heel is tender to moderate pressure. *(2)* Medial to lateral compression of the heel pad is painful. Grasping the fat pad from either side using the thumb and first finger is painful. *(3)* Sever's epiphysitis, calcaneal stress fracture, or true fracture of the calcaneus is characterized by focal tenderness and pain when compressing the bone from side to side. Using the thumb and first finger or cupping the hands together, medial to lateral compression of the calcaneus is nontender. *(4)* The plantar fascia is normal. The distal aspect of the heel at the origin of the plantar fascia is not more tender than the rest of the heel. *(5)* The tibiotalar and subtalar joints are normal. Ankle pronation and supination are normal and pain-free.

X-RAYS Plain x-rays of the ankle are normal.

SPECIAL TESTING No special testing is indicated.

DIAGNOSIS   The diagnosis is based on the characteristic findings on physical exam localized to the heel pad. Signs of plantar fasciitis, calcaneal bony lesions, and subtalar arthritis are absent.

TREATMENT   The goal of treatment is to protect the heel to allow the specialized fat of the heel pad to heal.

STEP 1   Examine the heel pad, and exclude plantar fasciitis, calcaneal bony lesions, and subtalar arthritis by exam.

Recommend cushioning for the heel with heel cups and a padded fatigue mat to stand on at work (p. 261).

Recommend padded arch supports (e.g., Spenco, Sorbothane) to be worn continuously in well-fitted shoes (p. 262).

Advise the patient to avoid tiptoeing or pressure across the ball of the feet (e.g., stairs, pedals, exercise equipment) and to limit standing and walking.

Recommend application of ice to the heel.

STEP 2 (3 TO 4 WEEKS FOR PERSISTENT CASES)   Reevaluate for plantar fasciitis, calcaneal bony lesions, or subtalar arthritis.

Limit weightbearing and continue heel cups.

PHYSICAL THERAPY   Physical therapy does not play a significant role in the active treatment of heel pad syndrome or in its prevention. Ice is used for the acute phase of the condition.

INJECTION   There is no injection for this condition.

SURGICAL PROCEDURE   There is no surgical procedure for this condition.

PROGNOSIS   Patients with an uncomplicated heel pad syndrome should have resolution of symptoms and signs within 2 to 3 weeks when treated with proper padding of the heel. Patients with persistent symptoms should be evaluated for subtle injury to the calcaneus (stress fracture or nondisplaced fractures), plantar fasciitis, or subtalar joint inflammation.

TIBIAL STRESS FRACTURE

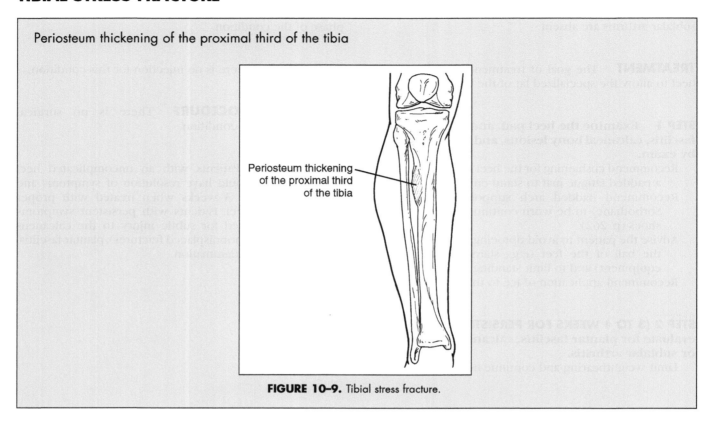

Periosteum thickening of the proximal third of the tibia

Periosteum thickening of the proximal third of the tibia

FIGURE 10–9. Tibial stress fracture.

DESCRIPTION   Stress fractures of the tibia result from repeated microtrauma to the proximal third of the bone, often occurring in the section of the tibia with the smallest cross-sectional area. The condition is seen almost exclusively in runners, professional ballet dancers, and military recruits, although patients with severe osteoporotic bones also are susceptible. Radiographically the periosteum of the tibia is thickened in the proximal third of the bone in runners compared with the middle third of the bone in ballet dancers. A true fracture line is seen rarely. Stress fracture must be distinguished from the more common shin splints, anterior compartment syndrome, and localized pain or paresthesia of the outer lower leg caused by lumbosacral radiculopathy.

SYMPTOMS   The patient complains of a deep pain along the anterior shin. The pain is aggravated by running and prolonged walking and standing. The patient often rubs the anterior portion of the shin when describing the condition and often complains incessantly how this has affected his or her ability to run or play tennis.

"When I hit 8 miles, I start to feel this achy pain in my shin."

"Doc, I think I have shin splints."

"My lower leg only hurts when I run."

"I've developed this tender area on my bone, right here (pointing to the anterior shin)."

EXAM   The patient is examined for tenderness along the anterior tibial surface and for signs of increased development and pressure in the anterior compartment of the leg.

EXAM SUMMARY

1. Patient may have a completely normal exam
2. Anterior tibial tenderness
3. Pain with torque placed across the tibia
4. Normal anterior compartment tension and painless stretch of the anterior tibialis muscle

(1) If the condition is mild, the exam can be completely normal. The tibia can have normal shape and size and be free of any localized tenderness. *(2)* With moderate to severe involvement, tenderness is localized over the affected bone, most commonly the anterior third of the tibia. *(3)* Only the most severe involvement has pain aggravated by placing torque across the bone, a valgus or varus pressure exerted by placing pressure at the knee

and ankle simultaneously. (4) Lastly, the anterior compartment just lateral to the tibia is nontender and of normal tension to palpation.

X-RAYS   Periosteal thickening over several centimeters is the classic change of tibial stress fracture. The thickening of the bone is the natural response to the microtrauma experienced by the tibia. A true fracture line is not seen. Plain x-rays of the tibia may remain normal for weeks, however, depending on the degree of trauma to the bone.

SPECIAL TESTING   Nuclear medicine bone scanning shows increased uptake over several centimeters along the cortex of the tibia. MRI shows early edema of the bone and periosteal thickening that precedes the changes on plain films of the tibia.

DIAGNOSIS   The definite diagnosis of tibial stress fracture requires special testing with either nuclear medicine bone scan or MRI. The physical findings are too nonspecific, and the changes on plain x-rays develop late in the course of the condition.

TREATMENT   The goals of treatment are to reduce the repetitive trauma experienced by the tibia by incorporating padding in well-supporting shoes and padding on the standing area at work (fatigue mats) and by altering exercise, emphasizing routines and activities with less weightbearing.

STEP 1   Examine the lower leg and ankle, palpate the dorsalis pedis and posterior tibialis pulses, measure the capillary fill times in the toes, and obtain plain films of the lower leg, including the knee joints.

Obtain a nuclear bone scan or an MRI if the diagnostic suspicion is high (worsening symptoms, high-end and competitive level activities, local tenderness along the anterior tibia).

Recommend decreased running and impact sport activities and replace with nonimpact bicycling, swimming, or rowing machine for 2 to 3 weeks.

Combine reduced activities and repeat radiographs of the tibia in 2 weeks if diagnostic suspicion is moderate.

Continue nonimpact muscle-toning exercises.

Recommend padded insoles or arch supports (e.g., Spenco, Sorbothane) to be worn continuously in well-fitted shoes (p. 262) during normal activities.

With improvement, gradually resume impact sport activities, increasing the time or distance by increments of 10% to 20% per week.

STEP 2 (3 TO 4 WEEKS FOR PERSISTENT CASES)   Recommend avoiding all impact sports activities for 2 to 3 weeks.

Resort to fixed immobilization with an air cast or short-leg walking cast (p. 260) for 2 to 3 weeks.

Consider repeat MRI if symptoms persist despite compliance with restriction.

Re-emphasize the use of padding in shoes during normal activities and for future prevention.

PHYSICAL THERAPY   Physical therapy does not play a significant role in the treatment of tibial stress fracture. ROM stretching exercises of the ankle are used only when treatment has involved casting.

INJECTION   No injection is indicated for this condition.

SURGICAL PROCEDURE   No surgical procedure is indicated for this condition.

PROGNOSIS   Stress fracture of the tibia is a reversible condition. Appropriate rest and avoidance of impact sports should allow complete healing of the traumatized bone.

GASTROCNEMIUS MUSCLE TEAR

Any of the muscles of the posterior leg can be
    severely strained or partially torn; the posterior leg
    muscles include:
At the knee:

Semimembranosus, semitendinosus
Biceps femoris, plantaris, and popliteus

In the calf:

Soleus and gastrocnemius

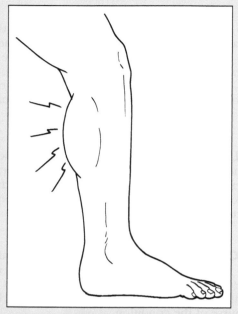

FIGURE 10–10. Gastrocnemius muscle tear.

DESCRIPTION   Gastrocnemius muscle tears usually
occur in the proximal third of the muscle and are nearly
always a result of trauma. Pain and tenderness are typically
focal. A palpable defect in the muscle accompanies the
larger tears. Bleeding or bruising typically is not apparent
initially and rarely at the site of injury. Bleeding dissects
down the leg along the tissue planes to the ankle, forming
the classic crescent sign at the malleolus. This soft-tissue
injury must be distinguished from a ruptured Baker
cyst and lower extremity deep venous thrombosis.

SYMPTOMS   The patient complains of calf pain or
lower leg pain after vigorous activities.

*"I have this really bad charley horse that just won't go
away."*

*"Several days ago I was playing basketball, and I came
down hard on my leg. I felt this really sharp pain in
my calf. Now my ankle is black and blue, but that's not
where it hurts."*

"Doc, my leg hurts and I have a hole in my muscle."

*"I had to run quickly to catch my bus, and I felt this
really sharp pain in my leg muscle."*

*"I think I have another blood clot. My calf muscle hurts
all the time just like it did with my phlebitis."*

EXAM   The patient is examined for local irritation and
tenderness of the intrinsic muscles of the calf.

EXAM SUMMARY

1. Local tenderness of the gastrocnemius muscle
2. Large tears have a persistent palpable defect in the
   muscle
3. Pain aggravated by resisting plantar flexion and
   stretching in dorsiflexion
4. Normal size and nontender Achilles tendon
5. Crescent sign posterior to the malleolus
6. Negative venous ultrasound for deep venous
   thrombosis

(1) Tenderness can be present anywhere along the
length of the gastrocnemius muscle, but tears occur most
commonly in the proximal third of the muscle. The size
varies according to the degree of tear and inflammatory
response. Diffuse tenderness is the rule in the acute
phase, which becomes more focal as healing progresses.
(2) Large tears may manifest a coin-sized defect, which
an athlete often points out to the examiner. *(3)* The
muscular pain typically is aggravated by forcing the foot
into dorsiflexion, stretching and tightening the muscle
injury. Pain is aggravated less predictably by resisting
plantar flexion of the foot isometrically. *(4)* No sign of
Achilles tendinitis is present in uncomplicated cases.
The size, shape, and compression of the tendon are
normal. *(5)* Within days large tears often present with
a crescent-shaped bruising located behind the malleolus
of the ankle, the crescent sign. Blood dissects down the
tissue planes of the leg to pool below the ankle. This is

a nonspecific sign, however. A ruptured Baker cyst, a torn plantaris muscle at the knee, or any lower leg bleeding can cause a crescent sign. (6) Lastly, patients with a previous history of deep venous thrombosis often confuse the symptoms of muscle injury with deep venous thrombosis. Their level of anxiety often dictates the clinician's choice of testing or treatment. With classic signs of muscle tear, a diagnostic ultrasound is unnecessary although frequently obtained to reassure the patient.

X-RAYS   Plain x-rays of the leg are normal.

SPECIAL TESTING   Special testing is unnecessary in routine cases. If the patient has significant risk factors for thrombosis (e.g., history of thrombosis, inactivity, obesity, recent cast or leg brace), a diagnostic ultrasound to exclude deep venous thrombosis is strongly recommended.

DIAGNOSIS   The diagnosis is based on the history of injury and the characteristic changes on exam of the lower leg muscles.

TREATMENT   The goals of treatment are to provide a sufficient interval of time with reduced activities and limited weightbearing to allow the muscle to heal.

STEP 1   Document the type of activity associated with the injury, thoroughly examine the lower calf muscles, and consider ordering a diagnostic ultrasound if the patient has significant risk factors for deep venous thrombosis.

If the injury is acute, advise ice, elevation, and compression with Coban tape, an Ace wrap, or both.

Running, walking, prolonged standing, and other weightbearing activities must be restricted for 1 to 3 weeks.

Crutches may be necessary in the first week.

Advise the patient to avoid tiptoeing or pressure across the ball of the feet (e.g., stairs, pedals, exercise equipment) completely and to limit standing and walking.

Recommend Achilles tendon-stretching exercises performed by hand pressure initially followed by wall stretches after the pain and local tenderness have abated (p. 292).

Advise a gradual return to regular activities.

Suggest an Ace wrap, athletic taping, or Lycra support to prevent recurrence.

PHYSICAL THERAPY   Physical therapy plays a minor role in the acute treatment and recovery phases of gastrocnemius tears.

PHYSICAL THERAPY SUMMARY

1. Ice, elevation, and compression are always applied for the acute injury
2. Touch-down weightbearing is used for larger tears (more extensive area of irritation, larger crescent sign, exquisite tenderness)
3. Achilles tendon-stretching exercises, passively performed, are indicated in the rehabilitation phase
4. Gradual toning of the muscle is recommended after the pain has subsided and flexibility has been restored

INJECTION   No injection is indicated for this condition.

SURGICAL PROCEDURE   No surgical procedure is indicated for this condition.

PROGNOSIS   Small muscle tears have the best prognosis. Large tears with a palpable defect on exam can be associated with distressingly recurrent symptoms. Overall strength is rarely compromised in either case. Vigorous activities placing stress through the damaged muscle can cause recurrent pain and bruising, however, immediately interfering with exercising and sports activities. Patients with recurrent episodes of pain and swelling require Ace wrapping and taping to reduce recurrences.

DIFFERENTIAL DIAGNOSIS OF FOOT PAIN

Diagnoses	Confirmations
Anatomic variation	
Pes planus and pes cavus	Exam
Pronation of the ankle	Exam
Metatarsalgia	
Tight extensor tendons or hammer-toe deformity (most common)	Exam
Morton's neuroma	Local anesthetic block
Rheumatoid arthritis	Exam; rheumatoid factor
Corns and calluses	Exam
Plantar warts	Exam
First metatarsophalangeal (MTP) joint	
Osteoarthritis—bunion	X-ray—foot series
Osteoarthritis—hallux rigidus	X-ray—foot series
Prebunion bursa	Local anesthetic block
Gout (podagra)	Synovial fluid analysis
Sesamoiditis	X-ray—sesamoid view
Swelling over the dorsum of the foot	
Extensor tenosynovitis	Exam
Cellulitis	Exam; complete blood count
Stress fracture of the metatarsals	X-ray; bone scan
Reflex sympathetic dystrophy	Bone scan
Dorsal bunion	X-ray—foot series
Bunionette of the fifth MTP joint	Exam; x-ray—foot series
Referred pain	
Lumbosacral spine radiculopathy	CT scan; MRI; electromyography
Tarsal tunnel syndrome	Nerve conduction velocity testing
Gastrocnemius tear	Exam

BUNIONS

Enter over the metatarsophalangeal joint medially at the distal metatarsal head.

Needle: ⁵/₈-inch, 25-gauge
Depth: ¹/₄ to ³/₈ inch (flush against the bone)
Volume: 0.5 mL of anesthetic and 0.25 mL of K40

NOTE: The injection is made under the synovial membrane adjacent to the bone, not in between the articular surfaces of the joint.

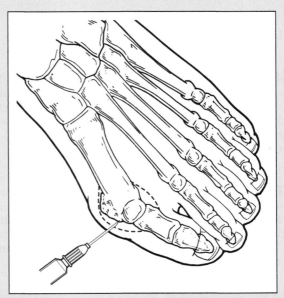

FIGURE 11-1. First metatarsophalangeal joint (bunion) injection.

DESCRIPTION   *Bunion* is the term used to describe the bony prominence and abnormal angle of the great toe, the hallmark sign of osteoarthritis of the first metatarsophalangeal (MTP) joint. Asymmetric pressure over the articular cartilage caused by shoes with a narrow toe box leads to loss of cartilage, angulation of the joint, and gradual subluxation of the extensor tendons. The asymmetric wear and tear on the joint leads to the typical valgus deformity. The condition develops over many years. Continued pressure over the medial joint line can cause acute arthritic flares or acute adventitial bursitis.

SYMPTOMS   The patient complains of abnormal-looking toes, problems with shoe wear, and pain in the great toe. The patient often rubs the top and bottom of the toe or simply stares with disgust at the deformity when describing the condition.

"I can't get a pair of shoes to fit comfortably now."

"I get this sharp pain in my big toe whenever I walk too far."

"My toe looks funny."

"Are these bunions? My grandmother had ugly toes too."

"My big toe aches all the time, especially when I bend it."

"I can't walk normally. My big toe doesn't bend very much anymore."

EXAM   The exam assesses degree of arthritic change, valgus angulation, and local inflammation. The involvement

of the first MTP joint is compared with the involvement of the overlying adventitial bursa.

EXAM SUMMARY
1. MTP joint tenderness and enlargement
2. Typical hallux valgus deformity
3. Crepitation on passive movement of the joint
4. Pain at the extremes of plantar flexion and dorsiflexion of the toe, performed passively
5. Limited range of motion (ROM) (rigidity)

(1) The MTP joint is tender and enlarged. Tenderness occurs along the medial joint line or over the entire joint if an acute arthritic flare is present. Joint enlargement is due to subluxation, osteophyte formation, and swelling. *(2)* The typical hallux valgus deformity is characterized by a prominent medial metatarsal head, an abnormal lateral angulation of the proximal phalanges, and, in advanced cases, the overlapping of the first and second toes. *(3)* Passive movement of the joint may cause crepitation. *(4)* Pain may be present at the extremes of plantar flexion and dorsiflexion, passively performed. *(5)* The ROM of the joint may be limited (hallux rigidus).

X-RAYS   Plain x-rays of the foot are recommended to confirm the diagnosis, to calculate the valgus angle, and to assess the degree of arthritic change. Progressive arthritic changes include asymmetric narrowing of the articular cartilage, bony osteophyte formation, subchondral bony sclerosis, and subchondral cyst formation. X-rays are always a prerequisite to surgical consultation.

SPECIAL TESTING   No special testing is indicated.

DIAGNOSIS   Advanced cases are diagnosed easily by simple inspection and exam. Moderate cases may require x-rays of the foot for confirmation. A regional anesthetic block is necessary occasionally to differentiate symptoms arising from the MTP joint, the adventitial bursa, or Morton's neuroma.

TREATMENT   The goals of treatment are to reduce joint inflammation, to protect the joint from pressure and impact, to realign the deformity, and to prevent any further arthritic change and valgus deformity. Shoes with wide toe boxes, toe spacers, and adhesive pads are the treatments of choice.

■ STEP 1   Educate the patient: *"This is an arthritis of the big toe. The most common cause is tight-fitting shoes."* **Strongly encourage the wearing of shoes with wide toe boxes.**

Demonstrate the use of a cotton or rubber spacer between the first and second toes (p. 263).

Recommend a thick felt ring over the medial joint (p. 262). Prescribe a bunion shield (p. 262).

Recommend padded insoles worn continuously to protect the joint against pressure from below.

Recommend applications of ice over the side and top of the toe for comfort.

Limit weightbearing activities, such as walking and standing.

Shorten the stride, decreasing the motion across the joint.

■ STEP 2 (4 TO 6 WEEKS FOR MODERATE CASES) Nonsteroidal anti-inflammatory drugs (NSAIDs) (e.g., ibuprofen [Advil, Motrin]) have limited benefit because of the poor penetration of the drugs into this small joint.

Re-emphasize the importance of loose-fitting shoes.

Perform a local intra-articular injection of K40.

Repeat the injection in 4 to 6 weeks if symptoms have not improved by at least 50%.

Perform passive stretching of the MTP joint to maintain flexibility after the acute symptoms have resolved.

■ STEP 3 (8 TO 10 WEEKS FOR CHRONIC CASES)   Consider a referral to an orthopedist or podiatrist if symptoms are persistent or if the deformity is great.

PHYSICAL THERAPY   Physical therapy does not play a significant role in the treatment of bunions. Ice

and elevation always are recommended for acute arthritic flares. Stretching exercises of the extensor and flexor tendons are important early in the condition before subluxation and deformity become permanent.

INJECTION   Local corticosteroid injection is used to control the symptoms of an acute inflammatory flare and to provide temporary relief for this progressive arthritic condition.

Positioning   The patient is placed in the supine position with the leg extended and the foot externally rotated.

Surface Anatomy and Point of Entry   The head of the first metatarsal (the medial prominence) and the medial MTP joint line are palpated and marked. The point of entry is adjacent to the joint line approximately $^1/4$ inch distal to the prominence.

Angle of Entry and Depth   The needle is inserted perpendicular to the skin and is advanced to the hard resistance of the bone ($^1/4$ to $^3/8$ inch).

Anesthesia   Ethyl chloride is sprayed on the skin. Local anesthetic is placed in the subcutaneous tissue (0.25 mL) and just outside the synovial membrane at $^1/4$ inch ($^1/4$ mL). All anesthetic should be injected outside the joint. The intra-articular injection is reserved for the corticosteroid because the joint accepts only small volumes.

Technique   A *medial approach* to the joint's synovial membrane is safest and easiest to perform. After placing the anesthetic just outside the synovial membrane, the first syringe is replaced with a second syringe containing the corticosteroid. The needle is advanced down to the periosteum of the bone. If the tip of the needle rests against the metatarsal bone, the injection flows under the synovial membrane and into the joint. Gentle pressure is required. *Note:* The needle is *not* advanced into the center of the joint.

INJECTION AFTERCARE

1. *Rest* for 3 days, avoiding all unnecessary weightbearing.
2. Recommend *loose-fitting, wide-toe-box shoes* with extra padding (double socks, felt ring, mole-foam) combined with a padded insole.
3. Use a *toe spacer* (e.g., cotton, foam) to improve alignment.
4. Use *ice* (15 minutes every 4 to 6 hours) and *acetaminophen (Tylenol ES)* (1000 mg twice a day) for postinjection soreness.
5. *Protect* the great toe for 3 to 4 weeks by avoiding all unnecessary walking and standing.
6. Recommend shortening the stride: *"Take extra time when walking to and from work."*
7. Begin *passive stretching* of the great toe in flexion and extension after the pain and swelling have been controlled, typically at 3 to 4 weeks.
8. Repeat *injection* with corticosteroid at 6 weeks if pain recurs or persists.
9. Request *plain x-rays* of the foot and a *consultation* with an orthopedic surgeon or podiatrist if two consecutive injections fail to control pain and swelling.

BUNION INJECTION

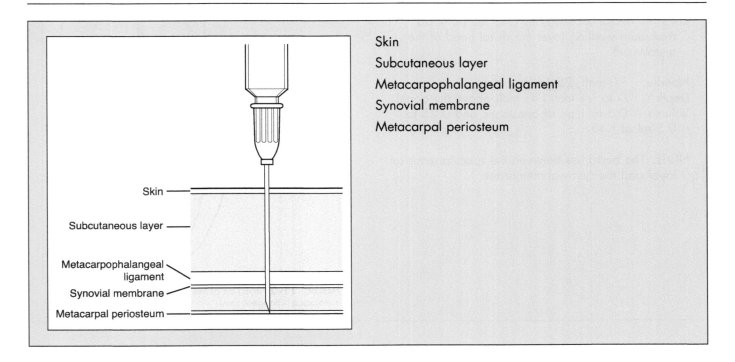

Skin

Subcutaneous layer

Metacarpophalangeal ligament

Synovial membrane

Metacarpal periosteum

Skin

Subcutaneous layer

Metacarpophalangeal ligament

Synovial membrane

Metacarpal periosteum

SURGICAL TREATMENT Bunionectomy includes osteotomy, realignment, and extensor tendon release to restore the normal alignment and appearance of the great toe. When the toe deformity (hallux valgus) is dramatic, ambulation is impaired, or arthritic flares have occurred frequently, surgery can be considered. Several surgical procedures are available, all of which strive to improve alignment, reduce medial joint line pressure, and improve function. The patient should be advised, however, that no one procedure is better than another, and that the toe may lack full ROM postoperatively. The patient must accept the risk of developing a functionally stiff joint.

PROGNOSIS When the wear-and-tear process begins, it tends to be relentlessly progressive. The patient should be advised that the underlying arthritis and deformity gradually worsen over the years. Prevention and protection cannot be overemphasized. To slow the process, the patient must be advised on the importance of wearing appropriate shoes with sufficient padding to protect against the pressure and impact of walking. Plain x-rays are useful to define the severity of the osteoarthritic changes affecting the great toe and the appropriateness of surgical referral. The patient must be made aware and must understand that all treatments, including surgery, are palliative.

ADVENTITIAL BURSITIS OF THE FIRST METATARSOPHALANGEAL JOINT

Enter the bursal sac medially over the point of maximum swelling (over the distal head of the metatarsal).

Needle: ⁵/8-inch, 25-gauge
Depth: ¹/4 to ³/8 inch (¹/8 inch above the bone)
Volume: 0.5 to 1 mL of anesthetic and 0.25 to 0.5 mL of K40

NOTE: The bursa lies between the subcutaneous fat layer and the synovial membrane.

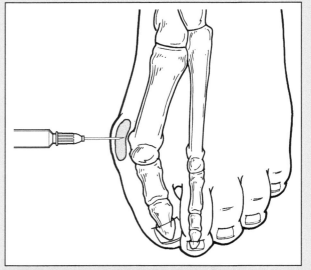

FIGURE 11–2. Injection of the adventitial bursa over the first metatarsophalangeal joint.

DESCRIPTION The bursa over the medial aspect of the first MTP joint becomes clinically important as the valgus deformity—the angle formed between the metatarsal and the proximal phalangeal bones—gradually increases. The repetitive pressure and friction of tight shoes over the medial aspect of the joint causes the bursal sac to become acutely inflamed. The inflammatory signs of swelling, redness, and tenderness are so dramatic that the condition often is misdiagnosed as acute podagra. The inflammation of this periarticular bursitis is restricted, however, to the medial aspect of the joint. By contrast, the inflammatory signs of acute gout affect the entire joint.

SYMPTOMS The patient complains of toe pain, swelling, and redness over the inner aspect of the toe.

"My big toe is swollen."

"I can't wear my shoes anymore. My big toe rubs on the inner side of my shoe."

"I have had to switch to sandals because my walking shoes rub too much on my big toe."

"I think I have gout."

"I've always had bunions, but now my toe has really begun to swell."

EXAM The exam assesses the degree of bursal inflammation, underlying arthritic change, and loss of ROM of the first MTP joint.

EXAM SUMMARY

1. Swelling and pain over the medial aspect of the MTP joint
2. Typical valgus deformity of the MTP joint (bunion deformity)
3. Mild pain when moving the MTP joint in flexion and extension (in contrast to gout)
4. Painless resisted flexion and extension of the MTP joint, isometrically performed

(1) Acute inflammation is present over the medial aspect of the first MTP joint. Swelling, redness, and warmth are present over a quarter-sized area. Tenderness is maximal over the medial aspect of the joint (as opposed to the diffuse tenderness over the entire MTP joint with gout). The inflammatory signs and local tenderness rarely extend beyond the confines of the bursal sac, unless a concurrent cellulitis is present (rare). *(2)* The typical bunion deformity, hallux valgus, is present. *(3)* The ROM of the joint is limited owing to arthritis of the underlying joint. Mild to moderate pain is present at the extremes of motion; this is in contrast to the severe pain and severe limitation of joint movement seen with acute podagra. *(4)* Isometrically resisted toe flexion and extension are painless. The extensor and flexor tendons of the foot are not involved.

X-RAYS X-rays of the foot are recommended. The underlying arthritic change at the MTP joint predominates.

Joint-space narrowing, bony spurs, and the valgus angulation are obvious changes and usually are advanced in degree. Soft-tissue swelling may be apparent on the anteroposterior projection. Calcification does not occur.

SPECIAL TESTING   No special testing is indicated.

DIAGNOSIS   The diagnosis is made by physical exam. The acute inflammatory change located medially, the presence of the typical valgus deformity, and the absence of signs of gouty arthritis strongly suggest the diagnosis. Local anesthetic block placed in the superficial tissue layers above the joint differentiates involvement of the bursa and acute gout or acute osteoarthritic flare of the MTP joint. When inflammatory change is extensive, the diagnosis must be confirmed by aspiration. Bursal fluid analysis (negative Gram stain, culture, and crystal analysis) is mandatory if infection is suspected.

TREATMENT   The goals of treatment are to reduce acute swelling and inflammation and to prevent recurrent bursitis by avoiding pressure and friction. Local corticosteroid injection is the preferred treatment for the acute inflammation. Wide-toe-box shoes and an adhesive padding placed over the bursa are used to protect the medial side of the joint from direct pressure and friction.

STEP 1   Obtain x-rays of the foot, aspirate the bursa if sufficient swelling is present, inspect the aspirate for blood and purulence, and send the aspirate for laboratory analysis (Gram stain, culture, crystals).

Perform a local injection of K40 if infection is unlikely (i.e., no penetrating trauma, no diabetes, no vascular insufficiency).

Recommend wide-toe-box shoes.

Recommend a felt ring or an adhesive bunion pad to reduce the direct pressure and friction over the medial aspect of the MTP joint (p. 263).

Ice over the medial joint is effective in controlling pain and swelling.

Suggest a bunion shield for advanced valgus deformity (p. 262).

Shorten the stride to reduce pressure and friction.

NSAIDs (e.g., ibuprofen) are ineffective owing to poor tissue penetration.

STEP 2 (4 TO 6 WEEKS FOR PERSISTENT CASES)   Repeat the injection in 4 to 6 weeks if the pain and swelling have not decreased by 50%.

Re-emphasize the importance of padding and proper shoes.

STEP 3 (8 TO 10 WEEKS IN THE RECOVERY PHASE)   Reinforce the need to wear well-fitting shoes and use a felt ring for prevention.

Consider surgical referral if the bunion deformity is severe and especially if bursitis has been difficult to treat.

PHYSICAL THERAPY   Physical therapy does not play a significant role in the treatment of this local musculoskeletal condition. Ice and elevation always are recommended for an acute inflammatory flare. Stretching exercises to preserve ROM are indicated for the underlying arthritis of the MTP joint.

INJECTION   Local anesthetic block is used to differentiate this periarticular condition from gout. Corticosteroid injection is used to control symptoms of acute inflammatory flare.

Position   The patient is placed in the supine position with the leg extended and the foot externally rotated.

Surface Anatomy and Point of Entry   The bursa lies directly over the medial prominence of the MTP joint. The point of entry is directly over the center of the bursa.

Angle of Entry and Depth   The needle is inserted perpendicular to the skin. The depth is no greater than $1/4$ to $3/8$ inch.

Anesthesia   Ethyl chloride is sprayed on the skin. Local anesthetic is placed in the subcutaneous tissue (0.25 mL).

Technique   A *medial approach* is preferred. After anesthetic is placed, the needle is advanced down to the hard resistance of the bone and withdrawn $1/4$ inch (the bursa is located just outside the joint capsule). Attempts to aspirate fluid are usually unsuccessful. If risk factors for infection are significant, and attempts to withdraw fluid are unsuccessful, the bursa should be flushed with sterile saline and sent for culture. Empirical antibiotics should be started before obtaining the final culture results. If infection is clearly ruled out, the bursa is injected with 0.25 to 0.5 mL of K40.

INJECTION AFTERCARE

1. *Rest* for 3 days, avoiding all unnecessary weightbearing.
2. Recommend loose-fitting, *wide-toe-box shoes* with extra padding (double socks, felt ring, mole-foam) combined with a padded insole.
3. Use a *toe spacer* (e.g., cotton, foam) to improve alignment.
4. Use *ice* (15 minutes every 4 to 6 hours) and *acetaminophen* (1000 mg twice a day) for postinjection soreness.
5. *Protect* the great toe for 3 to 4 weeks by avoiding all unnecessary walking and standing.
6. Recommend shortening the stride: *"Take extra time when walking to and from work."*
7. Begin *passive stretching* of the great toe in flexion and extension after the pain and swelling have resolved, typically at 3 to 4 weeks.
8. Repeat *injection* of corticosteroid at 6 weeks if pain recurs or persists.
9. Request *plain x-rays* of the foot and a *consultation* with an orthopedic surgeon or podiatrist if two consecutive injections fail to control pain and swelling.

METATARSOPHALANGEAL BURSITIS INJECTION

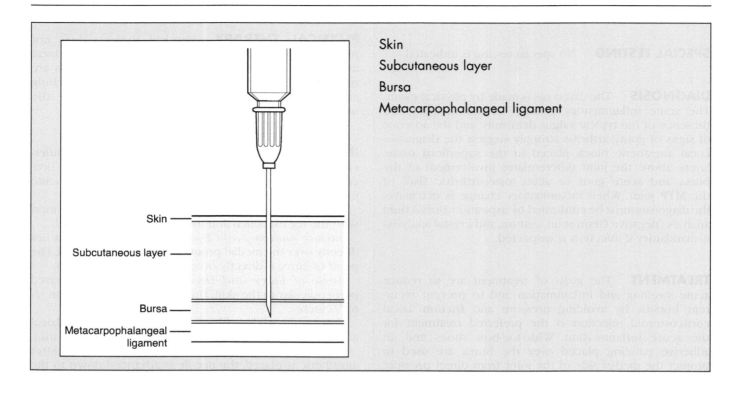

Skin
Subcutaneous layer
Bursa
Metacarpophalangeal ligament

Skin ——
Subcutaneous layer ——
Bursa ——
Metacarpophalangeal —— ligament

SURGICAL PROCEDURE Bursectomy is the treatment of choice, but usually is performed during the course of bunionectomy.

PROGNOSIS Local corticosteroid injection is effective in controlling the symptoms of an acute, inflammatory flare. Recurrent bursitis occurs in the setting of bunions with severe angulation deformity. Surgery usually is directed toward the underlying bunion. Bursectomy without surgical correction of the underlying bunion deformity is usually ineffective.

GOUT

Enter medially either on the metatarsal or on the phalangeal side of the joint line.

Needle: ⁵/₈-inch, 25-gauge for anesthesia or 21-gauge for aspiration
Depth: ³/₈ to ¹/₂ inch (depending on swelling)
Volume: 0.5 to 1 mL of anesthetic and 0.25 mL of K40

NOTE: Multiple attempts to enter the joint may be damaging; with the needle flush against the periosteum—under the synovial membrane—the needle is intra-articular; manual pressure may yield sufficient fluid for analysis.

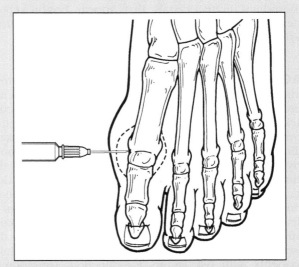

FIGURE 11–3. Injection and aspiration of acute gout (podagra).

DESCRIPTION Gout is an acute, crystal-induced, monarthric arthritis of the MTP joint of the great toe. Acute swelling, redness, and heat develop as an inflammatory response to precipitation of monosodium urate crystals in the synovial fluid. The synovial fluid becomes supersaturated with uric acid crystals as a result of overproduction of uric acid (e.g., hemolytic anemias, leukemia, psoriasis, and tumors with rapid cell turnover cause 10% of cases) or undersecretion of uric acid (e.g., renal disease, aspirin, niacin, and diuretics cause 90% of cases). Patients with recurrent gouty attacks should undergo laboratory evaluation to determine the cause of their altered metabolism. Gout also can affect the olecranon and prepatellar bursa, the tenosynovial sheaths of the dorsum of the foot and instep, and the other small joints of the foot.

SYMPTOMS The patient complains of severe toe pain, swelling, redness, and an inability to walk because of the pain.

"I woke up in the night with severe, sharp pain in my big toe."

"The pain in my toe was so bad that I couldn't stand having the sheet on my foot. Excuse me, doc, my slippers were the only shoes I could get on. There's no way I can wear shoes."

"My big toe is very red and swollen."

"Doc, I've got the gout in my big toe again."

"I can't put any weight down on my foot because of the severe pain in my big toe."

"There's no way I can walk. I can't bend my big toe."

"My arthritis has hurt in the past, but never like this."

EXAM The exam assesses the degree and extent of the inflammation affecting the first MTP joint.

EXAM SUMMARY

1. Acute swelling, redness, and heat arising from the MTP joint
2. Severe tenderness at the MTP joint
3. Pain aggravated by even the slightest movement of the joint

(1) The toe is swollen, red, and hot. The inflammation envelops the joint and may extend 1 inch proximally and distally, involving the soft tissues. The greatest degree of swelling is along the medial border of the joint. *(2)* Severe tenderness is present around the entire joint, with the greatest sensitivity medially (by contrast, the tenderness of adventitial bursitis is located only on the medial aspect of the joint). *(3)* Movement of the toe in any direction is extremely painful. The patient often exhibits great anxiety at the thought of moving the toe.

X-RAYS X-rays of the foot are optional in patients presenting with their first attack and recommended in patients with recurrent and chronic gout. Patients presenting with a first attack do not show bony or joint abnormalities. Patients with recurrent or chronic tophaceous gout may show periarticular or intra-articular erosions, round or oval erosions typically surrounded by a thin sclerotic margin.

SPECIAL TESTING The demonstration of monosodium urate crystals is the diagnostic test of choice. Light microscopy reveals the characteristic needle-shaped monosodium urate crystals that appear bright yellow under polarized light, also referred to as *negative birefringence*.

DIAGNOSIS The diagnosis of acute inflammatory monarthric arthritis of the first MTP joint is not difficult. There is difficulty, however, in differentiating the acute attack of gout from the much less common infective arthritis, two conditions with identical physical exam findings. A presumptive diagnosis of gout is much more likely if there has been a history of gouty attacks, if the serum uric acid is elevated, and if risk factors for infection (e.g., diabetes, vascular insufficiency, an absence of penetrating trauma) are absent. In addition, statistically, gout is at least 100 times more likely than infection. Absolute confirmation of the diagnosis requires showing the presence of urate crystals when analyzing the joint fluid. In patients with risk factors for infection, aspiration is mandatory to exclude infection.

TREATMENT The goal of treatment is to reduce rapidly the acute inflammation within the first MTP joint.

STEP 1 **Assess the patient's risk factors for infection (e.g., diabetes, vascular insufficiency, immunocompromise), aspirate the joint for synovial fluid analysis (crystals, cell count, Gram stain, and culture), obtain a serum uric acid level, and either proceed to local injection of corticosteroids or wait for the results of laboratory analysis.**

Recommend application of ice and elevation of the foot.

Eliminate low-dose aspirin, alcohol, diuretics (if possible), and any other drug that interferes with the secretion of uric acid.

Recommend avoiding pressure from shoes.

A prescription of any NSAID (e.g., ibuprofen) or colchicine or an injection of any of the corticosteroid derivatives effectively treats the severe inflammation.

STEP 2 (2 TO 4 DAYS ACUTE FOLLOW-UP) Measure the 24-hour urinary uric acid excretion to determine whether the patient is an overproducer or undersecretor.

If the patient is an overproducer of urates, perform an evaluation of the causes of urate overproduction.

Prescribe probenecid (for undersecretors) or allopurinol (for overproducers) for patients with recurrent attacks of gout.

Prescribe an NSAID or colchicine to protect against precipitating gout when initiating probenecid or allopurinol (1 month for recurrent acute gout and 6 months for chronic tophaceous gout).

STEP 3 (4 TO 8 WEEKS FOR LONG-TERM FOLLOW-UP) Recheck the uric acid to assess whether long-term preventive therapy has reduced the serum uric acid to the normal range.

Adjust the dosages of probenecid or allopurinol to keep the uric acid in the normal range.

PHYSICAL THERAPY Physical therapy does not play a significant role in the treatment of gout. Ice and elevation always are recommended. Passive stretching exercises in flexion and extension are used to restore ROM in the exceptional case that develops joint stiffness.

INJECTION Injection with local anesthetic is used to aspirate the joint for crystal analysis (see later). Corticosteroid injection is indicated when NSAIDs cannot be used because of peptic ulcer disease, concurrent use of warfarin (Coumadin), and renal failure. The technique used to aspirate is similar to the approach used to treat bunions (p. 211).

Special Technique A *medial approach* to aspirating the joint is the safest and easiest to perform. After placing the anesthetic just outside the synovial membrane, the needle is advanced to the periosteum of the metatarsal, and 0.25 mL of anesthetic is placed under the synovial membrane. With the needle held carefully in place, gentle manual pressure is exerted over the lateral and medial aspects of the joint to express one or two drops of synovial fluid for crystal analysis. Leaving the needle in place, 0.25 mL of K40 is injected into the joint. *Caution:* Do *not* advance the needle into the center of the joint. Damage to the articular cartilage can result.

PROGNOSIS NSAIDs and colchicine are effective in reducing the acute joint inflammation, usually within 1 to 2 days. Intra-articular corticosteroid injection also is effective and often reduces the pain, swelling, and erythema in a few hours. Either treatment effectively controls all symptoms and signs within 3 to 4 days. Long-term control of gout rests on prevention. Low-dose aspirin, alcohol, foods high in purine, and certain medications (most notably the diuretics and niacin) must be avoided. For patients with recurrent episodes of acute gout and patients with chronic gout, allopurinol or probenecid should be prescribed. Allopurinol—a xanthine oxidase competitive inhibitor—is the drug of choice for patients who are overproducers of uric acid. Probenecid is the drug of choice for prevention of gout in patients who are undersecretors of uric acid. Because 90% of patients with gout are undersecretors, probenecid is the logical choice for most patients. Patients who are found to be overproducers should be examined thoroughly for the specific cause of excess production of urates.

HAMMER TOES

Enter from above, midway between the metatarsophalangeal joints. After placing anesthetic in the dermis, advance the needle at a 45-degree angle down to the periosteum of the metatarsal head.

Needle: ⁵/₈-inch, 25-gauge
Depth: ³/₈ to ¹/₂ inch to the periosteum of the metatarsal head
Volume: 0.5 mL of anesthetic and 0.25 mL of K40

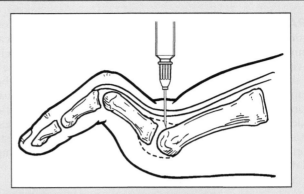

FIGURE 11–4. Injection of the acutely inflamed metatarsophalangeal joint as a part of hammer toes.

DESCRIPTION *Hammer toe* is the term used to describe the toe deformity caused by contracted extensor tendons of the foot. *Metatarsalgia* is the term used to describe painful MTP joints. As the tendons slowly lose their flexibility, the MTP joints gradually extend, and the proximal interphalangeal (PIP) joints gradually flex. The hammer-like deformity results. Pressure over these joints leads to plantar surface calluses and to dorsal surface corns, both of which consist of hypertrophic skin over the bony prominences. The hammer-toe deformity is the end result of years of tight, inflexible extensor tendons. Metatarsal pain can precede the deformity by years. Before the development of hammer toes, tight dorsal tendons can be shown on exam.

SYMPTOMS The patient complains of pain over the ball of the foot, calluses, or abnormal-looking toes.

"My toes are crooked."

"I can't bend my toes anymore."

"It's like walking on marbles. I have these thick calluses on the bottom of my feet."

"The skin over the top of my toes is starting to thicken."

"My toes are rubbing on my shoes."

"At the end of the day my toes ache. The whole ball of my foot hurts."

EXAM The extensor tendons of the toes are assessed for flexibility, the MTP joints are assessed for irritation and thickening, and the corns and calluses are documented.

EXAM SUMMARY

1. Tight extensor tendons, especially when the ankle is placed in plantar flexion
2. Tenderness directly over the MTP joints
3. Positive MTP squeeze sign
4. Corns and calluses
5. Hammer-toe deformity

(1) The hammer-toe deformity is characteristic of the end stage of this condition. Before developing this fixed contracture of the joint, all patients present with tight or partially contracted extensor tendons over the dorsum of the foot; this is best appreciated when placing the ankle in extreme plantar flexion. In this position, the patient experiences tightness, pain, or both. This tightness may be experienced just over the dorsum of the foot or up the anterior surface of the leg. *(2)* Individual MTP joints may be tender. Tenderness is best elicited by compressing the joint from above and below and rolling the MTP head between the fingers. *(3)* If the joints are particularly inflamed, the MTP squeeze sign is painful. In this maneuver, all the joints are compressed simultaneously by side pressure (medial to lateral), while holding the second, third, and fourth MTP joints in line with the opposite hand. *(4)* Corns over the top of the PIP joints and calluses below the MTP joint are seen as the condition progresses. These abnormalities antedate the development of the fixed hammer-toe deformity and are a direct result of the constant pressure over the MTP heads. The body attempts to protect the joints by developing hypertrophic skin over the bony prominences. *(5)* The typical hammer-toe

deformity is the final stage of the condition, when the joints become rigid.

X-RAYS X-rays of the foot are not recommended routinely. Although the lateral view shows the typical hammer-toe deformity in an advanced case, x-rays rarely provide additional information that could not be assessed on the basis of the physical exam. X-rays should be obtained in an atypical case (e.g., severe swelling, unusual coloration, unequal involvement of the toes). Dramatic tenderness and swelling in a symmetric pattern suggest rheumatoid arthritis. Excessive bony enlargement suggests degenerative changes at the MTP joints. Extensive swelling and discoloration suggest reflex sympathetic dystrophy or infection.

SPECIAL TESTING Bone scanning rarely is indicated. Joint aspiration is not possible.

DIAGNOSIS The diagnosis is based on a history of pain over the balls of the feet and an exam showing localized metatarsal tenderness and, in an advanced case, the typical hammer-toe deformity. The diagnosis is less evident when the typical deformity is not present. These early presentations often are labeled simply as metatarsalgia. These patients need to be examined closely for the painful tight extensor tendons.

TREATMENT The goals of treatment are to stretch the dorsal extensor tendons and to re-establish normal toe alignment. Passive stretching of the extensor tendons is the treatment of choice. When the classic hammer-toe deformity develops, however, surgical correction is preferred.

STEP 1 The stage of the condition is determined (early metatarsalgia versus advanced hammer-toe deformity), x-rays are obtained in an advanced case, and the number of MTP joints involved is documented.

Prescribe passive stretching exercises of the extensor tendons in a downward direction (manual stretching, picking up marbles, or grasping a towel).

Prescribe padded insoles to reduce the pressure over the metatarsal heads and to protect the MTP heads from developing calluses (p. 262).

Recommend wide-toe-box shoes.

Prescribe a hammer-toe crest (p. 263) placed under the four MTP joints for an advanced case with established deformity.

Pare the large corns and calluses with sharp dissection in the office, and recommend maintenance care at home with a pumice stone or hand-held file.

Suggest cotton ball, foam, or rubber spacers for padding between the toes.

Restrict walking, standing, and other weightbearing activities.

Shorten the stride to decrease the motion and stress across the joints.

STEP 2 (4 TO 6 WEEKS FOR PERSISTENT CASES) For patients with exquisitely painful MTP joints, perform a local injection of K40 at the most painful MTP head (limit injection to one to two toes).

Re-emphasize the importance of the stretching exercises.

STEP 3 (3 TO 4 MONTHS FOR CHRONIC CASES) Repeat the injection if joint inflammation persists.

Consider surgical referral for flexor tenotomy or arthroplasty if symptoms and deformity are persistent.

PHYSICAL THERAPY Physical therapy plays an essential role in the active treatment and prevention of hammer toes. The focus of therapy is passive and active stretching of the extensor tendons. After soaking the feet in warm to hot water for 15 minutes (a vibrating water massage appliance is ideal), the toes are held firmly at the MTP joints, and the toes are passively flexed downward in the direction of plantar flexion. Sets of 20 to 25 stretches are performed once or twice a day. Initially, these are performed with the ankle and foot in the neutral position. As flexibility improves, the ankle is plantar flexed more and more to accentuate the stretching. A pulling sensation should be felt in the anterior portion of the lower leg. After the passive stretching program, active stretching exercises are begun to increase the flexibility and prevent future problems. These active exercises include curling the toes up and down, grasping plush carpet with the toes, picking up marbles one by one, or picking up a small rolled-up towel.

INJECTION Treatment focuses on stretching exercises, padding, treatment of the secondary corns and calluses, and wide-toe-box shoes. Local corticosteroid injection is indicated most often for the acute inflammatory flare localized to one or two joints.

Positioning The patient is placed in the supine position with the leg extended and the foot plantar flexed.

Surface Anatomy and Point of Entry The heads of the MTP joints are palpated from above and below and marked. The point of entry is centered between the two MTP joint heads, approximately $1/2$ inch back from the web space.

Angle of Entry and Depth The needle is inserted into the skin at a 45-degree angle and is directed toward the most severely affected joint. The depth to the synovial membrane is $3/8$ to $1/2$ inch.

Anesthesia Ethyl chloride is sprayed on the skin. Local anesthetic is placed in the subcutaneous tissue (0.25 mL) and just outside the synovial membrane at $3/8$ inch (0.25 mL). All anesthetic should be kept outside the joint because it holds only a small volume.

HAMMER TOES INJECTION

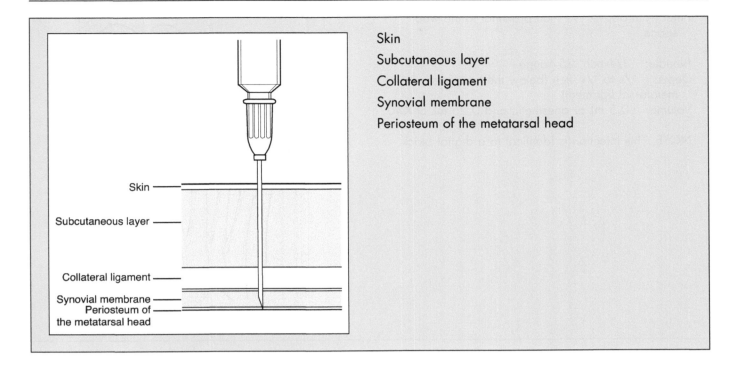

Skin

Subcutaneous layer

Collateral ligament

Synovial membrane

Periosteum of the metatarsal head

Skin
Subcutaneous layer
Collateral ligament
Synovial membrane
Periosteum of
the metatarsal head

Technique A *dorsal approach* is taken to the MTP joint. The 25-gauge needle is introduced midway between the MTP joints and advanced at a 45-degree angle down to the bone of the metatarsal head (typically $1/2$ inch down). Anesthetic is placed just outside the synovial membrane. The first syringe is removed and is replaced with the syringe containing the corticosteroid. The needle is advanced to the periosteum, and with the needle held flush against the bone, 0.25 mL of K40 is injected. An injection placed underneath the synovial membrane is an intra-articular injection.

INJECTION AFTERCARE

1. *Rest* for 3 days, avoiding all unnecessary weightbearing.
2. Recommend loose-fitting, wide-toe-box shoes with extra padding (double socks, padded insoles, padded arch supports when indicated, or a hammer-toe crest).
3. Use a toe spacer (e.g., cotton, foam) to improve alignment and to minimize pressure.
4. Use *ice* (15 minutes every 4 to 6 hours) and *acetaminophen* (1000 mg twice a day) for postinjection soreness.
5. *Protect* the toes for 3 to 4 weeks by avoiding all unnecessary walking and standing.
6. Recommend shortening the stride: *"Take extra time when walking to and from work."*
7. Begin *passive stretching* of the toes in flexion at 3 to 4 weeks (e.g., manual stretching, picking up marbles, grasping a towel, grabbing plush carpet).

8. Repeat *injection* at 6 weeks with corticosteroid if pain recurs or persists.
9. Request *plain x-rays* of the foot and a *consultation* with an orthopedic surgeon or podiatrist if two consecutive injections fail to control pain and swelling, the PIP joints have fixed contractures, and the patient is willing to undergo possible fusion.

SURGICAL PROCEDURE Arthroplasty is reserved for patients with fixed hammer-toe deformities, when the MTP and PIP joints have become rigid as a result of progressive extensor tendon contracture. The PIP joint is entered (capsulotomy), the extensor tendons are released (tenotomy), the collateral ligaments are severed, the distal end of the proximal phalanges is removed (arthroplasty), and the straightened toes are held in place for several weeks with Kirschner wires threaded through the center of the bones (fusion).

PROGNOSIS Daily stretching exercises of the dorsal extensor tendons combined with wide-toe-box shoes, padded insoles, hammer-toe crests, and cotton or rubber toe spacers are successful for the early stage of this condition (the painful metatarsalgia stage, before the toes have become irreversibly deformed). Stretching exercises performed regularly over months should reduce the painful metatarsalgia, prevent the formation of fixed tendon contracture, aid in reducing the reactive hypertrophic corns and calluses, and obviate the need for surgery.

MORTON'S NEUROMA

Enter from above, $^1/_2$ inch proximal to the web
  space.

Needle: $^5/_8$-inch, 25-gauge
Depth: $^5/_8$ to $^3/_4$ inch (below the transverse
  metatarsal ligament)
Volume: 0.5 mL of anesthetic and 0.25 mL of K40

NOTE: This injection is identical to a digital block.

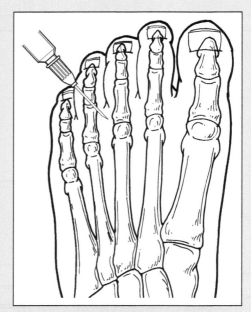

FIGURE 11–5. Morton's neuroma injection.

DESCRIPTION Morton's neuroma—interdigital neuroma—is a chronic irritation and inflammation of the digital nerve as it courses between the MTP heads. Pressure from below (walking or standing on hard surfaces with poorly padded shoes) and from the sides (tight shoes) causes the nerve to enlarge gradually; the pathologic changes consist of perineural thickening and fibrosis. The digital nerve between the third and fourth toes is affected most commonly. Predisposing factors include occupations that require constant standing with the MTP joints continually extended, advanced hammer-toe deformity, high heels, and hallux valgus.

SYMPTOMS The patient complains of pain between the toes or numbness along the sides of two adjacent toes.

"My two toes have gone numb."

"I have sharp pain between my toes."

"Certain tight shoes cause my toes to tingle."

"If I put all my weight on my right foot, I get a shooting pain through my toes."

"Sandals are the only shoes that feel comfortable."

"My third and fourth toes feel dead."

EXAM The space between the metatarsal heads is assessed for local tenderness, and the skin of the adjacent two toes is tested for loss of sensation.

EXAM SUMMARY

1. Maximum tenderness in the web space
2. Pain aggravated by the MTP squeeze sign
3. Passive ROM of the MTP joints that is painless
4. Loss of sensation along the inner aspects of the adjacent two toes (advanced cases)
5. Digital nerve block to confirm the diagnosis

(1) Local tenderness is greatest in the web space between the MTP heads; this is in contrast to the tenderness at the MTP heads in metatarsalgia. Firm pressure must be applied to elicit pain in the web space. *(2)* Pain can be reproduced by squeezing the MTP heads from either side (medial to lateral). This compression may cause an electric shock–like pain to shoot to the ends of the adjacent two toes. *(3)* Passive ROM of the MTP joints should be painless in an uncomplicated case. *(4)* Advanced cases may show a loss of sensation along the inner aspects of the adjacent two toes. Light touch or pain sensation may be decreased. *(5)* Finally, a digital nerve block should eliminate the local tenderness and pain with MTP squeeze.

X-RAYS X-rays of the foot are normal. No characteristic changes are seen on plain films.

SPECIAL TESTING Local anesthetic block is used to confirm the diagnosis.

DIAGNOSIS   A presumptive diagnosis is based on the pain and local tenderness in the web space between two adjacent MTP joints. Confirmation of the diagnosis requires relief with local digital nerve block placed just below the transverse metatarsal ligament. If the diagnosis is still in question, and the patient's symptoms are unrelieved with conservative care, surgical exploration may be indicated for definitive diagnosis.

TREATMENT   The goals of treatment are to reduce the pressure over the nerve and to eliminate the associated inflammation. The treatments of choice combine a padded toe spacer with soft insoles placed in wide-toe-box shoes.

STEP 1   Identify the maximum local tenderness, either over the metatarsal heads (metatarsalgia) or in the web space between the toes (neuroma), and assess the sensation of the adjacent two toes.

    Recommend wide-toe-box shoes to reduce the pressure on the nerve from the sides.

    Suggest soft, padded insoles to protect the nerve from pressure from below (p. 262).

    Demonstrate the use of a cotton or rubber spacer taped or placed between the affected toes (p. 263).

    Restrict all unnecessary weightbearing.

    Shorten the stride, decreasing the motion across the joints and reducing the pressure over the nerve.

    Avoid prescribing NSAIDs; they are ineffective owing to poor penetration into these tissues.

STEP 2 (4 TO 6 WEEKS FOR PERSISTENT CASES) Perform a local injection of K40.

    Re-emphasize the importance of proper shoes.

    Repeat the injection in 4 to 6 weeks if symptoms have not decreased by 50%.

STEP 3 (3 MONTHS FOR CHRONIC CASES)   Consider a referral to a podiatrist or an orthopedist for definitive surgery if two injections 6 weeks apart fail to control symptoms.

    Educate the patient: *"Some surgical procedures can cause permanent toe numbness."*

PHYSICAL THERAPY   Physical therapy does not play an important role in the treatment of Morton's neuroma.

INJECTION   Local anesthetic injection often is used to confirm the diagnosis. Local corticosteroid injection is indicated when padding, protection, and change in shoes fail to control symptoms.

Position   The patient is placed in the supine position with the leg extended and the foot plantar flexed to 30 degrees.

Surface Anatomy and Point of Entry   The heads of the MTP joints are palpated from above and below and marked. The point of entry is centered between the two MTP joint heads, approximately 1/2 inch back from the web space.

MORTON'S NEUROMA INJECTION

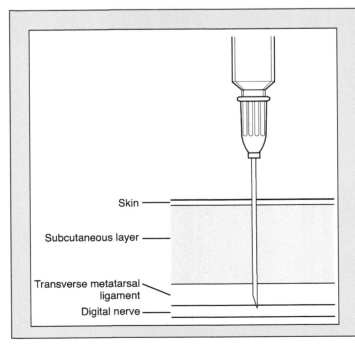

Skin
Subcutaneous layer
Transverse metatarsal ligament
Digital nerve

Angle of Entry and Depth The needle is inserted perpendicular to the skin and advanced down through the transverse metatarsal ligament (between the metatarsal heads). The depth is $3/8$ to $1/2$ inch to the transverse metatarsal ligament and $5/8$ to $3/4$ inch to the nerve.

Anesthesia Ethyl chloride is sprayed on the skin. Local anesthetic is placed in the subcutaneous tissue (0.25 mL), the transverse metatarsal ligament (0.25 mL), and just below the ligament (0.25 to 0.5 mL). If the injection is placed accurately under the transverse metatarsal ligament, the inner aspects of the adjacent toes should be numb.

Technique A *dorsal approach* is taken. The proximal phalangeal heads are palpated. The 25-gauge needle is inserted halfway between the MTP heads and advanced to the firm resistance of the transverse metatarsal ligament (subtle). After anesthetic is injected at this level, the needle is advanced through the ligament. Often a giving-way or popping sensation is felt. The patient is re-examined after 0.25 to 0.5 mL of anesthetic is injected. If the local tenderness and the MTP squeeze sign are relieved, K40 is injected.

INJECTION AFTERCARE

1. *Rest* for 3 days, avoiding all unnecessary weightbearing.
2. Recommend loose-fitting, *wide-toe-box shoes* with extra padding (double socks, padded insoles, and padded arch supports when indicated).
3. Use a *toe spacer* to improve alignment and minimize pressure.
4. Use *ice* (15 minutes every 4 to 6 hours) and *acetaminophen* (1000 mg twice a day) for postinjection soreness.
5. *Protect* the toes for 3 to 4 weeks by avoiding all unnecessary walking and standing.
6. Recommend *shortening the stride*: *"Take extra time when walking to and from work."*

7. Repeat *injection* at 6 weeks with corticosteroid if pain recurs or persists.
8. Request *plain x-rays* of the foot and a *consultation* with an orthopedic surgeon or podiatrist if two consecutive injections fail to control pain, and the patient is willing to undergo an operation that may result in permanent numbness.

SURGICAL PROCEDURE Patients with intractable symptoms can choose between transposition of the nerve, sclerosis with injection of ethyl alcohol, or the definitive neurectomy. The patient must be counseled on the postsurgical numbness that results when the nerve undergoes sclerosis or definitive removal.

PROGNOSIS Two consecutive corticosteroid injections with K40, 6 weeks apart, when combined with general foot care are effective in reducing the perineural inflammation and fibrosis around the digital nerve. The triamcinolone derivatives are the preferred injection for the treatment of Morton's neuroma due to greater effect on the perineural fibrosis. The triamcinolones have four to five times the antifibrosis effects compared with the prednisolone and betamethasone derivatives. The triamcinolones also are four to five times more likely to cause subcutaneous atrophy of fat—antilipolytic effect. Because the reduction of the perineural fibrosis is gradual, the condition should be observed for at least 2 months before proceeding to surgery. Nerve injuries take months to improve after the inflammation has been reduced and the offending irritation has been eliminated. A neurectomy can be considered for symptoms that persist over several months.

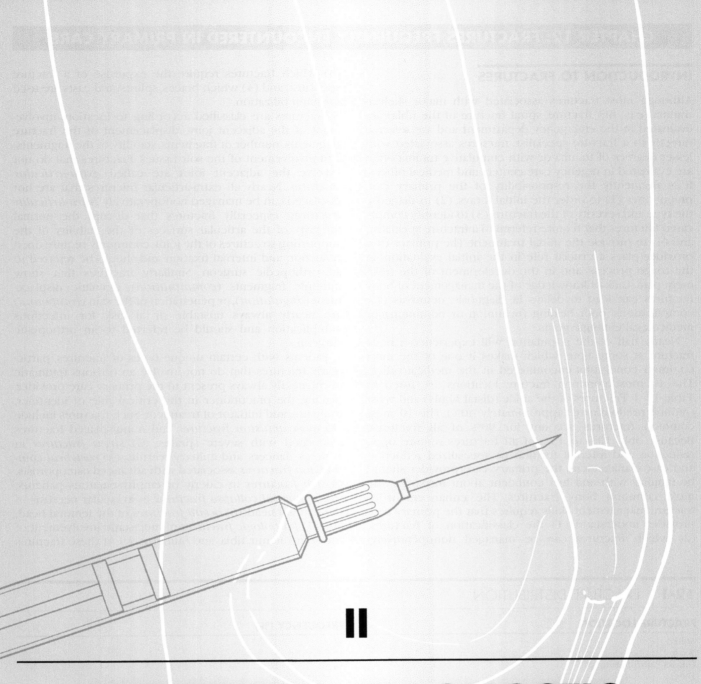

II

FRACTURES, DIAGNOSTIC PROCEDURES, AND REHABILITATIVE CARE

INTRODUCTION TO FRACTURES

Although most fractures associated with major skeletal trauma (e.g., hip fracture, spiral fracture of the tibia) are evaluated in the emergency department and are referred directly to a fracture specialist, fractures associated with lesser degrees of trauma or with cumulative trauma often are evaluated in urgency care centers and medical offices. It is frequently the responsibility of the primary care practitioner (1) to order the initial x-rays, (2) to diagnose the type and severity of the fracture, (3) to identify complicated fractures that require referral to a fracture specialist, and (4) to provide the initial treatment. The primary care provider plays a crucial role in the initial evaluation, in the triage process, and in the development of the treatment plan. Lack of knowledge of the management of bony fractures can lead to delays in diagnosis, neurovascular complications, poor healing (malunion or nonunion), or medicolegal entanglements.

Nearly half of the population will experience a bony fracture at some time, which makes it one of the most common conditions encountered in the medical office. The 10 most common fracture locations are listed in Table 12–1. Fractures of the ankle (distal fibula) and wrist (radius) predominate (approximately 40%). The 10 most common fractures account for 90% of all fractures. Because only 10% to 15% of all fractures require open reduction and internal fixation or specialized reduction and cast management, the primary care provider should be familiar with and feel confident about managing the most common bony fractures. The enhancement of fracture management skills requires that the primary care provider understand (1) the classification of fractures; (2) which fractures can be managed nonoperatively;

(3) which fractures require the expertise of a fracture specialist; and (4) which braces, splints, and casts are used for immobilization.

Fractures are classified according to location, involvement of the adjacent joint, displacement of the fracture fragments, number of fragments, stability of the fragments, and involvement of the soft tissues. Fractures that do not involve the adjacent joint are called *extra-articular fractures*. Nearly all extra-articular fractures that are not displaced can be managed nonoperatively. *Intra-articular fractures,* especially fractures that disrupt the normal integrity of the articular surfaces or the stability of the supporting structures of the joint, commonly require open reduction and internal fixation and should be referred to an orthopedic surgeon. Similarly, fractures that show multiple fragments (*comminution*), dramatic displacement (*angulation*), or penetration of the skin (*compound*) are nearly always unstable or at risk for infectious complication and should be referred to an orthopedic surgeon.

Patients with certain unique types of fractures, particularly fractures that do not involve an obvious traumatic event, nearly always present to the primary care provider, placing the practitioner in the critical role of identifier, evaluator, and initiator of treatment. Such fractures include (1) most *avulsion fractures* and nondisplaced fractures associated with severe sprains; (2) *stress fractures* in athletes, dancers, and military recruits; (3) *vertebral compression fractures* associated with advanced osteoporosis; (4) *rib fractures* in elderly or emphysematous patients; (5) *segmental collapse fractures* in avascular necrosis of the femoral head; (6) *occult fractures* of the femoral head; and (7) *pathologic fractures* of metastatic involvement of the spine, femur, tibia, and humerus. All of these fractures

12-1   FRACTURE DISTRIBUTION

FRACTURE LOCATION	FREQUENCY (%)
Ankle	23
Wrist	17
Fingers (tuft/phalanges)	14
Toes	7
Ribs	7
Knee (tibia/patella)	7
Clavicle	6
Elbow	6
Tarsus	3
Hip	2
Other	9

FRACTURES THAT ARE MANAGED OPERATIVELY

FRACTURE/DISLOCATION	REASON FOR ORTHOPEDIC REFERRAL
Fractures That Require Referral to Orthopedic Surgery	
Multifragment intra-articular	Risk of arthritis and malunion
Fracture/dislocations	Difficulty of reduction, risk of arthritis
Metastatic lesion of bone	Risk of pathologic fracture
Comminuted fractures	Risk of nonunion and angulation
Compound fractures	Risk of infectious complication
Fractures associated with neurovascular compromise	Soft-tissue injury

See Appendix for individual fracture management.

FRACTURES THAT ARE MANAGED NONOPERATIVELY

FRACTURE/DISLOCATION	NONOPERATIVE IMMOBILIZATION OR TREATMENT
General Categories of Fractures Managed Nonoperatively	
All stress fractures	Reduced running, standing, repetitive use
All nondisplaced extra-articular fractures	Casting for 3-6 weeks
Most small (flecks) avulsion fractures	Casting for 2-4 weeks
Some nondisplaced, single-fragment intra-articular fractures	Casting for 4-6 weeks
Humerus	
Fragment displacement <1 cm or angulation <45 degrees	Hanging cast plus pendulum-stretching exercises
Clavicle	
Nonarticular proximal third	Figure-eight splint or simple sling
Middle third	Figure-eight splint or simple sling
Nondisplaced distal third	Figure-eight splint or simple sling
Elbow	
Dislocation without fracture	Closed reduction with distal distraction
Nondisplaced radial head fracture	Simple sling and ROM exercises
Nondisplaced fracture of the radius or ulna	Long-arm cast with collar and cuff
Wrist	
Most distal radius fractures without foreshortening of the radius or with <20 degrees of angulation	Chinese finger-trap traction plus sugartong splint plus short-arm cast
Hand	
Boxer fracture of the fifth metacarpal with <40 degrees of angulation	Removable volar splint
Volar dislocation of the metacarpophalangeal joint with avulsion fracture <2-3 mm	Radial or ulnar gutter splinting
Extra-articular metacarpal fracture of the thumb without displacement in any plane	Thumb spica cast plus ROM exercises of the thumb
Dorsal dislocation of the metacarpophalangeal joint of the thumb if a single reduction succeeds	Dorsal hood splint
Gamekeeper's thumb, incompletely ruptured	Dorsal hood splint
Extra-articular fractures of the proximal and middle phalanges (nondisplaced and without rotation or angulation)	Buddy-tape plus ROM exercises
Acute boutonnière injury without avulsion fracture	Splinting of the proximal interphalangeal joint in extension plus ROM exercises of the finger joints
Dislocation of the proximal interphalangeal joint without volar lip fracture	Radial or ulnar gutter splinting for 2 weeks, then buddy-taping
All distal phalanx fractures	Stack splint
Most mallet fingers	Stack splint or dorsal aluminum splint in full extension
Mallet fractures, displacement <2-3 mm	Stack splint
Chest	
Rib fracture, without pulmonary injury	Wide bra, Ace wrap, or chest binder
Pelvis	
Nondisplaced, nonarticular, with minimal pain	Touch-down weightbearing crutches
Hip	
Hip fracture in a debilitated patient	Prolonged bed rest
Impacted fractures that are weeks old	Nonweightbearing crutches followed by touch-down weightbearing crutches
Stress fractures	Bed rest versus crutches versus reduced running
Avascular necrosis	Crutches
Knee	
Patellar, nondisplaced and intact quadriceps	Long-leg cast, well molded at the patella
Avulsion fracture at the joint line	Velcro straight-leg brace
Osteochondritis dissecans without mechanical locking or effusion	Straight-leg raises and observation
Tibial plateau rim, if <10 degrees	Long-leg cast
Tibia	
All tibial stress fractures	No running versus decreased running schedule
Most minimally displaced tibial fractures, if <1 cm leg shortening or <5-10 degrees of angulation	Long-leg casting with suprapatellar and medial tibial molding; neutral ankle position; knee flexed to 5 degrees
Fibula	
All fractures	Short-leg walking cast for pain control versus reduced standing and walking
Gastrocnemius	
Gastrocnemius tear	No running, reduced standing and walking, tape

Continued

FRACTURES THAT ARE MANAGED NONOPERATIVELY

FRACTURE/DISLOCATION	NONOPERATIVE IMMOBILIZATION OR TREATMENT
Ankle	
Isolated small avulsion fractures	Short-leg walking cast for 2-4 weeks
Nondisplaced single malleolar fractures	Jones dressing followed by a short-leg walking cast for 4-6 weeks
Stable bimalleolar fractures	Jones dressing followed by a short-leg walking cast for 4-6 weeks
Posterior process of the talus	Short-leg walking cast for 4-6 weeks
Lateral process of the talus, nondisplaced	Short-leg walking cast for 4-6 weeks
Calcaneus	
Most extra-articular fractures (except the displaced posterior process fracture)	Bed rest for 5 days, Jones dressing, short-leg walking cast with crutches and nonweightbearing, then gradual weightbearing
Talus	
Chips, avulsions, nondisplaced neck fractures	Short-leg walking cast for 8-12 weeks
Navicular	
All avulsion, stress, and tuberosity fractures (except with large fragments)	Short-leg walking cast for 4-6 weeks
Foot	
Heel-pad syndrome	Heel cups or padded insoles
All fifth metatarsophalangeal avulsion fractures	Short-leg walking cast for 2-4 weeks
Jones fracture of the fifth metatarsal, nondisplaced	Jones dressing followed by a short-leg walking cast for 3-4 weeks
Nondisplaced metatarsal fractures	Short-leg walking cast with crutches and nonweightbearing for 2-3 weeks, plus casting and weightbearing for an additional 2 weeks
All stress fractures of the metatarsals	Well-supported shoe plus limited standing and walking
Nearly all great toe fractures without comminution or soft-tissue injury	Taping plus a well-supported shoe versus short-leg walking cast for 2 weeks
Nearly all sesamoid fractures without comminution or soft-tissue injury	Short-leg walking cast for 3-4 weeks, then a well-supported shoe
Lesser toe fractures	Cotton ball between the toes plus taping

require a high index of suspicion for early diagnosis and often require confirmation by specialized radiographic testing.

The following section describes the fractures that affect the peripheral skeleton—the classification, the criteria for referral to an orthopedic surgeon, the general treatment plan for fractures that are managed surgically, and the details of treatment for fractures that are managed nonoperatively. The list is extensive but not comprehensive. If there is any question about the stability of the fracture, its intra-articular extension, or the optimal type or length of immobilization, referral to an orthopedic surgeon is recommended. More detailed descriptions of the management of any given fracture can be found in

FRACTURES OF THE HUMERUS

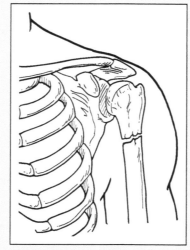

FIGURE 12-1. Fractures of the humerus.

Fractures of the humerus are classified according to location: proximal neck, shaft, and supracondylar. Proximal neck fractures are classified into two-part, three-part, and four-part fractures with or without dislocation of the shoulder joint (Neer classification). Humeral shaft fractures are classified by fracture line (spiral, transverse, longitudinal, comminuted) and by location relative to the pectoralis and deltoid insertions. Supracondylar fractures are grouped with fractures of the elbow; nearly all are referred to surgery (Sx).

standard texts of orthopedics. Lastly, associated soft-tissue injury must be assessed in all patients with bony fractures. The neurovascular status must be assessed distal to the site of the fracture. Pulse pressure and capillary fill times and light touch, two-point discrimination, and pain sensation must be assessed distal to the fracture site and compared side to side. In addition, the integrity of the muscular compartments of the forearm, thigh, and lower leg must be assessed and followed closely for signs of compromise with the fractures of the long bones in these areas.

FRACTURES OF THE HUMERUS: SHAFT AND PROXIMAL NECK

SUMMARY

Fractures of the humerus constitute approximately 2% of all fractures. The incidence increases with age and with osteoporosis (especially in the humeral neck). Humeral fractures are classified according to location: proximal neck, humeral shaft, and supracondylar. The proximal neck and humeral shaft fractures are grouped together, separate from the supracondylar fractures, because they usually are treated by nonoperative means. Supracondylar fractures are more complex, can involve the elbow joint, and may require open fixation (*Sx*).

SEQUENCE OF TREATMENTS

1. Order *x-rays*, classify the type of fracture, determine the degree of displacement or dislocation of the adjacent joints, and assess the integrity of the radial nerve by testing wrist strength.
2. Obtain *surgical orthopedic referral* (see later).
3. Immobilize in a *hanging cast* (p. 247) with collar and cuff appliance.
4. *Adjust* the length of the sling and its position at the wrist to correct for anterior or posterior bowing or valgus or volar angulation.

5. Begin daily finger stretches (p. 278) and Codman pendulum stretching exercise (p. 271) after the acute pain subsides.
6. Obtain weekly *x-rays* to assess for angulation, bowing, and callus formation.
7. Refer to *physical therapy* if frozen shoulder intervenes.
8. Begin *isometric toning exercises* at 6 to 8 weeks to restore full function of the shoulder (p. 272).
9. Limit *overhead reaching and positioning* if impingement signs are present and limit *lifting, pushing, and pulling* until full strength has been restored.

SURGICAL CONSULTATION Internal fixation is necessary for (1) shaft fractures that are open, severely comminuted, or transverse (where there is a higher degree of nonunion) and (2) neck fractures showing dislocation of the shoulder, fragment displacement greater than 1 cm, or fragment angulation greater than 45 degrees.

COMPLICATIONS Frozen shoulder (proximal neck fractures); chronic impingement (angulation of the greater tubercle); osteoarthritis of the shoulder (fracture/dislocation); radial nerve injury (lower-third shaft fractures); brachial artery injury (shaft fractures); nonunion (transverse and comminuted shaft fractures).

FRACTURES OF THE CLAVICLE

SUMMARY

Fracture of the clavicle is the most common fracture of childhood and is a common fracture in shoulder-girdle trauma in adults. These fractures are classified according to location (proximal-third, middle-third, and distal-third fractures), involvement of the adjacent articular cartilage of the supraclavicular joint or the acromioclavicular joint, and position of distal fractures relative to the

FRACTURES OF THE CLAVICLE

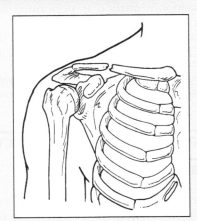

Fractures of the clavicle are classified according to location: proximal-third, middle-third, and distal-third fractures. Fractures of the proximal third are classified as nondisplaced, displaced, or intra-articular. All middle-third fractures are grouped together. Fractures of the distal third are classified according to displacement, location relative to the coracoclavicular ligaments, and whether the fracture line enters the acromioclavicular joint.

FIGURE 12–2. Proximal, middle, and distal third fractures of the clavicle.

coracoclavicular ligaments. Fracture of the middle third is the most common (80%). The second most common fracture is the interligamentous, nondisplaced fracture of the distal third (10%). Displacement of the fracture fragments depends on the pull of the sternocleidomastoid muscles (the proximal fragments are pulled superiorly) and the pectoralis major muscles (the distal fragments drop forward).

SEQUENCE OF TREATMENTS

1. Order *x-rays,* classify the type of fracture, and determine the degree of displacement or dislocation of the adjacent joints.
2. Refer to an orthopedic surgeon (see later).
3. Immobilize in a *simple sling* or *figure-of-eight splint* (p. 246).
4. Adjust the figure-of-eight splint to maintain close approximation of the fragments.
5. Codman exercises are unnecessary if the glenohumeral joint is not directly involved.
6. Begin *isometric toning exercises* in abduction and external rotation (rotator cuff tendons) at 4 to 6 weeks (p. 272).
7. Limit *overhead reaching and positioning* for the first 3 months, and limit *lifting, pushing, and pulling* until full strength has been restored to the rotator cuff tendons.
8. Gradually increase active general shoulder conditioning exercises at 3 months.

SURGICAL CONSULTATION Surgery must be considered in the case of any fracture associated with first-rib, pneumothorax, or neurovascular injury (<3%); in distal-third fractures with displacement (because of the greater risk of nonunion); and in nonunion that includes shoulder dysfunction or chronic pain.

COMPLICATIONS Complications include dislocation of the acromioclavicular or supraclavicular joint; head and neck injuries (displaced fractures); first-rib fracture; pneumothorax (3%); brachial plexus injury (caused by severe and forceful blows in a downward direction); subclavian vessel or internal jugular vein injuries (caused by rare, severe blows); nonunion, which is rare; and malunion with cosmetic deformity, which is common.

DISTAL HUMERAL FRACTURES: SUPRACONDYLAR FRACTURE

SUMMARY

Supracondylar fractures of the distal humerus are categorized as elbow fractures or dislocations and can be classified further as extension or flexion types, depending on the force of the injury. The most common injury is a fall on the outstretched hand. Because the fracture can extend into the elbow joint and involve either the brachial artery or the median nerve, referral to an orthopedic surgeon is

strongly advised (*Sx*). Nondisplaced or minimal fractures that do not enter the elbow joint can be treated with a *posterior splint* for 1 to 2 weeks, followed by early range of motion (ROM) exercises of the elbow.

DISTAL HUMERAL FRACTURES: INTERCONDYLAR FRACTURE

SUMMARY

Intercondylar fractures should be referred immediately to an orthopedic surgeon (*Sx*). The T-configuration or Y-configuration fractures of the distal humerus are the most difficult to manage of fractures of the upper extremity. Open reduction with rigid internal fixation is the preferred treatment to optimize the alignment and continuity of the articular surfaces of the elbow.

ELBOW DISLOCATION WITHOUT CONCOMITANT FRACTURE

SUMMARY

Elbow dislocation occurs mostly in the young (10 to 20 years old) and in the elderly. The elbow usually dislocates posteriorly. Neurovascular evaluation of the brachial artery, median nerve, and ulnar nerve is mandatory before proceeding to reduction. Closed reduction involves distraction with or without hyperextension to unlock the olecranon, followed by anterior translation. Open reduction is rare.

REDUCTION

1. The patient is to be in a *prone position*.
2. The *arm is hung* over the side of the exam table with *weight* applied to the wrist or with *traction* applied by the examiner.
3. With constant traction, and as the olecranon is felt to slip distally, the elbow is gently flexed.
4. The *ROM* of the elbow in flexion to 30 degrees and in supination/pronation is performed to ensure the stability of the reduction.
5. A *posterior splint* (p. 250) is applied for 2 to 3 weeks.
6. Gentle, *passive ROM* exercises are performed within 1 to 2 weeks to prevent contracture.
7. With improving motion, *isometric toning exercises* of elbow flexion and extension are begun.

NONDISPLACED RADIAL-HEAD FRACTURE

SUMMARY

The preferred management of nondisplaced radial-head fracture with a *sling* (p. 246) and ROM exercises is a classic example of the application of early physical therapy. This approach can be combined with aspiration of the hemarthrosis and intra-articular injection of local

→ anesthetic (p. •••) to assist in early exercising. Associated injuries to the medial collateral ligament, interosseous membrane, and wrist should be excluded. Displaced radial head fractures should be referred to an orthopedic surgeon for radial head excision (*Sx*).

NONDISPLACED FRACTURES OF THE SHAFTS OF THE RADIUS AND ULNA

SUMMARY

Fixed immobilization in a *long-arm cast* (p. 250)—axilla to metacarpals—with a collar and cuff suspension at the proximal forearm is the treatment of choice for a non-displaced fracture. Displaced fractures must be evaluated by an orthopedic surgeon (*Sx*). Open reduction and fixation is the preferred method of counteracting the opposing muscular forces, restoring the proper length of the bones, and achieving axial and rotational alignment. Similarly, open reduction and internal fixation is the preferred treatment for a Monteggia fracture in an adult (displaced fracture of the ulna with radial head dislocation).

FRACTURES OF THE DISTAL RADIUS

SUMMARY

Of the variety of fractures that affect the wrist, Colles fracture is the most common. Nondisplaced fractures and displaced fractures that are readily reduced and stable can be managed with casting for 3 to 6 weeks. Colles fractures that are reducible but unstable, comminuted, or intra-articular and Smith fractures and Barton fractures may require open reduction and internal fixation (*Sx*). These fractures should be managed by an orthopedic surgeon.

SEQUENCE OF TREATMENT FOR COLLES FRACTURES

1. Order *x-rays,* classify the type of fracture, determine the degree of displacement or dislocation of the adjacent joints, and assess the integrity of the median nerve.
2. Refer to an *orthopedic surgeon* (see later).
3. Perform hematoma, axillary, or Bier block *anesthesia.*
4. Perform closed reduction using *finger-trap traction* (p. 252) with proximal brachial countertraction.
5. Repeat *x-rays* to ensure a slightly volar tilt and restoration of the length of the radius.
6. Use a *sugar-tong splint* (p. 250) for the first 48 hours to allow room for swelling.
7. After 48 hours, replace the splint with a *short-arm cast* (p. 249) for undisplaced fractures or a *long-arm cast* (p. 249) with slight flexion and ulnar deviation for displaced fractures (if unstable, refer to surgery).
8. Repeat *x-rays* at 4 to 6 weeks to assess for healing.
9. Use a *Velcro wrist splint with a metal stay* (p. 249) for 3 to 4 weeks after immobilization.
10. Start passive ROM exercises of the wrist in dorsiflexion and volar flexion after fixed immobilization.

SURGICAL PROCEDURE   Pin fixation or open reduction is necessary for a fracture that remains unstable despite closed reduction, for a Barton fracture/dislocation, for a comminuted fracture, and for a displaced fracture (especially an intra-articular fracture).

FRACTURES OF THE DISTAL RADIUS

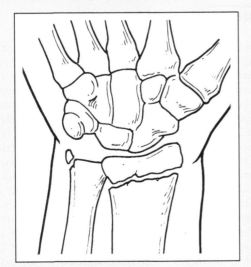

Fractures of the distal radius are classified according to the direction of angulation of the radius and whether the radiocarpal joint, radioulnar joint, or both are involved. Colles fracture involves the distal 2 cm of the radius, is angled dorsally, and may or may not involve the joints. Smith fracture is identical to Colles fracture except for the volar angulation. Barton fracture is a fracture/dislocation with the predominant finding of wrist dislocation by clinical criteria and x-ray results.

FIGURE 12-3. Fractures of the distal radius: Colles, Smith, and Barton.

COMPLICATIONS Intra-articular and extra-articular fractures that result in a foreshortened or angled radius (>5 mm or >20 degrees) have a greater incidence of poor ROM of the wrist, osteoarthritis of the wrist, and median nerve damage.

NAVICULAR FRACTURE AND SEVERE WRIST SPRAIN

See Chapter 4 for details of management of navicular fracture and severe wrist sprain.

METACARPAL FRACTURES

SUMMARY

Fractures of the metacarpals are classified according to location—head, neck, shaft, and base. These fractures are difficult to manage because of fracture angulation, fragment rotation (especially oblique fractures of the shaft), inherent instability after reduction, and postfracture stiffness that can occur as a result of improper immobilization. For these reasons, open reduction and pin fixation are suggested (*Sx*). The Boxer fracture of the fifth metacarpal neck can be treated nonoperatively, however. If the fracture is not comminuted, angulation is less than 40 degrees, and the patient is willing to accept a deformity on the back of the hand, good function results from 4 weeks of wearing a removable *ulnar gutter splint* (p. 250).

VOLAR DISLOCATION OF THE METACARPOPHALANGEAL JOINTS

SUMMARY

Dislocation of the metacarpophalangeal joints involves injury to the lateral collateral ligaments and is an uncommon condition. Immobilization with a *radial or ulnar gutter splint* (p. 250) is the preferred treatment unless an avulsion fracture greater than 2 to 3 mm is present. In the case of a large avulsion fracture, pin fixation is the preferred surgical procedure. Often a patient presents with similar symptoms weeks to months after an injury to the metacarpophalangeal joint. Intra-articular corticosteroid injection combined with 3 weeks of immobilization using a radial or ulnar gutter splint is effective, although symptoms may persist for 9 to 12 months.

EXTRA-ARTICULAR METACARPAL FRACTURES OF THE THUMB

SUMMARY

Transverse or oblique fractures of the shafts of the metacarpal (totally extra-articular in all views) can be treated with closed reduction with good results. The fracture is immobilized for 4 weeks in a well-molded *thumb-spica cast* (p. 251) and followed by passive ROM exercises of the thumb. Metacarpal fractures that involve the carpometacarpal joint are inherently unstable and must be managed surgically (see later).

INTRA-ARTICULAR METACARPAL FRACTURES OF THE THUMB

SUMMARY

Comminuted metacarpal fractures or fractures that involve the carpometacarpal joint are inherently unstable and must be managed surgically (*Sx*). A Bennett fracture is a fracture/dislocation of the base of the metacarpal and is unstable because of the dorsal and radial pull of the abductor pollicis longus. A Rolando fracture is a comminuted fracture of the base of the thumb and is even more unstable than Bennett fracture. Both fractures should be managed by an orthopedic surgeon because of the difficulty in maintaining anatomic reduction without internal pin fixation.

DORSAL DISLOCATION OF THE META-CARPOPHALANGEAL JOINT OF THE THUMB

SUMMARY

If a single attempt at closed reduction is unsuccessful, an orthopedic surgeon should be consulted. Closed reduction is impossible with a trapped volar plate.

GAMEKEEPER'S THUMB, COMPLETE RUPTURE

See Chapter 4 for details of management of gamekeeper's thumb.

FRACTURES OF THE PROXIMAL AND MIDDLE PHALANGES

SUMMARY

Fractures of the phalanges are classified by location, configuration (transverse or oblique), and the effects of the fracture on the rotation and foreshortening of the digit. Most of these fractures can be managed nonsurgically. Extra-articular fractures that do not exhibit displacement, rotation, or angulation can be treated with *buddy-taping* (p. 252) and active ROM exercises. Nearly all transverse fractures can be managed in this fashion. In addition, small chip fractures of the collateral ligaments, dorsal chip fractures of the central slip of the extensor tendon at the base of the middle phalanx, and nondisplaced marginal fractures of the base of the proximal phalanx can be managed with buddy-taping. Transverse fractures at the base or neck of the proximal phalanx, nearly all spiral oblique fractures, and all comminuted and condylar (intra-articular) fractures must be evaluated by an orthopedic surgeon for possible open reduction and internal fixation (*Sx*). All phalangeal fractures must be assessed for late complications, including malrotation, lateral deviation, recurvatum angulation, shortening, intra-articular malunion, nonunion, tendon adherence, joint stiffness, and nail-bed interposition.

ACUTE BOUTONNIÈRE INJURY

SUMMARY

Finger injuries leading to an acute boutonnière deformity—tissue disruption of the central slip of the extensor tendon combined with tearing of the triangular ligament on the dorsum of the middle phalanx—can be treated by closed reduction as long as no bony chip fracture is present. The proximal interphalangeal joint is immobilized in full extension with a *proximal interphalangeal splint*, and active and passive ROM exercises are performed daily. As with all finger and thumb injuries, postimmobilization stiffness must be guarded against.

DISLOCATIONS OF THE PROXIMAL INTERPHALANGEAL JOINT

SUMMARY

There are three types of dislocation of the proximal interphalangeal joint: dorsal, volar (rare), and rotatory (uncommon). The dorsal or volar plate injury (with or without a small volar avulsion fracture) is the most common type of dislocation and is the result of hyperextension of the joint. Reduction is accomplished by closed means. The proximal interphalangeal joint is immobilized with a *proximal interphalangeal splint* (p. 253) for 2 weeks (≤15 degrees of flexion) or with *buddy-taping* (p. 252) for 3 to 6 weeks. Buddy-taping has the advantage of allowing early active motion (guarding against residual joint stiffness), while preventing hyperextension. ROM exercises are continued for several weeks after immobilization. Surgical consultation is strongly recommended for dorsal dislocations associated with volar lip fractures involving more than 20% of the articular surface and for nonreducible dislocations (*Sx*).

FRACTURE OF THE DISTAL PHALANX

SUMMARY

Fractures of the distal phalanx are classified as longitudinal, transverse, or crushed-eggshell types. These account for 50% of all hand fractures. Simple protective splinting for 3 to 4 weeks using a *fingertip guard or Stack splint* (p. 253) is combined with specific treatment of the soft-tissue injuries (e.g., laceration, subungual hematoma). The splint should not be placed close to the proximal interphalangeal joint to avoid joint stiffness.

MALLET FRACTURES

SUMMARY

With Mallet fracture, the extensor tendon has avulsed a large fragment of bone (greater than one third of the articular surface) from the dorsal articular surface of the distal interphalangeal joint. Management is controversial. Open reduction and fixation is advocated by some surgeons if the avulsed fragment is large, volar subluxation is present, and the fragment has been displaced more than 2 to 3 mm (*Sx*).

RUPTURE OF THE EXTENSOR TENDON: MALLET FINGER

SUMMARY

The mallet finger deformity can result from stretching or partially tearing the extensor tendon or from complete rupture or rupture with avulsion fracture of the distal phalanx. Treatment consists of splinting the distal interphalangeal joint in full extension or slight hyperextension for 1 to 2 months, using a *dorsal aluminum splint* and tape (p. 253) or a *Stack splint* (p. 253). The patient should be advised that function may be impaired in 30% of cases, especially in patients older than age 60 and in patients with rheumatoid arthritis or peripheral vascular disease, if treatment is delayed more than 4 weeks, and if immobilization lasts less than 4 weeks. Patients with large avulsion fractures should be evaluated by an orthopedic surgeon (*Sx*).

RUPTURE OF THE EXTENSOR TENDON OF THE THUMB: MALLET THUMB

SUMMARY

Mallet thumb results from a rupture of the extensor pollicis longus insertion. Treatment with interphalangeal joint splinting and operative repair provide similar results (*Sx*).

RUPTURE OF THE FLEXOR DIGITORUM PROFUNDUS TENDON

SUMMARY

Rupture of the flexor digitorum profundus tendon is an uncommon injury caused by forced hyperextension of the distal interphalangeal joint. Early operative repair is the treatment of choice (*Sx*).

COMPRESSION FRACTURE OF THE VERTEBRAL BODY

SUMMARY

Compression fracture of the vertebral body is the most common fracture of the spine. The leading causes are structural weakness secondary to osteoporosis, trauma, and metastatic disease. The lower thoracic vertebrae and the lumbar vertebrae are the sites most often affected. Metastatic disease always should be suspected if the fracture occurs above T7.

COMPRESSION FRACTURE OF THE VERTEBRAL BODY

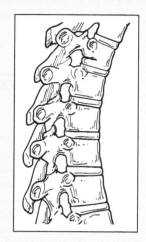

FIGURE 12–4. Wedge-shaped compression fracture of the vertebral body.

Osteoporosis and trauma are the most common causes of vertebral body compression fracture; metastatic cancer and osteomyelitis are much less common causes. Trauma and osteoporosis most often affect the lower thoracic spine and lumbar vertebrae. As a general rule, if a compression fracture occurs above T7, metastatic disease or infection must be excluded.

SEQUENCE OF TREATMENTS

1. Order *x-rays* of the spine, obtain baseline *laboratory values* (complete blood count, calcium, alkaline phosphatase, and erythrocyte sedimentation rate), and evaluate the *neurologic status* of the patient.
2. Obtain a *neurosurgical consultation* if angulation exceeds 35 degrees, if the fracture is unstable, or if neurologic compromise is present.
3. Prescribe adequate *analgesia* for this painful condition.
4. Recommend *bed rest* for 3 to 5 days for a patient with acute and severe pain.
5. Educate the patient: *"The fracture may take several months to heal."*
6. Prescribe a *lumbosacral corset* (p. 254) or a three-point brace (p. 255) if pain control has been difficult to achieve.
7. Follow *alkaline phosphatase, calcium, and complete blood count* to assess healing.
8. Perform *bone densitometry* to assess the degree of bone loss.
9. Prescribe *calcium, vitamin D, or hormonal replacement* with estrogen and progesterone.
10. Gradually *increase the level of activities* after the acute pain has subsided, and strongly encourage an *aerobic exercise* program.

SURGICAL PROCEDURE Fracture stabilization is performed for severely angulated or unstable fractures.

COMPLICATIONS Depending on the underlying cause, the number of fractures, their locations, and their effects on the underlying neurologic structures, vertebral body compression fractures can be complicated by chronic pain (in the case of multiple fractures), neurologic impairment (epidural metastasis, epidural abscess, or severe collapse), pulmonary insufficiency (multiple fractures), chronic osteomyelitis, and overlying skin ulceration (multiple fractures leading to an exaggerated kyphosis).

RIB FRACTURE

SUMMARY

Rib fractures are classified as nondisplaced ("cracked") or displaced. Fractures result from blunt trauma to the chest or from severe paroxysms of coughing. Nondisplaced fractures should be suspected if the patient has localized chest wall pain that is aggravated by direct palpation over the rib, deep breathing, coughing or sneezing, or chest wall compression. If the fracture is not a result of blunt trauma, and the patient does not have generalized osteoporosis, a pathologic fracture should be suspected.

SEQUENCE OF TREATMENTS

1. The lungs should be auscultated carefully for diminished lung sounds, and the soft tissues should be palpated for crepitance.
2. Order *x-rays* of the chest and rib in selected patients.
3. Apply *ice* directly over the rib.
4. Prescribe an *antitussive* if appropriate or use acetaminophen with codeine compound (Tylenol with Codeine) to control pain and cough.
5. Educate the patient: *"A fractured rib may take several weeks to heal."*
6. Perform an *intercostal nerve block* with local anesthesia for severe localized pain.
7. Suggest a well-fitted bra, a snug jogging bra, an Ace wrap, or a *rib binder* to provide chest wall support.
8. Advise the patient that overmedication or excessive chest-wall binding can lead to local areas of lung collapse or pneumonia.

RIB FRACTURE

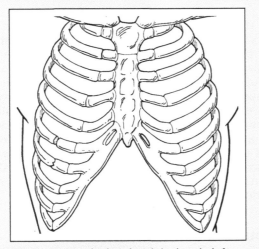

Rib fractures are encountered commonly in primary care. Nondisplaced fractures can be managed with chest wall splinting, analgesics, and antitussives as indicated. Greater attention must be paid to patients with displaced rib fractures. The entire bony thorax, great vessels, and pulmonary tree and parenchyma must be assessed for additional injury.

FIGURE 12–5. Nondisplaced and displaced rib fractures.

SURGICAL PROCEDURE   No surgical procedure is indicated.

COMPLICATIONS   Blunt trauma of a sufficient degree to the chest can cause damage to the internal organs, great vessels, or other structures of the thorax (sterno-clavicular joint, sternum, and vertebral bodies). The patient must be observed closely for progressive respiratory distress (pneumothorax or hemothorax). A patient with significantly compromised lung function secondary to emphysema, asthma, or other illness may require temporary hospitalization.

PELVIC FRACTURES
SUMMARY

The successful management of a fractured pelvis requires the combined clinical skills of the primary care provider, the orthopedic surgeon (Sx), and the urologist. Blunt trauma severe enough to fracture the sacrum, ilium, ischium, or pubic bones often leads to injury of the under-lying organ system. Life-threatening hemorrhage; urologic injury to the bladder, urethra, or ureters; or gastrointestinal injury to the colon must be assessed quickly for possible emergent treatment. After the patient has been stabilized medically, specific x-rays should be obtained to determine the severity and classification of the injury. The x-rays should include cervical spine, chest, posteroanterior pelvis, and inlet and outlet views of the pelvic ring. If the acetabulum is involved, special iliac and obturator views or a CT scan of the entire pelvis must be obtained. With these x-rays, fractures can be classified according to the degree of pelvic ring disruption, the involvement

of the acetabulum, and the degree of displacement and instability of the bony fragments in the vertical and rotational directions. Hospitalization, sling traction, and close observation for the first 24 to 48 hours, including hemodynamic monitoring, is combined with early pin placement for external fixation or open reduction and internal fixation (Sx). Unstable patients with ongoing retroperitoneal hemorrhage should be evaluated by pelvic angiography and treated with embolization.

HIP FRACTURES AND FRACTURES OF THE FEMUR
SUMMARY

Fractures of the femur are divided into fractures involving the hip joint and fractures of the femur. Hip fractures are subdivided further into impacted, occult, avascular necrosis, stress, and nondisplaced and displaced neck fractures. Fractures of the femur are subdivided further into intertrochanteric, trochanteric process, subtrochanteric, shaft, and supracondylar fractures (although the last-mentioned traditionally is grouped with fractures of the knee). All of these fractures are treated surgically (internal fixation, hemiarthroplasty, or total hip replacement) with the exception of certain impacted and occult fractures, stress fractures of the femoral neck, and avascular necrosis. The primary care physician must be able to diagnose and initiate the early treatment of these four fractures (see later).

EMERGENCY DEPARTMENT TREATMENT FOR HIP FRACTURE   The patient presents with a displaced femoral neck fracture with a foreshortened leg that is externally rotated. Transfers should be made with great attention to support of the extremity. The patient must be evaluated for a cardiovascular event that could have caused the fall. Appropriate intravenous analgesia should be provided. Traction should be applied at 5 to 10 lb, depending on the size of the patient and the bulk of the quadriceps. Consultation with an orthopedic surgeon should be made emergently.

METASTATIC INVOLVEMENT OF THE FEMUR AND TIBIA

SUMMARY

Metastatic involvement of the weightbearing bones of the lower extremity poses a special management problem. Secondary fracture through these bones has a disastrous effect on a patient's quality of life and can create a potential medicolegal dilemma for the provider. Protected weightbearing, radiation therapy, and prophylactic intramedullary rod placement are used to prevent secondary fracture. If metastatic disease is identified by bone scanning, the patient should be placed on limited weightbearing immediately. Plain x-rays of the pelvis, femur, and tibia are obtained to determine the compromise of the cortical structural bone, and urgent referral is made to an orthopedic surgeon (*Sx*) and radiation oncologist. These patients must be followed regularly and closely.

AVASCULAR NECROSIS OF THE HIP

See Chapter 8 for details of management.

OCCULT FRACTURE OF THE HIP

SUMMARY

The diagnosis of hip fracture is straightforward in most cases. A nondisplaced or incomplete fracture of the femur may elude early detection, however. This occult fracture occurs as a result of a fall. Elderly patients with advanced osteoporosis are at particular risk. The diagnosis must be suspected when the hip exam discloses severe pain and extreme guarding with hip rotation. Plain x-rays do not show an obvious fracture line when advanced osteopenia is present. Weightbearing must be restricted until the diagnosis is confirmed or excluded by studies. To avoid the medicolegal issues of delay in diagnosis or inappropriate management, weightbearing must be restricted to avoid completing the fracture.

SEQUENCE OF TREATMENTS

1. *Examine* the patient's tolerance of weightbearing and the severity of pain with passive internal and external rotation.
2. Order an anteroposterior pelvis *x-ray*.
3. If the diagnosis is suspected, weightbearing must be *restricted acutely* by using crutches or by strict bed rest.
4. Order an MRI to evaluate for a subtle occult fracture.
5. Obtain an urgent *consultation* with an orthopedic surgeon.
6. Repeat *plain x-rays* in 2 to 3 weeks.
7. Resume weightbearing when rotation of the hip is pain-free, and significant healing has been shown on plain x-rays.

OCCULT FRACTURE OF THE HIP

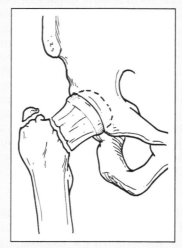

Occult fracture of the hip must be suspected if any of the following is true:

1. A fall has occurred, and the patient is elderly and is known to have osteoporotic bones.
2. Weightbearing is impossible because of moderate to severe hip pain.
3. Internal and external rotation of the hip causes moderate to severe hip pain on exam.

Note: Plain x-rays of the hip do not show true fracture lines because the bones are too osteoporotic.

FIGURE 12–6. Occult fracture of the hip.

SURGICAL PROCEDURE   Although debilitated patients can be treated with prolonged bed rest, physical therapy ROM exercises, and gradual weightbearing, there is a substantial risk of medical complications, such as pneumonia, deep venous thrombosis, and stasis ulceration. For this reason, early percutaneous fixation of the hip and total hip replacement are the treatments of choice. The patient and the patient's family should be advised of the morbidity associated with prolonged confinement to bed.

COMPLICATIONS   The risk of full weightbearing (conversion of an occult fracture into a displaced fracture) is so great that percutaneous pinning is performed in all but severely debilitated patients. Patients treated with combined bed rest and limited weightbearing are at risk for deep venous thrombosis and infectious complications.

FRACTURES OF THE KNEE: TIBIAL PLATEAU AND DISTAL FEMUR

SUMMARY

Owing to the diversity of fractures that occur at the knee (tibial plateau) and the distal femur (supracondylar), the intra-articular extension of a sizable proportion of the fractures, the associated injuries to the supporting ligaments, and the need for specialized traction and cast-bracing, most patients with these fractures should be referred to an orthopedic surgeon for management (*Sx*). Fractures that can be treated nonoperatively include avulsion fractures at the joint line (medial collateral and lateral collateral ligament injuries), nondisplaced osteochondritis dissecans fractures that do not cause mechanical locking, minimally depressed tibial plateau rim fractures (depression <10 degrees), and certain patellar fractures (see later).

FRACTURES OF THE PATELLA

SUMMARY

Patellar fractures are classified as transverse, stellate, longitudinal, marginal, or, rarely, osteochondral. More than half of patellar fractures are transverse, and most of these are the result of a direct blow to the patella that is magnified by the tremendous pull of the quadriceps mechanism. Most show little or no separation of the fragments owing to the intact medial and lateral quadriceps muscle "expansions." Nonoperative treatment with *long-leg casting* (p. 258) and gradual restoration of weightbearing is the treatment of choice for nondisplaced fractures. Surgery involves cerclage wiring or lag-screw internal fixation for displaced fragments or total patellectomy for severely comminuted fractures (*Sx*).

SEQUENCE OF TREATMENTS

1. *Aspirate* the hemarthrosis.
2. *Assess the quadriceps mechanism* by asking the patient to lift the leg against gravity; this can be determined more accurately after aspiration of the hemarthrosis and intra-articular anesthesia.
3. Refer to an *orthopedic surgeon* if the quadriceps mechanism is ruptured, or the fragments are separated by more than 2 to 3 mm.
4. Immobilize with a *long-leg cast* (p. 258) for 4 to 6 weeks.
5. Allow partial weightbearing until the pain is significantly decreased, then full weightbearing.
6. Perform *straight-leg-raising exercises* (p. 289) as soon as the pain has lessened.
7. *Restrict* squatting and kneeling, and avoid repetitive bending for 3 to 6 months.
8. Obtain bilateral *sunrise x-rays* at 1 year to assess for early osteoarthritic changes.

OSTEOCHONDRITIS DISSECANS OF THE MEDIAL FEMORAL CONDYLE

SUMMARY

Osteochondritis dissecans is an osteochondral fracture (bone and cartilage) at the site of attachment of the posterior cruciate ligament on the lateral aspect of the medial condyle. As to its exact cause, direct trauma, ischemia, and true avulsion are theorized. Patients present with nonspecific knee complaints or with mechanical locking resulting from an associated loose body. Patients with large fragments, persistent knee effusion, and mechanical locking should be referred to an orthopedic surgeon to consider posterior cruciate ligament repair, drilling of the fragment (to stimulate revascularization), or repair of any other associated injuries to ligaments or meniscal cartilage (*Sx*).

TIBIAL SHAFT FRACTURES

SUMMARY

Most tibial shaft fractures should be managed by an orthopedic surgeon (*Sx*). Fractures with no less than 1 cm of shortening, 5 degrees of varus or valgus angulation, or 10 degrees of anteroposterior or rotational angulation can be managed nonoperatively. After closed reduction using intravenous sedation, a *long-leg cast* (p. 258) with suprapatellar and medial tibial molding is applied. The foot and ankle are kept in the neutral position, and the knee is flexed to 5 degrees. Healing time averages 5 months. Cast wedging is used to correct any postreduction angulation. When adequate callus formation is noted on x-rays, the cast can be replaced with a patellar tendon bearing cast or brace to complete the healing process. During the recovery period, the patient must be monitored carefully for deep venous thrombosis, anterior compartment syndrome, and distal ischemia.

TIBIAL STRESS FRACTURE

See Chapter 10 for details of management.

COMBINED TIBIAL AND FIBULAR SHAFT FRACTURES

SUMMARY

A combined tibial and fibular fracture should be referred to an orthopedic surgeon because of the presence of instability, angulation, and greater degrees of soft-tissue injury (*Sx*).

ISOLATED FIBULAR SHAFT FRACTURE

SUMMARY

Isolated fibular shaft fracture is much less common than the combined tibial and fibular fracture. It usually occurs as a result of a direct blow. Immobilization is used for pain control only. The fracture can be treated with a shortened stride, decreased weightbearing activities, or immobilization with a *short-leg walking cast* (p. 260). Fixed immobilization with casting is recommended when weightbearing pain is troublesome.

GASTROCNEMIUS MUSCLE TEAR

See Chapter 10 for details of management.

FRACTURES OF THE ANKLE

SUMMARY

Fractures of the ankle are probably the most difficult of all fractures to manage, in part because of the complexity of the ankle joint, but also because of the diversity of fractures that can occur. Various combinations of injuries to ligaments and interosseous membranes and bony fractures are possible. Classification is based on the injury pattern, the particular bones and ligaments that have been injured, the degree of fragment displacement, and the degree of incongruity of the articular surface. The Henderson system identifies malleolar, bimalleolar, and trimalleolar fractures. Lauge-Hansen classifies according to injury forces, that is, the supination-adduction injury pattern corresponds to the classic turned-in ankle sprain. Danis-Weber classifies the fractures according to the location of the fibular fracture relative to the syndesmosis, which correlates well with fracture instability.

The goal of the primary care physician is to diagnose the extent of the injury accurately by assessing the severity of the injury, the radiographic abnormalities, and the stability of the fracture and joint. The posteroanterior, lateral, and mortise x-rays are used to define the number and locations of the fractures. Measurements of the tibiofibular line, talocrural angle, talar tilt, and medial clear space from these views are used to determine fracture stability and displacement. Angle measurements on stress views of the ankle are used to determine ligamentous injuries. CT scans are used to define complex fracture patterns.

Small-fragment avulsion fractures, nondisplaced single malleolar fractures, and stable bimalleolar fractures can be treated nonoperatively. Initially, a *Jones compression dressing* with plaster splint reinforcement (p. 261) is used until swelling begins to resolve. Subsequently a *short-leg walking cast* (p. 260), fracture brace, or walking boot (p. 259) is prescribed. Weightbearing is limited until pain has decreased, and fracture healing is documented. Most fractures at the syndesmosis, all fractures above the syndesmosis, and fractures with significant displacement (radiographically, by line measurement or stress views) should be placed in a Jones dressing. The patient

FRACTURES OF THE ANKLE

Using the mortise view, ankle alignment and stability are assessed by the following measurements:

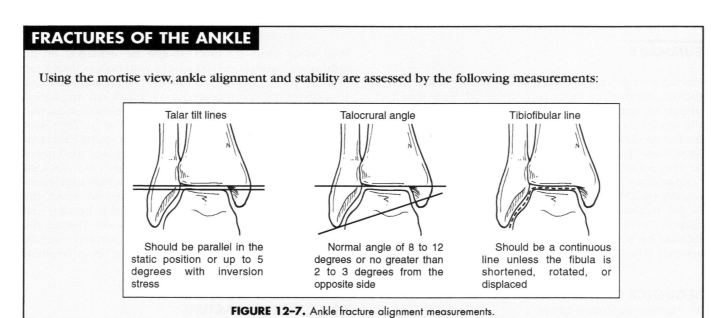

Talar tilt lines	Talocrural angle	Tibiofibular line
Should be parallel in the static position or up to 5 degrees with inversion stress	Normal angle of 8 to 12 degrees or no greater than 2 to 3 degrees from the opposite side	Should be a continuous line unless the fibula is shortened, rotated, or displaced

FIGURE 12–7. Ankle fracture alignment measurements.

should be given crutches and referred to an orthopedic surgeon (*Sx*).

FRACTURES ACCOMPANYING SEVERE ANKLE SPRAIN

SUMMARY

Inversion injury with extreme equinus positioning can cause a *fracture of the posterior process of the talus,* which must be distinguished from the os trigonum, an accessory bone that is located posterior to the talus. This stable fracture can be treated with a compressive dressing or a *short-leg walking cast* (p. 260) for 4 to 6 weeks. Inversion injury with the ankle dorsiflexed can cause a *fracture of the lateral process of the talus.* A mortise view or posteroanterior tomograms are necessary to show the fracture line. Small and minimally displaced fragments can be treated with a *short-leg walking cast* (p. 260) for 4 to 6 weeks. If the fragment is large, surgical referral for internal fixation is required (*Sx*). Inversion injury with rotation can cause excessive pressure on the peroneus brevis tendon and result in an *avulsion fracture of the base of the fifth metatarsal.* Small and minimally displaced fragments can be treated with a *short-leg walking cast* (p. 260) for 4 to 6 weeks. Malleolar fractures also are common with severe ankle sprains.

FRACTURES OF THE CALCANEUS

SUMMARY

The calcaneus is the tarsal bone that is most commonly fractured. Most fractures result from vertical falls and twisting injuries. Fractures are classified as extra-articular or intra-articular. Extra-articular fractures are subdivided further into anterior, tuberosity, medial process, sustentacular, and body fractures. Radiographically, posteroanterior, lateral, axial-calcaneal, and oblique views are combined with CT scans to define the location and intra-articular extension of the fragments. Most extra-articular fractures can be treated nonoperatively. After 5 to 6 days of strict bed rest with leg elevation to control swelling (including hospitalization in selected cases) and a *Jones compression dressing* (p. 261) for 2 to 3 days, a *short-leg walking cast* (p. 260) is applied. Ambulation is restricted to nonweightbearing crutches until union is definitely seen on repeat x-rays (typically, several weeks). Subsequently, weightbearing is graduated through partial to full weightbearing, as tolerated. Surgical referral is indicated for nonunion of the anterior process fracture, for displaced posterior process fractures (to restore the integrity of the Achilles tendon), and for all intra-articular fractures (*Sx*). Intra-articular fractures heal unpredictably. The clinician must apprise the patient of the potential of long-term complications, including subtalar joint pain, subtalar post-traumatic arthritis, peroneus tendinitis, bone spur formation, calcaneocuboid osteoarthritis, or entrapment of the medial and lateral plantar nerves.

FRACTURES OF THE TALUS

SUMMARY

The incidence of talus fractures is second only to that of calcaneal fractures. Classically, these are the result of hyperdorsiflexion injuries, as in hitting the brakes. Fractures are classified as chips, avulsions, or nondisplaced or displaced neck fractures. Surgical referral is advisable for the displaced neck fracture, which often is accompanied by subtalar joint dislocation, because a favorable outcome demands a perfect reduction of the articular cartilage (*Sx*). The remaining fractures respond to 8 to 12 weeks of immobilization with a *short-leg walking cast* (p. 260) in a slightly equinus position for the first month, followed by 1 to 2 months in the neutral position. As soon as union is documented on repeat x-rays, ROM exercises can be started. Despite perfect reduction, healing can be complicated by avascular necrosis of the body in 50% of cases.

FRACTURES OF THE NAVICULAR

SUMMARY

The *cortical avulsion fracture of the dorsal navicular* occurs adjacent to the talus and is the result of a twisting injury. Unless the fragment is large, these fractures should be treated with 4 to 6 weeks of a *short-leg walking cast* (p. 260). The *tuberosity fracture* occurs medially and often is confused with the accessory navicular bone. If the tuberosity is not displaced, a *short-leg walking cast* (p. 260) in neutral position for 4 to 6 weeks is the preferred treatment. The *navicular stress fracture* occurs in young athletes. Plain x-rays are difficult to interpret. If a long-distance runner has persistent local tenderness and difficulties with arch pain, a bone scan can be ordered to identify this uncommon stress fracture.

HEEL PAD SYNDROME

See Chapter 10 for details of management.

FRACTURES OF THE MIDTARSALS

SUMMARY

Midtarsal fractures are rare because of the rigidity of the midfoot.

CHARCOT, OR NEUROPATHIC, FRACTURES

SUMMARY

Patients with impaired sensation resulting from peripheral neuropathy are at risk for fracture and for impaired fracture healing. Often such patients present with localized swelling and erythema that is disproportionate to the average amount of reactive soft-tissue change for that particular fracture. The midfoot is often the site of these fractures. Nonunion and malunion of the fracture are common because of the delay in diagnosis.

ACCESSORY BONES OF THE FEET

SUMMARY

The accessory bones occur in a variety of locations. Radiographically, they are sharply defined, well-circumscribed, oval or round ossifications adjacent to the tarsal or metatarsal bones. They are significant only from the standpoint of their being frequently misinterpreted as fractures. Their specific locations and distinctive anatomic features should differentiate them from avulsions and small-fragment fractures of the bones of the feet.

FRACTURES OF METATARSALS 1 THROUGH 4

SUMMARY

A metatarsal fracture is caused most often by a direct blow to the top of the foot. Such fractures are classified according to the mechanism of injury (stress fractures), the location (base, neck, or shaft), the direction of the fracture line (transverse or spiral), and the displacement. Nondisplaced fractures of the neck or shaft of metatarsals 2 through 4 can be treated with ice, elevation, analgesia, and a *short-leg walking cast* (p. 260). Nondisplaced fractures of the first metatarsal are treated similarly, but with the addition of a 2- to 3-week period of non-weightbearing casting followed by a short-leg walking cast to complete the 5-week immobilization. Displaced metatarsal fractures should be referred to an orthopedic surgeon for reduction (*Sx*).

STRESS FRACTURES OF THE METATARSALS: MARCH FRACTURE

SUMMARY

Athletes, military recruits, and patients with osteoporosis who walk and stand for prolonged periods are at risk for the microfracturing of the metatarsal bones. The diagnosis should be suspected if the exam of the foot shows dramatic swelling over the dorsum of the foot, local tenderness of the metatarsal, and pain when the metatarsals are squeezed from either side. Plain x-rays may show periosteal thickening, but that is a late finding. Nuclear medicine bone scanning shows the abnormality in the early stages.

SEQUENCE OF TREATMENTS
1. *Wide-toe-box shoes* lessen the side-to-side pressure.
2. *Padded insoles* (p. 262) worn continuously lessen the effects of impact.
3. *Weightbearing,* both walking and standing, must be restricted until the pain has dramatically lessened.
4. Walking with a *shortened stride* lessens the impact on the bones.
5. Persistent symptoms can be treated with a *short-leg walking cast* (p. 260).
6. *Surgical consultation* is indicated if the bone fails to heal with restrictions and protection, or if a completed fracture occurs with angulation.

ACCESSORY BONES OF THE FEET

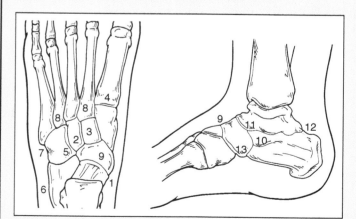

The accessory bones of the feet are significant because they can mimic fractures.

1. Os trigonum
2. Os sustentaculum
3. Talus accessorius
4. Os subcalcis
5. Os tibiotibiale
6. Calcaneus secundarium
7. Os supranaviculare
8. Os supratalare
9. Os tibiale externum
10. Os intercuneiforme
11. Os peroneum
12. Os vesalianum
13. Os intermetatarseum

FIGURE 12–8. The accessory bones of the feet in the differential diagnosis of foot fractures.

METATARSAL STRESS FRACTURES (MARCH FRACTURE)

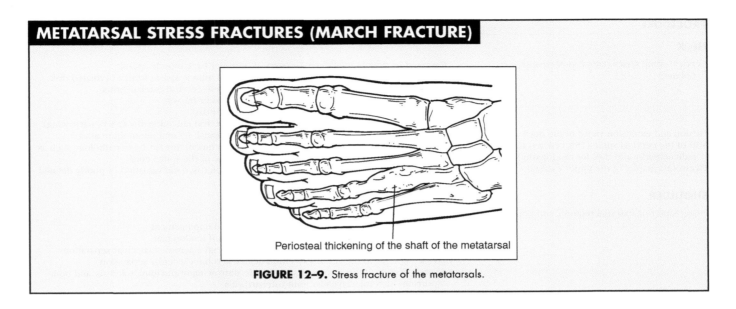

Periosteal thickening of the shaft of the metatarsal

FIGURE 12–9. Stress fracture of the metatarsals.

SURGICAL PROCEDURE   Open reduction and internal fixation is necessary for the rare case of complete fracture with displacement or angulation.

FRACTURES OF THE FIFTH METATARSAL BONE

SUMMARY

Fractures of the fifth metatarsal are unique. Severe inversion injuries of the ankle can cause the avulsion of a fleck of bone from the most proximal portion of the metatarsal. The peroneus brevis tendon detaches a small portion of cortex when the ankle is turned in. A *short-leg walking cast* (p. 260) is the treatment of choice. Immobilization should be continued for 3 to 4 weeks to allow the tendon to reattach securely to the metatarsal. Jones fracture involves the tuberosity of the base of the metatarsal. It should not be confused with a transverse fracture of the base, which has a much different prognosis. Jones fracture commonly is located within 3/4 inch of the most proximal portion of the metatarsal. It usually is treated with a *bulky Jones dressing* (p. 261) for the first 24 to 36 hours and nonweightbearing followed by a *short-leg walking cast* (p. 260) for 3 to 4 weeks. A transverse fracture of the shaft of the fifth metatarsal is treated with a *short-leg walking cast.* There is a high incidence of delayed union and of nonunion of this fracture despite proper immobilization.

TURF TOE: STRAIN OF THE GREAT TOE

SUMMARY

Hyperextension of the first metatarsophalangeal joint causes stretching of and strain on the capsule of the joint and the plantar plate of the great toe. Occasionally a capsular avulsion fracture occurs. Treatment includes *buddy-taping* of the joint (p. 264), stiff shoes, and a stiff orthosis for 2 to 3 weeks.

FRACTURES OF THE GREAT TOE

SUMMARY

Fracture of the proximal phalanx of the great toe occurs as a result of direct trauma (dropped objects) or a stubbing injury. Most fractures show minimal displacement. Treatment includes *buddy-taping* (p. 264), stiff shoes, or a *short-leg walking cast* (p. 260) with a toe plate for 2 weeks. Displaced intra-articular fractures can be reduced with *finger traps* (p. 252), then treated in the same fashion as the nondisplaced fractures.

FRACTURES OF THE SESAMOID BONE

SUMMARY

Fractures of the sesamoid bone (medial-aspect fractures occur much more frequently than lateral-aspect fractures) must be distinguished from the congenital bipartite sesamoid. True fractures have rough edges, are transverse in direction, and eventually show callus formation. Bipartite sesamoid fractures occur bilaterally and have smooth, sharply bordered edges. Most fractures occur as a result of direct trauma, avulsion forces, or repetitive stress. Treatment with a *short-leg walking cast* (p. 260) for 3 to 4 weeks is followed by a stiff shoe and a metatarsal bar or pad.

FRACTURES OF THE TOES

SUMMARY

Fractures of the lesser toes are reduced easily with manual pressure or with finger traps. *Buddy-taping* (p. 264) to the adjacent larger toe with cotton placed in the toe web is the treatment of choice. The patient should wear wide-toe-box shoes until the toe has healed.

CHAPTER 13: RADIOLOGY AND PROCEDURES

PROCEDURE	FINDINGS—SIGNIFICANCE

NECK

Cervical spine series (lateral, posteroanterior, oblique)	"Reversed or straightened curve"—cervical or upper back muscle spasm
	Localized straightening of the cervical curve—local muscle spasm from a herniated disk
	Facet joint and vertebral body spurring and sclerosis—cervical osteoarthritis
	Subluxation of 2 vertebral bodies—spondylolisthesis or fracture
	Large anterior osteophytes causing "a lump in the throat"
	Dumbbell-shaped foraminal encroachment from cervical radiculopathy (>50% narrowing)
Flexion and extension views of the neck	Odontoid subluxation from rheumatoid disease (normal 3.5 mm odontoid to atlas)
MRI of the cervical spine (75% ordered for radiculopathy and 20% for myelopathy)	Common findings: herniated disk, foraminal encroachment disease, bony pathology such as osteomyelitis and metastases, and intrinsic disease of the spinal cord
Electromyography of the upper extremity	Denervation associated with nerve root compression (used in evaluation of poorly defined arm pains)

SHOULDER

Posteroanterior, external rotation, and Y-outlet views	Calcification—rotator cuff or bicipital tendinitis
	Greater tubercle sclerosis and erosion—subacromial impingement
	Superior migration of the humeral head—rotator cuff tendon tear
	Acromioclavicular joint width >4-5 mm—second-degree acromioclavicular separation
	Clavicle superior to the acromion—third-degree acromioclavicular separation
	Squared-off ends of the acromion and clavicle, narrowing of the joint, sclerosis, and bone spurring—acromioclavicular joint osteoarthritis
	Anterior or posterior position of the humerus—dislocation
	Bony pathology
Axillary view (best view for measuring the glenohumeral joint space)	Glenohumeral joint narrowing, sclerosis, and spur formation are characteristics of glenohumeral osteoarthritis
Acromial arch view	Narrowing, irregularity of the acromion or acromioclavicular joint spur encroachment—subacromial impingement
Weighted views of acromioclavicular joint	Acromioclavicular joint space >4-5 mm—second-degree acromioclavicular shoulder separation
Arthrography with or without CT	Contracted glenohumeral space—frozen shoulder
	Dye leaking into the subacromial bursa—rotator cuff tendon tear
	Irregularities of the glenohumeral joint—osteoarthritis or rheumatoid disease
	Irregularity of the glenoid labrum—labral tear
MRI	Separation/irregularity of the rotator cuff tendon—"tear"
Subacromial lidocaine injection test for rotator cuff tendinitis	75% pain relief and >75% of external rotation and abduction strength—uncomplicated rotator cuff tendinitis
	Poor pain relief, <75% strength—rotator cuff tendon tear

ELBOW

Posteroanterior and lateral	Triceps calcification—incidental finding
	Radial head and ulnar osteophytes, joint-space narrowing, sclerosis—osteoarthritis
MRI	Irregularity of the articular cartilage—osteochondritis dissecans with or without loose bodies
Nerve conduction velocity of the ulnar nerve	Slowing—cubital tunnel syndrome
Bursal aspiration	Crystals—gout or pseudogout
	Gram-positive cocci—*Staphylococcus aureus*
	Bloody or serous effusion—traumatic bursitis

WRIST

Posteroanterior, lateral, and oblique	Radiocarpal joint-space narrowing, sclerosis of the radius, irregular shape to the navicular, and increased gap between the navicular and the lunate—radiocarpal osteoarthritis
	Sclerosis of the navicular—avascular necrosis of the navicular
	Sclerosis of the lunate—avascular necrosis of the lunate or Kienböck's disease
	Calcification of the triangular cartilage—pseudogout
	Abnormal alignment of the carpal bones—subluxation of the navicular or lunate
	Increased gap between the lunate and navicular—subluxation, carpal dissociation
	Loss of the uniform 1-mm spacing between the carpal bones—rheumatoid arthritis or osteoarthritis
Coned down view of the navicular	Cortical irregularities or fracture line—navicular fracture
Carpal tunnel view	Subluxation of the lunate causing carpal tunnel syndrome
Nerve conduction velocity of median nerve	Slowing of the nerve—carpal tunnel (30% false negative)

THUMB

Posteroanterior, lateral, and oblique	Sclerosis, narrowing, spurring, and subluxation of carpometacarpal joint—carpometacarpal osteoarthritis
	Asymmetric narrowing, sclerosis, spurring of metacarpophalangeal joint—osteoarthritis

HAND

Posteroanterior, lateral, and oblique	Asymmetric joint-space narrowing, osteophytes, and ("soft-tissue technique") bony sclerosis of the distal interphalangeal or proximal interphalangeal joints—osteoarthritis
	Punctate calcification in the soft tissues of the metacarpophalangeal joints—foreign body reaction to gravel, corticosteroid injection
	Juxta-articular osteoporosis of the metacarpophalangeal or proximal interphalangeal joints—early rheumatoid arthritis

Symmetric joint-space narrowing and periarticular erosions—advanced rheumatoid arthritis

Asymmetric erosive change of the proximal interphalangeal joint without juxta-articular osteoporosis or dramatic joint-space narrowing—chronic tophaceous gout

Fluffy periosteal elevation of the proximal phalanges—correlation with sausage digit of Reiter's disease

"Pencil-and-cup" deformity of destructive arthritis—psoriasis

Unilateral juxta-articular osteoporosis—Sudeck's atrophy of bone; reflex sympathetic dystrophy

LUMBOSACRAL SPINE

Posteroanterior and lateral

Loss of the normal lumbar lordosis—paraspinal muscle spasm
Sclerosis and narrowing of the facet joints—osteoarthritis; spinal stenosis
Wedge-shaped vertebral body—compression fracture
S-shaped curve—scoliosis
S-shaped curve with rotation—rotatory scoliosis
Anterior displacement of one vertebral body over another—spondylolisthesis
Bony pathology

Oblique views

Missing pars intra-articularis (the neck of the Scotty dog)—spondylosis or spondylolisthesis

Flexion and extension views

Increased movement of the vertebral bodies—spondylolisthesis instability

MRI

As for CT with greater detail of nerve and cord integrity and of postoperative cases with scar tissue

CT (many indications and uses—75% for radiculopathy, 20% for metastatic workup, 5% for advanced arthritis)

Bulging disk compressing the spinal nerve, lateral recess narrowing, fragmented disk lodged in the lateral recess—radiculopathy
Narrowing of spinal canal—spinal stenosis
Bony pathology

Bone scanning

Increased uptake is nonspecific in osteoarthritis, bony pathology, osteomyelitis

Myelography

Replaced by CT and MRI

HIP

Posteroanterior and lateral (order standing posteroanterior view of both hips on 1 cassette)

Joint-space narrowing between superior acetabulum and femoral head, bony sclerosis and a variable degree of superior acetabular osteophytes—osteoarthritis
Migration of the femoral head into the pelvis—protrusio acetabuli
Sclerotic line and "stepoff" at proximal one third of the head of the femur—avascular necrosis (late)
Calcification over the lateral femur—trochanteric or gluteus medius bursa (uncommon)
Various bony abnormalities

Frog-leg view

Alternate view of femoral head

Standing anteroposterior pelvis with level measurement of leg-length discrepancy

Widening and irregularity of the symphysis pubis—osteitis pubis or diastasis

Oblique views of the pelvis

Bony sclerosis of the sacrum and ileum, bony erosions, widening of the joint—sacroiliitis
Bony sclerosis of the iliac side of the sacroiliac joint—osteitis condensans ilii (benign)

Lateral views of the coccyx

Abnormal anterior angulation of the coccyx—post-traumatic coccygodynia

Bone scanning

Diffuse uptake—arthritis, infection
Uptake in proximal third of the femoral head—avascular necrosis or various bony abnormalities

MRI

Irregularity of the proximal third of the femoral head—avascular necrosis (90% of all hip MRI)

KNEE

Posteroanterior and lateral (order bilateral standing views on 1 cassette)

Medial joint-space narrowing (normal 1 mm wider than the lateral)—early osteoarthritis
Asymmetric narrowing, increased tibial sclerosis, and tibial or femoral osteophytes—advanced osteoarthritis
Narrowing of the medial joint space, valgus angle of the knee <8 to 9 degrees—osteoarthritis
Meniscal calcification—chondrocalcinosis
Defect in the femoral condyle—osteochondritis dissecans
Linear calcification of the medial collateral ligament—Pellegrini-Stieda syndrome (old medial collateral ligament injury)
Various bony abnormalities
Calcification in the joint—loose body
Calcification outside the joint—flabella

Merchant view of the patella ("sunrise" view)

Patella does not sit in the center of the patellar femoral groove—subluxation or frank dislocation
Asymmetric joint-space narrowing, patellar sclerosis and patellar pole osteophytes—patellofemoral osteoarthritis

Tunnel view

Well-circumscribed calcified body between the femoral condyles—loose body

MRI of the knee

Irregularities of the menisci—tears, congenital defects
Irregularities of the articular cartilage—arthritis, osteochondritis dissecans
Disrupted cruciate ligaments—torn anterior or posterior cruciate

Arthrography

Supplanted by MRI

Ultrasound

Popliteal mass—Baker's cyst or popliteal artery aneurysm

Bursa aspiration

Crystals—gout, pseudogout
Gram-positive cocci—S. aureus
Serous or bloody aspirate—traumatic bursitis

Arthroscopy, diagnostic

For confirming meniscal, patellar, or cruciate pathology seen on MRI

Continued

PROCEDURE	FINDINGS—SIGNIFICANCE
ANKLE	
Posteroanterior, lateral, and mortise views (many indications and uses)	Joint-space narrowing, sclerosis, and hypertrophic osteophytes—tibiotalar arthritis
	Calcification of the Achilles tendon—nearly always asymptomatic
	Calcification posterior to the Achilles tendon insertion—pre-Achilles bursitis
	Calcaneal heel spur—possible plantar fasciitis
	Fleck of calcium off the proximal fifth metatarsal—avulsion fracture of peroneus longus—severe ankle sprain
	Well-circumscribed calcified bodies adjacent to the tarsal bones—sesamoid bones, which are rarely symptomatic
	Talar bone irregularities in the severely sprained ankle—lateral process fracture of the dome of the talus, posterior process fracture, and others
Varus stress x-ray of the talus	Shift and subluxation with stress—chronic lateral instability of the ankle
Oblique views of the ankle	Tarsal bones fusion—tarsal coalition
Nerve conduction velocity of the posterior tibialis nerve	Slowing of nerve transmission—tarsal tunnel syndrome
FOOT	
Posteroanterior, lateral, and oblique	Of the first metatarsophalangeal joint, sclerosis and asymmetric narrowing—bunions
	Abnormal angulation of the metatarsophalangeal and proximal interphalangeal joints—hammer toes
	Juxta-articular osteoporosis of the metatarsophalangeal joints and proximal interphalangeal joints—rheumatoid arthritis
	Thickened cortex of the third or fourth metatarsal shafts—stress fracture
	Hypertrophic spurring at the first metatarsal first cuneiform—dorsal bunion
	Calcification of the posterior one third of the calcaneus—calcaneal stress fracture
	Diffuse osteoporosis of the bones of the foot—reflex sympathetic dystrophy
	Bony erosion with an "overhanging margin"—gout
Standing lateral foot	Flattening of the longitudinal arch—pes planus—versus high arch—pes cavus
Sesamoid view of the big toe	Irregularities of the sesamoid bones—bipartite sesamoid bone versus fracture

NECK

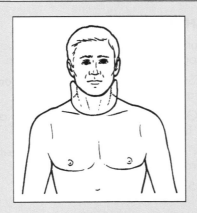

SOFT CERVICAL COLLAR

USE: Cervical strain, whiplash, fibromyalgia, tension headaches

ADVANTAGES: Inexpensive, easy to put on, reasonably comfortable

DISADVANTAGE: Does not restrict neck motion sufficiently

COST: $8.00 to $9.00

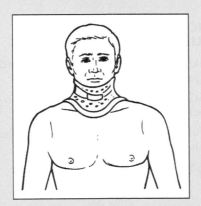

PHILADELPHIA COLLAR

USE: Neck trauma transport, herniated disk, postoperative recovery

ADVANTAGES: Much improved restriction of neck motion, some vertical stretch

DISADVANTAGES: Cost, uncomfortable, slightly more difficult to put on

COST: Soft, $35.00 to $40.00; hard, $60.00 to $65.00

WATER BAG CERVICAL TRACTION

USE: Cervical radiculopathy, cervical strain, whiplash, fibromyalgia

COST: $40.00 to $45.00

PULSATING WATER MASSAGER/ELECTRIC HAND MASSAGER

USE: Cervical strain, tension headaches

COST: $35.00 to $45.00

SHOULDER

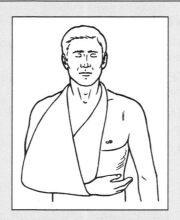

SIMPLE SHOULDER SLING

USE: Acute bursitis, acute tendinitis, glenohumeral dislocation, acromioclavicular separation

FRACTURES: Humerus, clavicle, radial head; postoperative recovery

ADVANTAGES: Inexpensive, easy to put on, can be made at home

DISADVANTAGES: Insufficient immobilization, can lead to frozen shoulder

COST: $5.00 to $10.00

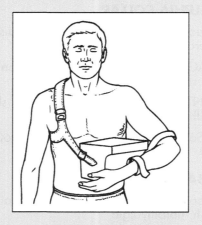

ABDUCTION PILLOW SHOULDER IMMOBILIZER

USE: Rotator cuff tendon tear, recovery from rotator cuff surgery

ADVANTAGE: Excellent immobilization in a position of abduction

DISADVANTAGES: Hard to put on, can lead to frozen shoulder, expensive

COST: $50.00 to $65.00

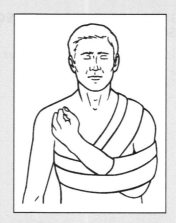

SLING AND SWATHE BANDAGE

USE: Glenohumeral dislocation, severe acromioclavicular separation

FRACTURE: Upper humerus

ADVANTAGES: Better control of motion and pain, inexpensive

DISADVANTAGES: Requires a technician, cannot be removed easily by the patient

COST: $4.00 to $5.00

SHOULDER *(Continued)*

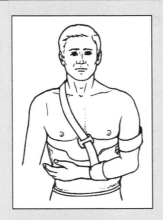

SHOULDER IMMOBILIZER

USE: Acromioclavicular separation, glenohumeral dislocation

FRACTURE: Humeral neck

ADVANTAGES: Easy to put on, relatively inexpensive, much less bulky, can be worn under clothing

DISADVANTAGE: Frozen shoulder in a susceptible patient

COST: Universal, $19.00 to $22.00; Velcro, $31.00 to $33.00

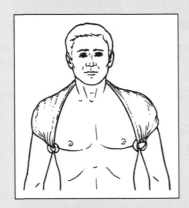

FIGURE-OF-EIGHT STRAP

USE: Acromioclavicular separation, dislocation

FRACTURE: Clavicle

ADVANTAGES: Inexpensive, easy to apply, can be worn under clothing

DISADVANTAGE: Axillary irritation

COST: $11.00 to $15.00

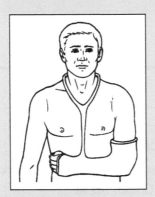

HANGING CAST

USE: No medical orthopedic indications

FRACTURES: Humeral surgical neck, humeral shaft

ADVANTAGE: Provides downward traction on the fractured elements

DISADVANTAGES: Heavy and bulky compared with a simple sling, more expensive, uncomfortable, requires a technician

COST: $65.00 to $100.00

ELBOW

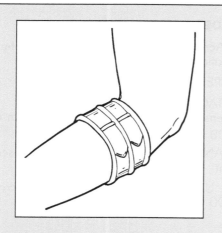

TENNIS ELBOW BAND

USE: Lateral epicondylitis, extensor carpi radialis strain, brachioradialis strain

ADVANTAGES: Decreases the tension coming back to the tendon, inexpensive, easy to put on, not restrictive

DISADVANTAGES: Does not decrease the aggravation resulting from wrist use, probably works only for mild cases

COST: $10.00 to $18.00

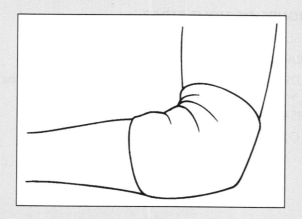

NEOPRENE PULL-ON ELBOW BRACE

USE: Olecranon bursitis, arthritis of the elbow, poorly healing olecranon process fracture, cubital tunnel

ADVANTAGES: Inexpensive, easy to put on, can be worn under clothing

DISADVANTAGE: None

COST: $8.00 to $18.00

WRIST

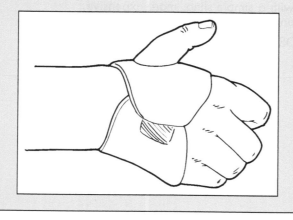

SIMPLE VELCRO WRIST SUPPORT

USE: Sprained wrist, weightlifting support

FRACTURE: Carpal bones

ADVANTAGES: Inexpensive, lightweight, easy to put on

DISADVANTAGE: Very little wrist support or restriction in wrist motion

COST: $9.00 to $10.00, up to $25.00

WRIST *(Continued)*

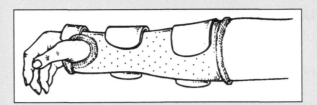

VELCRO WRIST SPLINT WITH METAL STAY

USE: Lateral and medial epicondylitis, carpal tunnel syndrome, severe wrist sprains, radiocarpal arthritis, dorsal ganglion

ADVANTAGES: Good restriction of wrist motion, relatively inexpensive, lightweight, easy to put on

DISADVANTAGES: Can cause pressure over the thumb and a temporary numbness of the local cutaneous nerve, may not restrict wrist motion sufficiently for specific conditions

COST: $22.00 to $35.00

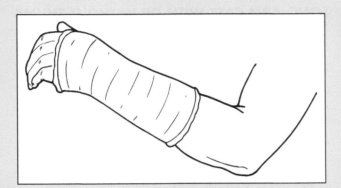

SHORT-ARM CAST WITH OR WITHOUT THUMB SPICA

USE: Lateral and medial epicondylitis, metacarpal subluxation

FRACTURES: Colles, navicular, miscellaneous forearm

ADVANTAGES: Best support and restriction of the wrist, cannot be removed

DISADVANTAGES: Bulky, heavy, susceptible to water damage, not universally available, requires a technician

COST: Plaster, $30.00 to $32.00; fiberglass, $65.00 to $70.00

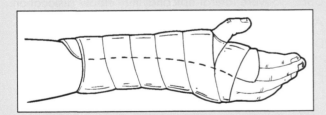

RADIAL GUTTER SPLINT

USE: No medical orthopedic indications

FRACTURES: Nondisplaced metacarpals, numbers 2 and 3, nondisplaced phalanges, numbers 1 and 2

ADVANTAGES: More lightweight than a short-arm cast, can be removed, more convenient

DISADVANTAGE: Does not provide strict immobilization

COST: Plaster, $21.00 to $23.00; fiberglass, $39.00 to $40.00

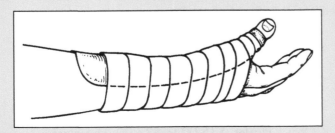

DORSAL HOOD SPLINT

USE: De Quervain's tenosynovitis, carpometacarpal arthritis

ADVANTAGES: Removable, lightweight

DISADVANTAGES: Requires a technician, not as durable as the Velcro splints

COST: Plaster, $15.00 to $16.00; fiberglass, $28.00 to $30.00

WRIST *(Continued)*

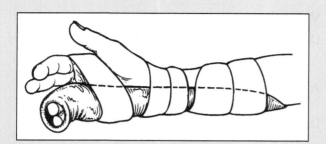

ULNAR GUTTER SPLINT

USE: Ulnar collateral ligament strain, triangular cartilage injuries

FRACTURES: Boxer, nondisplaced phalanges, numbers 4 and 5

ADVANTAGES: Removable, lightweight

DISADVANTAGES: Requires a technician, not as durable as Velcro splints

COST: Plaster, $21.00 to $23.00; fiberglass, $39.00 to $40.00

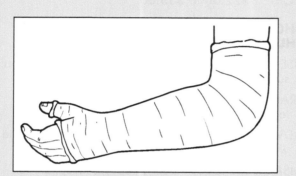

LONG-ARM CAST WITH OR WITHOUT THUMB SPICA

USE: No medical orthopedic indications

FRACTURES: Navicular, complicated Colles, nondisplaced radius and ulnar shaft

ADVANTAGE: Securely holds the forearm and wrist in a fixed position

DISADVANTAGES: Cumbersome, requires a technician, expensive

COST: Plaster, $33.00 to $37.00; fiberglass, $61.00 to $68.00

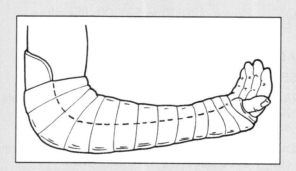

POSTERIOR SPLINT

USE: Severe lateral epicondylitis, elbow dislocation

ADVANTAGES: Removable, relatively lightweight

DISADVANTAGES: Requires a technician, may not restrict motion sufficiently

COST: $40.00 to $44.00

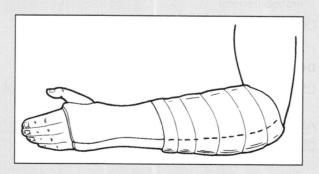

SUGAR-TONG SPLINT

USE: No medical orthopedic indications

FRACTURES: Colles, distal radius (*Note:* this is a temporary splint only)

ADVANTAGES: Allows swelling in the first few days, easy to recheck the fracture

DISADVANTAGES: Insufficient immobilization compared with a short-arm cast, expensive to put on two casts

COST: Plaster, $35.00 to $37.00; fiberglass, $65.00 to $67.00

WRIST *(Continued)*

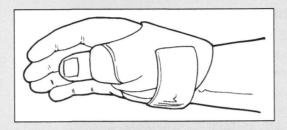

PADDED SHELL VELCRO THUMB SPLINT OR VELCRO THUMB SPICA SPLINT

USE: Carpometacarpal arthritis, de Quervain's tenosynovitis, gamekeeper's thumb

ADVANTAGES: Lightweight, comfortable, relatively inexpensive

DISADVANTAGE: May not restrict motion sufficiently

COST: $26.00 to $28.00

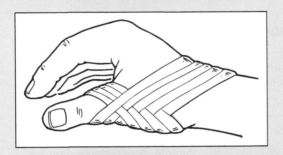

THERMOPLASTIC MOLDED THUMB SPLINT

USE: Carpometacarpal arthritis, gamekeeper's thumb

ADVANTAGES: Custom-fitted, excellent support and immobilization

DISADVANTAGES: Requires a technician, may be overly limiting to the patient, relatively expensive

COST: $25.00 to $26.00

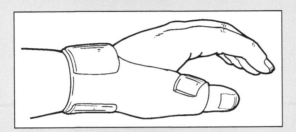

TAPING FOR OSTEOARTHRITIS OF THE THUMB

USE: Carpometacarpal arthritis, gamekeeper's thumb

ADVANTAGES: Very inexpensive, permits some use without much aggravation, can be applied by the patient whenever needed

DISADVANTAGES: Does not last, must be reapplied, easily soiled

COST: $1.00 to $2.00

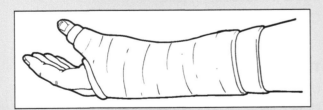

THUMB-SPICA CAST

USE: Carpometacarpal arthritis, de Quervain's tenosynovitis, gamekeeper's thumb

FRACTURES: Navicular, trapezial, metacarpal, number 1

ADVANTAGES: Best immobilization for the thumb, cannot be removed by the patient

DISADVANTAGES: Bulky and heavy, cannot be wet, requires a technician, expensive

COST: Plaster, $60.00 to $66.00; fiberglass, $109.00 to $121.00

WRIST (Continued)

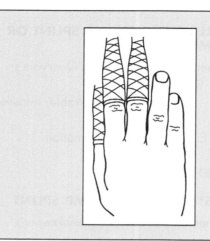

CHINESE FINGER-TRAP TRACTION

USE: No medical orthopedic indications

FRACTURES: Colles, proximal phalanges (finger or toe)

ADVANTAGE: Gradual, even distribution of tensions

DISADVANTAGE: Skin irritation

COST: $25.00 (reusable)

HAND

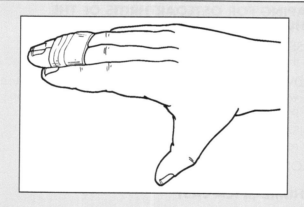

BUDDY-TAPING

USE: Simple finger sprains, trigger finger osteoarthritis of the finger joints, de Quervain's tenosynovitis

FRACTURES: Nondisplaced phalanges, tendon avulsion fractures, tuft, distal interphalangeal dislocation

ADVANTAGES: Simple, inexpensive, can be applied by the patient, reasonable immobilization

DISADVANTAGES: None

COST: $1.00 to $2.00

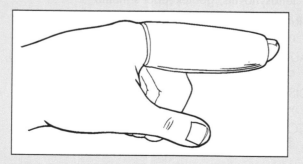

TUBE SPLINTS

USE: Simple finger sprains

FRACTURES: Nondisplaced phalangeal

ADVANTAGES: Simple to put on, comfortable

DISADVANTAGES: Expensive, may not sufficiently restrict motion

COST: $15.00 to $16.00

HAND (Continued)

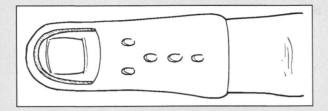

STACK SPLINTS

USE: Mallet finger

FRACTURES: Tuft

ADVANTAGES: Inexpensive, easy to put on

DISADVANTAGES: None

COST: $4.00 to $5.00

DORSAL SPLINT

USE: Mallet finger, minor finger sprains, proximal interphalangeal dislocation, mallet thumb

ADVANTAGES: Easy to put on, inexpensive

DISADVANTAGES: None

COST: $4.00 to $5.00

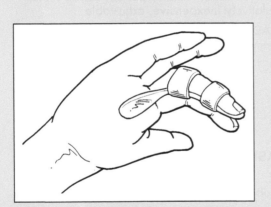

METAL FINGER SPLINT

USE: Severe proximal interphalangeal or distal interphalangeal sprains

FRACTURES: Tuft

ADVANTAGES: Better immobilization of the proximal interphalangeal joint, inexpensive

DISADVANTAGES: Difficult to keep on, may irritate the palm

COST: $5.00 to $7.00

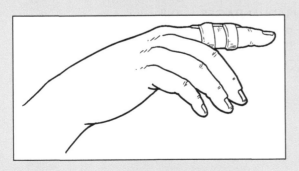

PROXIMAL INTERPHALANGEAL JOINT SPLINT IN EXTENSION

USE: Acute boutonnière injury

ADVANTAGES: Simple, inexpensive

DISADVANTAGES: Finger stiffness, range of motion exercises are not performed concurrently

COST: $2.00 to $3.00

LUMBOSACRAL REGION

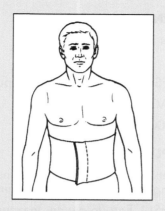

NEOPRENE WAIST WRAP

USE: Uncomplicated lumbosacral strain, facet syndrome, weightlifting

ADVANTAGES: Easy to put on, inexpensive, comfortable, can be worn easily under clothing, easily adjusted

DISADVANTAGES: Insufficient support and immobilization

COST: $12.00 to $25.00

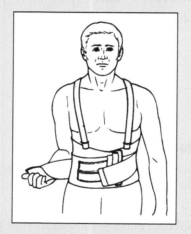

VELCRO LUMBOSACRAL CORSET

USE: Lumbosacral strain, uncomplicated lumbosacral compression fracture, osteoarthritis, ankylosing spondylitis, recovery phase of lumbosacral radiculopathy, facet syndrome, prevention

ADVANTAGES: Easily put on, comfortable, relatively inexpensive, adjustable

DISADVANTAGES: Insufficient support and immobilization

COST: $25.00 to $32.00

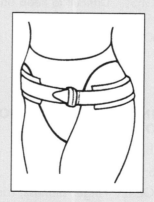

ELASTIC SACROILIAC BELT

USE: Sacroiliitis, iliolumbar syndrome, osteitis pubis, recovery phase of pelvic fracture

ADVANTAGES: Easy to put on, inexpensive, can be worn under clothing, easily adjusted

DISADVANTAGES: Difficult to keep on if overweight, limited usefulness, variable patient response

COST: $12.00 to $14.00

LUMBOSACRAL REGION *(Continued)*

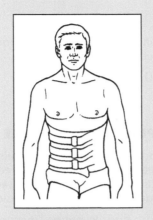

LUMBOSACRAL ELASTIC BINDER WITH HEATED PLASTIC SHIELD

USE: Chronic low back pain, lumbosacral compression fracture, lumbosacral radiculopathy (healing phase)

ADVANTAGES: More support, maintains the lumbosacral spine in extension, more limitation of flexion

DISADVANTAGES: Expensive, requires a technician to form the shield, uncomfortable

COST: $125.00 to $140.00

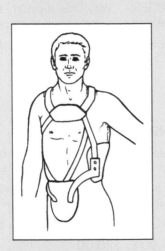

THREE-POINT EXTENSION BRACE (JEWITT)

USE: Compression fractures, kyphosis from any cause

ADVANTAGES: Offers the greatest restriction of all braces, best control of movement

DISADVANTAGES: Expensive, bulky and obtrusive, uncomfortable, not well tolerated, must be readjusted by a professional

COST: $250.00 to 300.00

HIP

CRUTCHES

USE: Any severe hip pain, especially avascular necrosis, severe bursitis, severe flare of arthritis, suspected metastatic disease involving the femur

COST: $20.00 to $25.00 to rent

KNEE

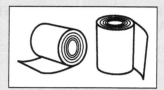

ACE WRAP

USE: Any minor knee problem, rib fractures, hamstring pull, gastrocnemius injury

COST: $3.00 to $5.00

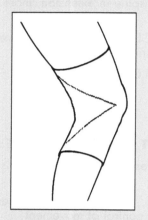

NEOPRENE PULL-ON KNEE BRACE

USE: Osteoarthritis, prepatellar bursitis, first-degree medial collateral ligament or lateral collateral ligament strain, Osgood-Schlatter disease, rheumatoid arthritis, bland knee effusions

ADVANTAGES: Easy to put on, inexpensive, simple

DISADVANTAGES: Very little support, slips, hard to fit on obese patients, may restrict venous flow

COST: Simple, $8.00 to $10.00; patellar cutout, $20.00 to $25.00

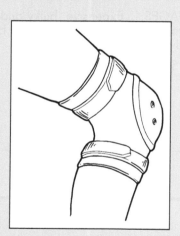

VELCRO KNEE PADS

USE: Prepatellar bursitis, infrapatellar bursitis, patellofemoral syndrome, osteoarthritis

ADVANTAGES: Plastic metal cup anterior is very protective, inexpensive, easy to put on

DISADVANTAGE: May restrict venous blood flow

COST: $15.00 to $20.00

Metal-hinged braces: Lenox-Hill, $800.00 to $900.00; Off-loader brace, $800.00 to $900.00

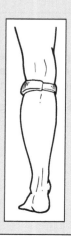

PATELLAR STRAP

USE: Patellofemoral syndrome, patellar tendinitis, patellofemoral osteoarthritis, patellar subluxation, patellar dislocation

ADVANTAGES: Simple, inexpensive, easy to put on and adjust

DISADVANTAGES: May not provide enough correction of the abnormal patellofemoral tracking, may restrict venous blood flow

COST: $15.00 to $16.00

KNEE *(Continued)*

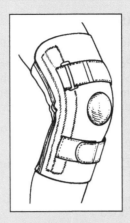

VELCRO PATELLAR RESTRAINING IMMOBILIZER

USE: Patellofemoral syndrome, patellar subluxation, patellar dislocation, patellofemoral osteoarthritis, first-degree medial collateral ligament or lateral collateral ligament strains, medial compartment osteoarthritis

ADVANTAGES: Improved patellofemoral tracking, easy to put on, patient acceptance

DISADVANTAGES: Moderately expensive, hard to fit on obese patients

COST: $35.00 to $60.00

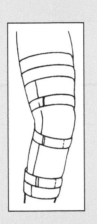

VELCRO STRAIGHT LEG BRACE

USE: Acute knee injury, second-degree or third-degree medial collateral ligament or lateral collateral ligament strains, patellar tendinitis, medical management of a meniscus tear

ADVANTAGES: Excellent protection and immobilization of the knee, easily put on

DISADVANTAGES: Relatively expensive, bulky, cannot wear under clothing, affects normal walking gait

COST: 18-inch, $45.00 to $52.00; 24-inch, $64.00 to $73.00

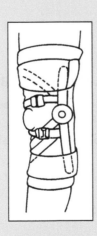

METAL-HINGED BRACES (MCDAVID KNEE GUARD, LENOX-HILL DEROTATIONAL BRACE, DON JOY REHABILITATION BRACE)

USE: Ligament instability (especially the acromioclavicular ligament), postoperative acromioclavicular ligament repair, third-degree medial collateral ligament or lateral collateral ligament instability, osteoarthritis with angulation, hyperextension laxity

ADVANTAGES: Excellent and adjustable control of the knee motion and immobilization, better varus/valgus protection

DISADVANTAGES: Very expensive, custom-made, not readily available

COST: $900.00 to $1200.00

KNEE (Continued)

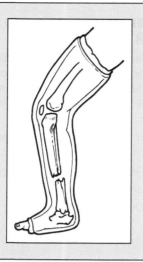

LONG-LEG CAST

USE: No medical orthopedic indications

FRACTURES: Patellar, uncomplicated tibial plateau, minimally displaced tibial/fibular shaft, medial collateral ligament or lateral collateral ligament avulsion, nondisplaced osteochondritis

ADVANTAGE: Excellent protection and immobilization of the knee

DISADVANTAGES: Relatively expensive, bulky, affects normal walking gait

COST: Cylinder, $42.00 to $50.00; thigh to ankle, $60.00 to $70.00

ANKLE

ATHLETIC TAPING FOR ANKLE SPRAIN

USE: Ankle sprain, mild ankle arthritis

ADVANTAGES: Inexpensive, permits some use without much aggravation, can be applied by the patient whenever needed

DISADVANTAGES: Does not last, must be reapplied, easily soiled

COST: $2.00 to $3.00

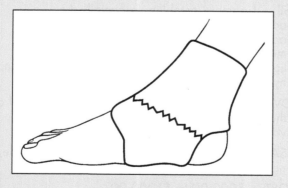

NEOPRENE PULL-ON ANKLE BRACE

USE: Minor sprains, minor degrees of pronation, mild osteoarthritis

ADVANTAGES: Simple, inexpensive, relatively easy to put on

DISADVANTAGES: Hard to wear in a shoe, not supportive

COST: $8.00 to $10.00

ANKLE *(Continued)*

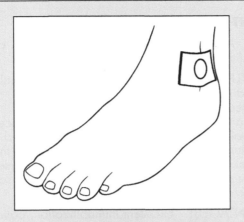

NEW SKIN/MOLESKIN

USE: Achilles tendinitis, pre-Achilles bursitis, bursitis over bunion, dorsal bunion, blisters, abrasions

ADVANTAGES: Easy to apply, inexpensive, can be custom cut to shape and size

DISADVANTAGES: None

COST: $2.00 to $3.00

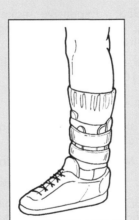

VELCRO ANKLE BRACE

USE: Recurrent ankle sprain, osteoarthritis of the ankle, moderate pronation, posterior tibialis tenosynovitis, peroneus tenosynovitis, tarsal tunnel

ADVANTAGES: Easy to put on, relatively inexpensive, better support than a neoprene pull-on

DISADVANTAGE: Does not provide adequate support for some conditions

COST: $30.00 to $52.00

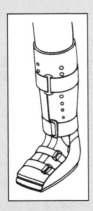

ROCKER-BOTTOM PLASTIC ANKLE IMMOBILIZER

USE: Achilles tendinitis, severe ankle sprain, posterior tibialis tenosynovitis, peroneus tenosynovitis, severe plantar fasciitis, stress fracture of the foot

ADVANTAGES: Excellent support and restriction of the ankle, removable, comfortable

DISADVANTAGES: Expensive, bulky, interferes with driving a car

COST: $55.00 to $130.00 (varies depending on vendor)

ANKLE (Continued)

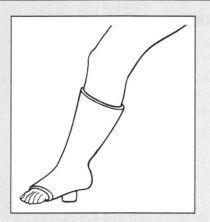

SHORT-LEG WALKING CAST

USE: Achilles tendinitis, severe ankle sprain, plantar fasciitis, severe flare of ankle arthritis

FRACTURES: Tibial stress, nondisplaced bimalleolar, nondisplaced fibular, avulsion of the lateral malleolus, calcaneal stress, extra-articular calcaneal, posterior process and lateral process of the talus, navicular, avulsion or nondisplaced fracture of the talus, avulsion of the base of the fifth metatarsal, nondisplaced fracture of metatarsal 1 through 4, Jones fracture of the fifth metatarsal, march, sesamoid, great toe

ADVANTAGES: Excellent immobilization, patient cannot remove it

DISADVANTAGES: Expensive, makes driving unsafe, bulky, may throw off walking gait, cannot be wet, requires a technician

COST: Plaster, $51.00 to $54.00; fiberglass, $94.00 to $100.00

UNNA BOOT

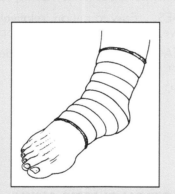

USE: Venous stasis ulcer, moderate ankle sprain, poorly healing wounds

FRACTURES: Minimally displaced fibular

ADVANTAGES: Lightweight, requires a technician

DISADVANTAGES: Does not immobilize or protect the ankle sufficiently, cannot be wet

COST: $25.00 to $30.00 (versus athletic tape, $4.00 to $5.00)

FOOTDROP NIGHT SPLINT, READY-MADE ANKLE-FOOT ORTHOSIS, CUSTOM-MADE ANKLE-FOOT ORTHOSIS

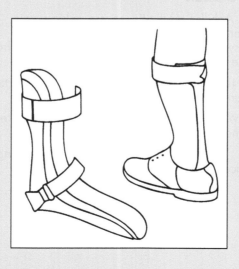

USE: Stroke, Charcot-Marie-Tooth disease, polio or postpolio, any cause of footdrop, plantar fasciitis

ADVANTAGES: Protects against flexion contractures, improves gait, prevents falls

DISADVANTAGE: Mild skin irritation

COST: Over-the-counter, $15.00 to $30.00; custom-made, $40.00 to $65.00

ANKLE *(Continued)*

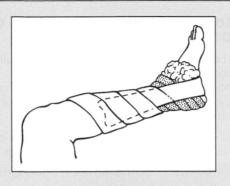

JONES DRESSING WITH OR WITHOUT POSTERIOR SPLINT REINFORCEMENT

USE: No medical orthopedic indications

FRACTURES: Ankle, calcaneal, navicular, Jones, metatarsal

ADVANTAGES: Allows expansion for acute swelling and reinspection of the fracture, lighter in weight than a fixed cast

DISADVANTAGE: Not rigid enough to hold a reduction

COST: $40.00 to $50.00

FOOT

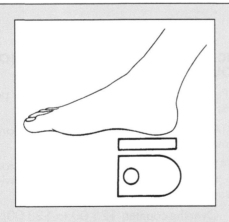

HEEL CUSHIONS

USE: Heel pad syndrome, plantar fasciitis/spur, calcaneal stress fracture, ankle arthritis

ADVANTAGES: Inexpensive, effective cushioning of the heel, transferable from shoe to shoe, does not wear out

DISADVANTAGE: Does not correct an arch problem or alignment problem of the ankle

COST: $3.00 to $5.00

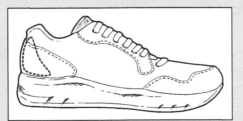

HEEL CUPS

USE: Heel pad syndrome, plantar fasciitis/spur, calcaneal stress fracture, severe epiphysitis, hip or knee osteoarthritis

ADVANTAGES: Inexpensive, effective cushioning of the heel, transferable from shoe to shoe

DISADVANTAGE: Does not correct an arch problem or alignment problem of the ankle

COST: $5.00 to $8.00

FOOT *(Continued)*

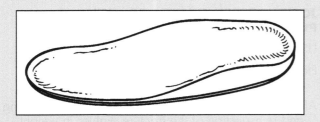

PADDED INSOLES (SCHOLLS, SPENCO, OR SORBOTHANE)

USE: Heel pad syndrome; hammer toes; calluses; metatarsalgia; rheumatoid disease of the metatarsophalangeals; Morton's neuroma; ankle, knee, or hip osteoarthritis; healing phase of stress fractures of the foot

ADVANTAGES: Excellent cushioning of the entire foot, inexpensive, transferable from shoe to shoe

DISADVANTAGE: Do not have arch supports

COST: $12.00 to $25.00

PADDED INSOLES WITH ARCH SUPPORTS

USE: Plantar fasciitis, pes cavus, pes planus, pronated ankles, tarsal tunnel

ADVANTAGES: Soft padding plus arch support, relatively inexpensive, transferable from shoe to shoe

DISADVANTAGE: Not enough arch support to correct moderate to severe arch abnormalities

COST: $22.00 to $25.00

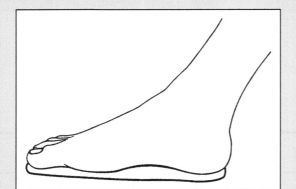

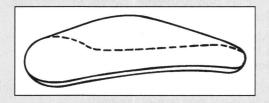

PLASTIC ORTHOTIC ARCH SUPPORTS (OVER-THE-COUNTER OR CUSTOM-MADE)

USE: Persistent plantar fasciitis, pes cavus, pes planus, ankle pronation, tarsal tunnel

ADVANTAGE: Can correct any degree of arch abnormality

DISADVANTAGES: Expensive, must be custom-made, time delay to obtain, hard surface without any padding

COST: Over-the-counter, $25.00 to $28.00; custom-made, $75.00 to $100.00

BUNION SHIELDS

USE: Bunions

ADVANTAGES: Provides protection to the soft tissues and the joint, inexpensive

DISADVANTAGE: Hard to fit into shoes

COST: $5.00 to $15.00

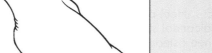
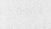

FOOT *(Continued)*

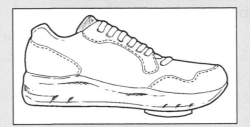

METATARSAL BAR

USE: No medical orthopedic indications

FRACTURES: Nondisplaced phalangeal, nondisplaced metatarsal, stress fracture of the metatarsal

ADVANTAGE: Reduced pressure over the forefoot

DISADVANTAGES: Shoes have to be altered, may throw off normal walking gait, can be expensive if many shoes are adjusted

COST: $20.00 to $25.00

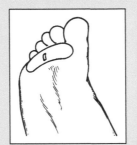

HAMMER-TOE CRESTS

USE: Hammer toes

ADVANTAGES: Easy to put on, inexpensive

DISADVANTAGE: Mildly uncomfortable

COST: $14.00 to $16.00

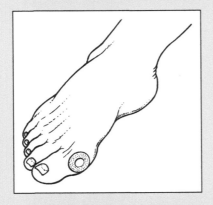

FELT RINGS

USE: Bunion of the first metatarsophalangeal, dorsal bunion, corns, calluses, hammer toes, pre-Achilles bursitis

ADVANTAGES: Easy to apply, inexpensive

DISADVANTAGE: Skin rash from the adhesive (rare)

COST: $3.00 to $4.00

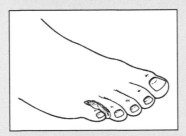

TOE SPACERS, COTTON OR PLASTIC

USE: Morton's neuroma, interdigital soft corns, bunions, any toe deformity

ADVANTAGES: Easy to apply, inexpensive

DISADVANTAGES: None

COST: Cotton, $1.00 to $2.00; rubber, $3.00 to $4.00

FOOT *(Continued)*

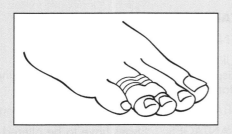

BUDDY-TAPING OF THE TOES

USE: Any toe deformity, hammer toes, turf toe

FRACTURES: Phalanges numbers 2 through 5

ADVANTAGES: Easy to apply, inexpensive

DISADVANTAGES: None

COST: $1.00 to $2.00

INTRODUCTION

Physical therapy treatments—passive stretching exercises, isometric toning exercises, ultrasound, local massage, phonophoresis, and thermal applications—play an essential role in the complete management of the soft-tissue injuries and bony fractures that affect the skeleton. Physical therapy is especially important for the conditions that have a strong element of *mechanical dysfunction* compared with the degree of inflammation and the conditions that are associated with *disuse atrophy*. The Codman pendulum-stretching exercise is the treatment of choice for the subacromial impingement that accompanies rotator cuff tendinitis. The gluteus medius–stretching exercise is fundamental to reducing the direct pressure of the tendons that accompanies trochanteric bursitis. Passive stretching exercises in abduction and external rotation are essential to restoring full range of motion (ROM) to the glenohumeral joint in cases of frozen shoulder. Each condition demands a unique set of treatments.

Physical therapy treatments must be recommended at the appropriate *time* and at the appropriate *stage* of recovery. Stretching exercises to restore full ROM after severe ankle sprain are started after 2 to 4 weeks of immobilization. The acute inflammation and pain must be arrested and the ligament securely reattached to the bone before ROM exercises are begun. Similarly, isometric toning exercises to restore the strength of the rotator cuff tendons cannot be started until the inflammation of the rotator cuff tendon has been nearly resolved. Ideally the optimal timing and extent of these treatments should be determined individually. The decision to initiate any physical therapy treatment must be assessed by the primary care provider and should be based on (1) the phase of recovery; (2) the patient's ability and willingness to carry out a home exercise program; and, most important, (3) the patient's tolerance of the specific exercise, as determined by the health care provider in the office. Performing the exercise in the office engenders greater confidence in the provider's treatment plan, provides hands-on explanation of the exercise, and allows the provider to assess the patient's understanding and tolerance of the exercise.

The recommendations in this book should serve as guidelines for prescribing physical therapy. The timing of these treatments, the frequency of performance, and the number of repetitions represent averages. Any specific physical therapy treatment must be adjusted according to the individual patient's understanding, cooperation, and tolerance. The information that follows represents general recommendations for physical therapy.

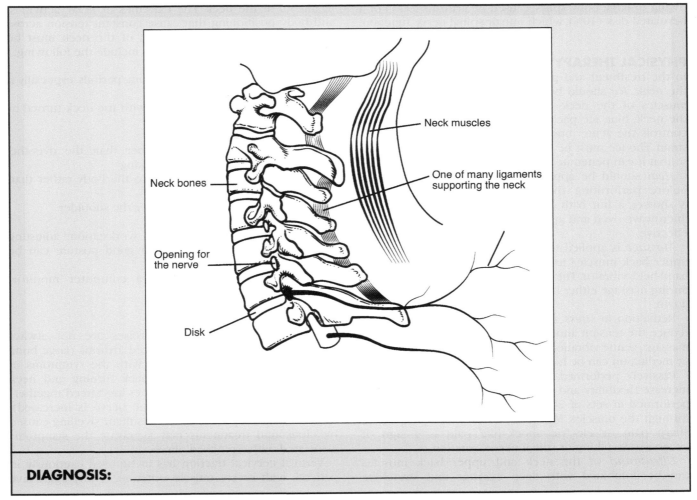

Neck muscles

One of many ligaments supporting the neck

Neck bones

Opening for the nerve

Disk

DIAGNOSIS: _____

GENERAL CARE OF THE NECK

ANATOMY The neck comprises *seven neck bones* (vertebrae) connected together by a network of ligaments and muscles, all of which serve to protect the spinal cord and the spinal nerves. Seven pairs of spinal nerves exit the spinal column and travel down the neck through the shoulder and into the lower arm. Each nerve must pass by one of the disks and through an opening (foramen) formed by two adjacent neck bones.

CONDITIONS Everyone develops a problem in the neck at some time. Arthritis is a universal problem that develops with age. Gradual stiffness, especially when turning from side to side, and the forward positioning of the head are common manifestations. Neck strain—muscular irritation in the neck and upper back—is an exceedingly common condition caused by tension, emotional strain, and poor posture. Many patients suffer recurrent neck stiffness, headaches, and pain from another common cause—whiplash. A rapid-deceleration injury as a result of a motor vehicle accident or a heavy blow to the head can cause permanent damage to the neck's supporting ligaments and muscles. Some patients develop symptoms down the arm that result from a pinched nerve owing to large bony spurs, caused by arthritis (90%) or a herniated disk (10%), which impair spinal nerve function.

PHYSICAL THERAPY Physical therapy is fundamental to the treatment and prevention of conditions affecting the neck. *Ice* should be applied directly to the affected muscles of the neck. An iced towel wrapped around the neck, blue ice packs, or a simple ice bag effectively controls the acute muscle spasms that accompany neck strain. The ice must be left in place for 15 to 20 minutes so that it can penetrate to the deeper tissues.

Heat should be applied to the muscles of the neck before performing the passive stretching exercises. A shower, a hot bath, and a moist towel warmed in a microwave oven and applied for 10 to 15 minutes all are effective.

Massage is applied to both sides of the neck and the upper back muscles using hand pressure or an electric, hand-held vibrator. The neck muscles should be relaxed during massage either by supporting the head or by lying down.

Reduction in *stress* and improvement in *posture* help reduce the tension and pressure in the neck. Upper back massage, gentle vibration with heat, relaxation techniques, or meditation can be helpful in selected cases.

Passively performed *stretching exercises* are used to increase flexibility and preserve motion. Each exercise is performed in sets of 20, gradually increasing the stretch through the muscles. Mild discomfort is to be expected. Sharp pain or electric shock–like pain is a sign of excessive stretching or spinal nerve irritation.

Ultrasound of the neck and upper back muscles can be combined with deep massage and stretching exercises. Neck strain and whiplash respond well to this combination.

Vertical cervical traction is reserved for chronic whiplash, chronic neck strain, and arthritis associated with a pinched nerve. Vertical stretching of the neck muscles and ligaments must be started gradually and increased slowly.

Good Body Mechanics The following recommendations emphasize correct posture, neutral neck positions, and preventive measures:

- Sitting with the shoulders back
- Sleeping with the head aligned with the torso: on the back with a small pillow or on the side with enough pillows to keep the head straight
- Using seat belts and an air bag
- Using arm rests to keep the shoulders slightly shrugged
- Taking periodic breaks from desktop work
- Avoiding continuous sitting or standing
- Choosing a chair with good lumbar support

Activity Limitations The preferred activities and body positions emphasize neutral neck position and a minimum of tension across the supporting muscles and ligaments of the neck. The extremes of ROM, activities, and body positioning that cause constant tension across the upper back and at the base of the neck must be minimized or avoided. Limitations include the following:

- Not doing overhead work for long periods, especially if looking up is necessary
- Not sleeping on the stomach with the neck turned or rotated
- Avoiding stressful situations
- Relying on the hip belt rather than the over-the-shoulder straps when backpacking
- Carrying heavy objects close to the body rather than with outstretched arms
- Not carrying a heavy purse over the shoulder
- Avoiding continuous sitting
- Avoiding slumping over the workstation; adjusting the level of the work so that good posture can be maintained
- Avoiding looking down at a computer monitor; adjusting it to eye level

Precautions Stretching exercises are not always tolerated by patients with advanced arthritis (large bone spurs), with limited mobility, or with the symptoms of a pinched nerve. Extremes of neck turning and neck extension can be painful (the bones are forced together) or harmful (the pressure over the nerve is increased). Likewise, the deep heating and resultant swelling caused by ultrasound treatments may aggravate the symptoms associated with a pinched nerve.

Vertical cervical traction has to be used cautiously in patients with severe muscle irritation. Overly aggressive traction (too much weight or too long a period of traction) may aggravate the underlying muscular irritability. A neck x-ray must be obtained before any vertical traction stretching program is begun.

PHYSICAL THERAPY SUMMARY

1. Ice applied directly to an acute muscle spasm
2. Heat and massage for chronic muscle spasms
3. Neck muscle-stretching exercises, passively performed
4. Stress reduction
5. Posture improvement
6. Ultrasound
7. Vertical cervical traction

NECK MASSAGE

Heat your upper back and the neck for 15 minutes. Lie down on your stomach with your head aligned with your body. (Place a pillow under your chest and neck.) Ask your partner to press firmly with circular motions along the side of your neck and over the upper back muscles.

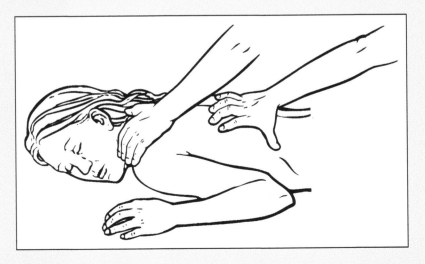

STRETCHING EXERCISES FOR THE NECK

Heat your neck and upper back in a bathtub, in a shower with a water massage, or with moist towels heated in a microwave oven. Gently stretch the muscles in sets of 10 to 15, with each held for 5 seconds. Expect mild, achy muscle pain, but not sharp or electric shock–like pain. Relax the muscles in your neck during the exercises. Perform these exercises in the morning to relieve stiffness and just before sleeping.

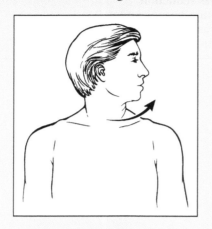

Neck Rotation
Slowly turn your head to the right. Place tension on your chin with your fingertips. Hold for a few seconds and return to the center. Repeat to the left.

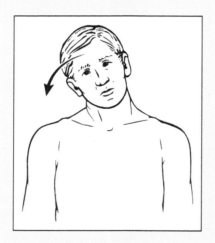

Neck Tilting
Tilt your head to the right, trying to touch your ear to the tip of your shoulder. Place tension on the temple with your fingertips. Hold for a few seconds and return to the center. Repeat to the left.

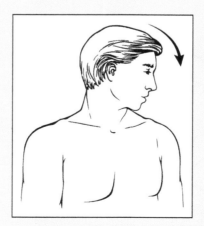

Neck Bending
Try to touch your chin to your chest. Hold for a few seconds and return to the neutral position. Breathe in gradually and exhale slowly with each exercise. Relax the neck and back muscles with each neck bend.

HOME CERVICAL TRACTION

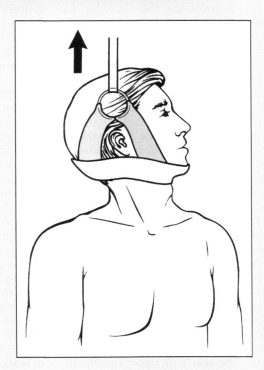

Home traction using a cervical water bag traction unit can be started after an evaluation by a physical therapist. Traction is begun using 4 to 5 lb of water weight for 5 minutes, which is increased slowly to 12 to 15 lb for 10 minutes. Each week, the weight or time or both are increased by 1 to 2 lb or 1 to 2 minutes or both. The neck muscles should be relaxed. Heat application before treatment is advised.

Note: Traction can aggravate some conditions, particularly some disk herniations. If symptoms worsen, stop the traction and re-evaluate. Arthritis of the neck may have to be treated three times a week for an indefinite period.

GENERAL CARE OF THE SHOULDER

ANATOMY   The shoulder is a ball-and-socket joint formed by the upper arm bone (the humerus), the cap of the shoulder (the acromion process), and the bony socket (the glenoid of the scapula). It has many moving parts, as follows:

One major joint—the ball-and-socket joint
Three auxiliary joints—the end of the collar bone (the acromioclavicular joint), the joint of the collar bone and the breast plate (the supraclavicular), and the wing over the ribs (the scapulothoracic)
Eight major tendons—the rotator cuff tendons (four), biceps, triceps, deltoid, and pectoralis
One major lubricating bursal sac—the subacromial bursa
Four major ligaments—three over the end of the collar bone and one encircling the ball-and-socket joint

CONDITIONS   There are many causes of shoulder pain, including tense neck and upper back muscles, a pinched nerve in the neck, shoulder strain or separation, tendinitis, bursitis, and arthritis. Tendinitis of the rotator tendons and frozen shoulder resulting from disuse account for two thirds of all problems, however. Shoulder separation occurs at the end of the clavicle. Arthritis at the end of the clavicle occurs to some degree or another in everyone, but only a small percentage of patients develop symptoms from it. Arthritis of the ball-and-socket joint is infrequent.

PHYSICAL THERAPY   Physical therapy plays a major role in the active treatment and rehabilitation of conditions involving the shoulder. *Ice* applications can be used as the initial anti-inflammatory treatment for any shoulder condition. The response is unpredictable, however. The shoulder joint and its supporting structures (the rotator tendons) are located deep in the tissues, 1 to $1^1/_2$ inches below the skin.

Deep *heat* and *massage* are used to increase the blood flow to these tissues and prepare the shoulder for stretching. The shoulder is heated in a shower or warm bath for 10 to 15 minutes. Total body heating is preferable to local heat (a moist heating pad or a towel warmed in a microwave oven) because of the depth of the tissues.

The *weighted pendulum-stretching exercise* has a dual function in the active treatment of the shoulder. Its primary role is to stretch gently the tendon space between the ball-and-socket joint and the cap (see later). Its secondary role is to prevent frozen shoulder by providing passive movement of the shoulder joint. The muscles of the shoulder are relaxed, allowing the weight to open the shoulder and provide room for the shoulder bursa and the rotator tendons. A weight of 5 to 10 lb is held in the hand; a filled gallon milk jug weighs 8 lb, but any weight that can be held easily in the hand will do. The arm is kept vertical and close to the body, avoiding further tendon impingement. The exercise is begun as a pure stretch, dangling the arm. With improvement, the arm is allowed to swing freely, but no farther than 1 foot in any direction. The exercise is performed after heating for 5 minutes once or twice a day.

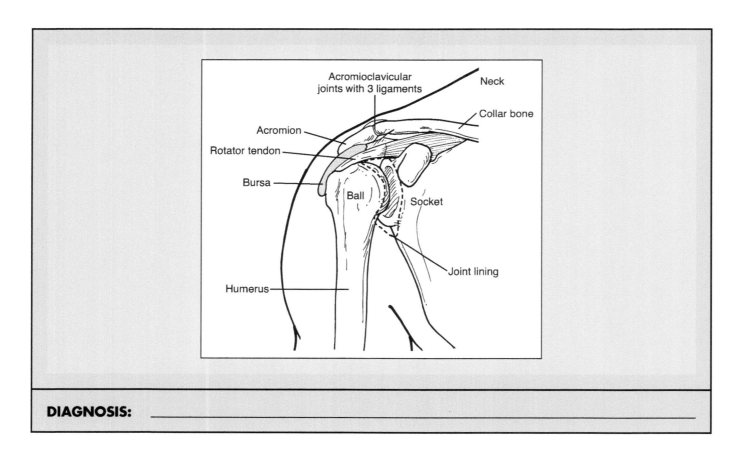

DIAGNOSIS: _____

Muscle toning exercises for the supporting tendons are used to strengthen and tighten the joint. These exercises always should follow the weighted pendulum-stretching exercises. Rotation and lifting exercises are performed in sets of 20, each held 5 seconds with moderate tension. Flexible rubber tubing, bungee cords, or large rubber bands provide the necessary resistance. These exercises are increased gradually to restore the strength of the weakened tendons and muscles and put them in balance with their shoulder counterparts. Mild soreness should be expected. Sharp or severe pain may indicate a flare of the underlying condition.

Good Body Mechanics   Safe activities and positions involve keeping the arm down and in front of and close to the body. A good rule of thumb is to perform all activities with the elbow held at the sides, as follows:

- Lifting objects close to the body
- Weight training with light weights below shoulder level
- Sidestroke or breaststroke when swimming
- Side-arm or underhand ball throwing
- Volleying rather than serving in tennis
- Desktop writing and assembly with good posture

Activity Limitations   Activities and positions that require repetitive reaching out, up, or back are to be minimized or avoided altogether:

- Overhead reaching
- Throwing
- Sleeping with the arm over the head
- Sleeping directly on the shoulder
- Leaning on the elbows, jamming the shoulder
- Lifting heavy objects with the arms extended
- Heavy pushing and pulling
- Serving and the overhead smash in tennis
- Overhead military press
- Incline bench press
- Chin-ups and push-ups
- The crawl and backstroke when swimming
- Archery, pulling a 90-lb bow

Associative Conditions   Reductions in stress and improvements in posture help reduce the pressure over the ball-and-socket joint, the shoulder tendons, and the bursa. Upper back and neck massage, gentle vibration with heat, relaxation techniques, and meditation may be helpful in selected cases.

PENDULUM STRETCH EXERCISES FOR THE SHOULDER

Before exercise or heavy work, shoulders should be stretched in a downward direction. This exercise provides greater space for the rotator cuff and the bicep tendons, allowing them to work more effectively and efficiently. Regular use of pendulum exercises can increase the space under the cap of the shoulder by 1/4 inch.

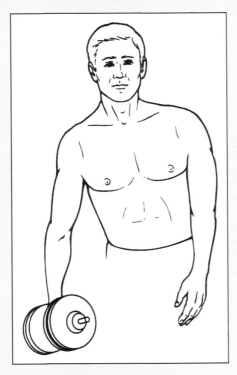

Weighted Pendulum Stretch
Heat the shoulder with moist towels or in a hot bath or hot shower. A weight of 5 to 10 lb is held lightly in the hand (a filled gallon container weighs 8 lb). The muscles of the shoulder are to be relaxed. The arm is kept vertical and close to the body (bending over too far may cause pinching of the rotator cuff tendons). The arm is allowed to swing back and forth or in a small-diameter circle (≤1 inch in any direction). A properly performed stretching exercise may cause a deep achy pain, either in the armpit or down the inner aspect of the arm. This exercise can be performed just as effectively while sitting.

This exercise is helpful for shoulder tendinitis (rotator cuff and biceps tendinitis), shoulder bursitis, frozen shoulder, and rotator cuff tendon tears. It is not appropriate for shoulder separation/strain or upper back/neck muscle strain.

STRENGTHENING EXERCISES FOR THE ROTATOR CUFF TENDONS

The rotator cuff tendons are the weakest and most susceptible to injury of the eight major tendons in the shoulder. Isometric exercises are necessary to improve the strength of these tendons. These exercises balance the strength of the shoulder muscles. Flexible rubber tubing, bungee cords, or large rubber bands are used to develop muscle tone and strength. First, the shoulder is heated, then it is prepared by stretching, using the weighted pendulum swing exercise. After a 2- to 3-minute rest, sets of 15 to 20 exercises, each held 5 seconds, should be performed daily.

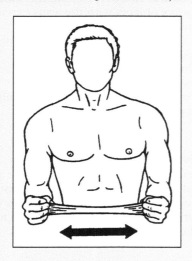

Outward Rotation Isometric

The elbows are held at 90 degrees, close to the sides. The rubber bands are grasped with the hands. The forearms are rotated outward only 2 to 3 inches and held 5 seconds. The forearms swing out like a door.

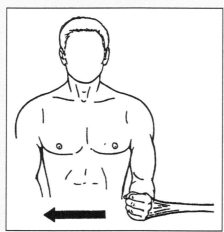

Inward Rotation Isometric

The elbow is held at 90 degrees, close to the side. The rubber bands are hooked onto a door handle and grasped with the hand. The forearm is rotated inward only 2 to 3 inches and held 5 seconds. The forearm swings in like a door.

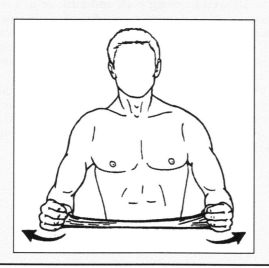

Lifting Isometric

The elbows are bent to 90 degrees. The rubber bands are placed near the elbows. The arms are lifted up only 4 to 5 inches away from the body and held 5 seconds.

These exercises are used for shoulder tendinitis, shoulder bursitis, and rotator cuff tendon tears and are begun 3 to 4 weeks after the acute inflammation has resolved. Ideally the outward and inward rotation strength should be restored before moving on to the lifting exercise. *Note:* If begun too soon, these exercises may result in a flare of the underlying condition. During the healing process, heavy work must be restricted.

STRETCHING EXERCISES FOR A FROZEN SHOULDER

These exercises, performed once or twice a day for several months, should loosen the tightened shoulder lining and restore normal ROM. First, heat the shoulder for 15 to 20 minutes and perform a 5-minute pendulum swing. Next, perform sets of 10 to 20 of the following three exercises. A mild muscle-type pain along the front or side of the shoulder is to be expected. Severe discomfort is unusual and suggests overstretching.

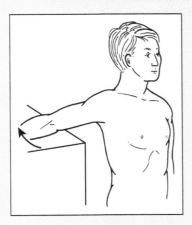

Armpit Stretch

Use your good arm to lift the arm onto a shelf, a dresser, or any object about breast high. Gently bend at the knees, opening up the armpit. Try to push the arm up just a little bit farther with each stretch.

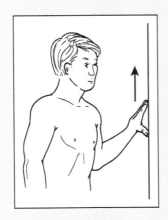

Finger-Walk Up the Wall

Face a wall about three quarters of an arm's length away from it. Using only your fingers (*not* your shoulder muscles) raise your arm up to shoulder level. Repeat this exercise.

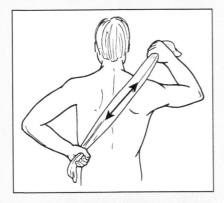

Towel-Stretch Behind the Back

Take a 3-foot-long towel, grasp it with both hands, and hold it at a 45-degree angle. Use the upper, good arm to pull the arm toward the lower back. This can be repeated with the towel in the horizontal position.

Precautions Weighted pendulum-stretching exercises should be avoided if there is any history or suggestion of dislocation or partial dislocation of the ball-and-socket joint. Likewise, these exercises should be used with caution by patients with a history of shoulder separation at the clavicular joint. Either condition can be aggravated by downward traction! Isometric toning exercises must be properly prescribed to be beneficial. Chronic shoulder tendinitis or shoulder tendinitis complicated by a torn tendon can be aggravated by overly aggressive toning. It is always safest to start out with low tension and increase gradually as tolerated

PHYSICAL THERAPY SUMMARY

1. Heat and massage
2. Weighted pendulum-stretching exercises, performed with relaxed shoulder muscles
3. Muscle-toning exercises in lifting and turning out
4. Activity limitations
5. Stress reduction

GENERAL CARE OF THE ELBOW

ANATOMY   The elbow works like a simple door hinge. It is formed by the two forearm bones (the *radius* and *ulna*) and the upper arm bone (the *humerus*). It is capable of moving in only two directions, bending and straightening (*flexing* and *extending*). Forcing the arm backward (*hyperextension*) causes the ulna to break or the elbow joint to dislocate. Movement at the elbow always affects the wrist joint. Conditions affecting the elbow often cause problems at the wrist and vice versa. Elbow anatomy includes the following:

One major joint—the hinge joint
One companion joint—the wrist
Four major tendon groups—the biceps (in front), the triceps (in back), the muscles that extend the wrist and fingers up (on the outside), and the muscles that flex the wrist and fingers down (on the inside)
One major lubricating bursal sac—the olecranon bursa over the back of the elbow
Two major ligaments—the hinge ligaments on the outside and inside of the elbow

CONDITIONS   Tendinitis is the most common condition to affect the elbow. Tennis elbow is an inflammation of the outer tendon; it is 10 times more common than golfer's elbow, an inflammation of the inner tendon. Both conditions result from heavy use of the wrist and forearm muscles. Bursitis occurs over the back of the elbow and is caused by direct pressure in most cases (draftsman's elbow). Arthritis of the elbow is uncommon and is almost always the result of a previous injury.

PHYSICAL THERAPY   Physical therapy plays a major role in the rehabilitation of elbow tendinitis and conditions that interfere with the normal ROM of the elbow joint (arthritis, fractures, chips of the joint cartilage). The elbow joint and its supporting tendons (the wrist extensors on the outside and the wrist flexors on the inside) are located just under the surface. Local applications of *ice* for 10 to 15 minutes three to four times a day are effective in controlling pain and inflammation.

Phonophoresis with a hydrocortisone gel applied directly over the inner and outer tendons of the elbow is effective in reducing the mild to moderate inflammation that accompanies elbow tendinitis. The superficial location of the tendons allows good penetration of the medication, leading to a reduction in the degree of local swelling and heat.

Muscle toning exercises involving gripping and wrist motion are fundamental to restoring full support to the elbow and wrist. A graduated program of exercises is necessary. It should begin at the lowest tolerated level of gripping and be followed by a stepwise increase in the toning of the forearm muscles responsible for the maintenance of forearm tone, wrist strength, and elbow support. The importance of performing these exercises in sequence cannot be overemphasized. They should be taken just to the edge of discomfort over several weeks to improve the strength of the elbow and wrist gradually without inciting recurrent tendon inflammation.

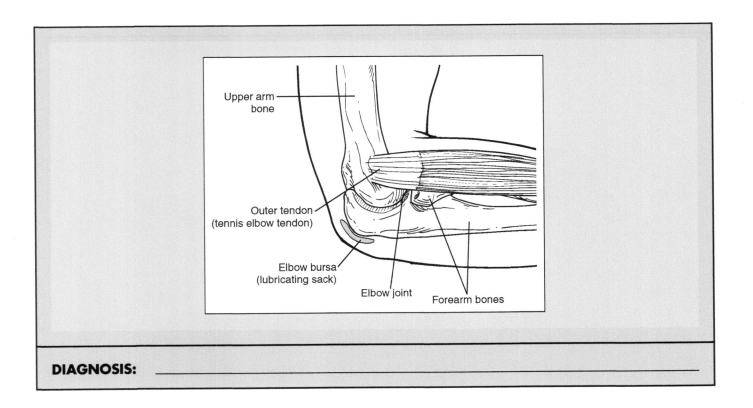

DIAGNOSIS: _____

TENNIS ELBOW–STRENGTHENING EXERCISES

These exercises are begun 2 to 3 weeks after the acute pain and local tenderness have subsided. They strengthen the muscle and the tendon, reducing the risk of recurrent tendinitis. Muscle soreness in the forearm (2 to 3 inches down from the elbow) is common. If sharp or intense pain is felt in the outer elbow, the exercises should be discontinued (possibly indicates recurrence of injury).

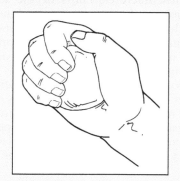

Grip Strengthening

Gripping exercises always should precede wrist isometrics. Begin with a small, compressible rubber ball (e.g., an old tennis ball or silicone ball). Grip firmly but not hard. Perform 20 to 25 mild squeezes, holding each for 5 seconds. With increasing strength, advance to a spring-loaded metal gripper.

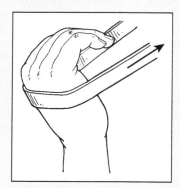

Wrist Isometrics

After 2 to 3 weeks of gripping exercises, isometric strengthening of wrist bending can be started. Perform 15 to 20 sets per day. Keep the wrist in a neutral position while pulling on a large rubber band, bungee cord, or flexible rubber tubing. Achy pain should be felt in the forearm, but sharp pain over the elbow may indicate recurrent tendinitis.

These exercises are preventive measures. In addition to these exercises, switch to a two-handed backhand, use power tools, wear a tennis-elbow band, try to lift objects with two hands, and emphasize lifting with the palms up.

Good Body Mechanics   A healthy elbow joint requires a healthy wrist joint, well-toned and strong biceps and triceps muscles that move the joint, and well-toned and strong forearm muscles that support the elbow and the wrist. The use of good body mechanics includes the following:

- Lifting objects close to the body with the elbow in a partially flexed position
- Keeping the wrist in a neutral position when performing repetitive forearm work or weight training
- Using wrist supports when weightlifting
- Using leverage to reduce the effects of torque (e.g., a cheater bar when using a torque wrench, keeping the elbow close to the body)
- Avoiding tight gripping; increasing the gripping surface of tools with gloves or padding
- Using a hammer with extra padding to reduce tension and impact
- Holding heavy tools with two hands
- Using the double backhand in tennis
- Applying grip tape or oversized grips to golf clubs

Activity Limitations   Activities that cause impact and tension at the wrist and forearm cause the greatest aggravation of the elbow, including the following:

- Lifting with the elbow fully extended
- Doing heavy work, unless gripping strength is good, and the forearm muscles are well toned
- Leaning on the elbows
- Allowing unprotected repetitive impact and tension

Associative Conditions   Poorly toned forearm muscles and a poorly supported, weak wrist contribute substantially to injuries of the elbow. Similarly the most important means of protecting the elbow is to maintain the strength of the gripping muscles and the muscles that support the wrist.

PHYSICAL THERAPY SUMMARY

1. Local applications of ice over the tendons or the joint
2. Phonophoresis with a hydrocortisone gel
3. Gripping exercises, performed initially with half grips and gradually increasing
4. Toning exercises of wrist extension (tennis elbow) or wrist flexion (golfer's elbow)

GENERAL CARE OF THE WRIST AND HAND

PHYSICAL THERAPY   Physical therapy plays a major role in the prevention of carpal tunnel syndrome, trigger finger, and the scarring that occurs in the palms of the hands (Dupuytren's contracture).

STRETCHING OF THE WRIST AND HAND TENDONS

These stretching exercises help to rehabilitate and prevent trigger finger, thickened palms (Dupuytren's contracture), and carpal tunnel syndrome. They are begun 3 to 4 weeks after acute pain and inflammation have resolved. The hand and wrist are heated for 15 to 20 minutes. The wrist and fingers are bent back using very light finger pressure.

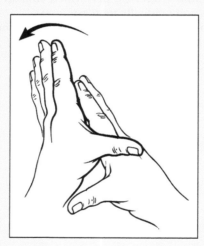

Wrist Stretching
Bend the wrist back as far as is comfortable. Enhance the stretch with gentle, constant tension against the fingers. A pulling sensation should be felt in the forearm. Perform sets of 15 to 20 per day.

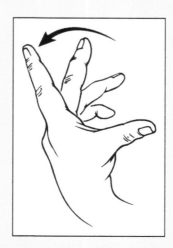

Finger Stretching
Massage the palm and base of the fingers with lanolin cream for 5 minutes. Stretch the affected fingers back with gentle finger pressure. Perform sets of 15 to 20 per day.

Gradual stretching exercises should be performed over several months to prevent a recurrence or to slow down the progression of the problem. In addition, avoid vibrating tools, heavy gripping and grasping of tools, and any tools that place pressure over the wrist or the palm tendons.

GENERAL CARE OF THE BACK

ANATOMY   The lower back (the lumbosacral spine) consists of *five back bones* (vertebrae) connected together by a network of ligaments and muscles, all of which protect the spinal cord and spinal nerves. Five pairs of spinal nerves exit the spinal column and travel down the back through the pelvis and buttocks and into the lower legs. Each nerve passes by one of the spinal disks and through a bony passage formed by the two adjacent back bones.

CONDITIONS   Back problems are exceedingly common. Everyone develops some degree of arthritis and at least one episode of low back strain. Poor posture, excessive weight, lack of exercise, and improper lifting all contribute to acute lumbar strain. Some patients develop symptoms down into the leg because of a pinched nerve. The most common cause of a pinched nerve in the lower back is a herniated disk.

PHYSICAL THERAPY   Physical therapy is essential to all phases of treatment of the low back. In the *first few days and weeks* of an acute back condition, *cold, heat, massage, and gentle stretching exercises* are used to treat muscle irritation and spasm.

Cold, heat, and cold alternating with heat are effective in reducing pain and muscle spasm. Some patients respond to one better than another. A bag of frozen corn, an iced towel from the freezer, or an ice pack should be left in place for 15 to 20 minutes three to four times a day. Moist heat is preferable and is used similarly.

Massage of the lower back muscles is effective in reducing muscle spasm. It always should be performed on a comfortable surface while the patient is lying on the stomach. Hand pressure or pressure from an electric vibrator is applied from the lower rib cage to the top of the pelvis. Up-and-down and circular motions are performed on both sides. Massage is especially effective just before going to bed.

Low back muscle *stretching exercises* are performed to restore lost flexibility. These exercises are especially important for patients with scoliosis, fractured vertebrae, or other structural back disorders. Side-bends, knee-chest pulls, and pelvic rocks are designed to stretch the low back muscles, the buttocks muscles, and the sacroiliac joints. These exercises are begun after the most intense muscle spasms have resolved (usually days). Initially, they

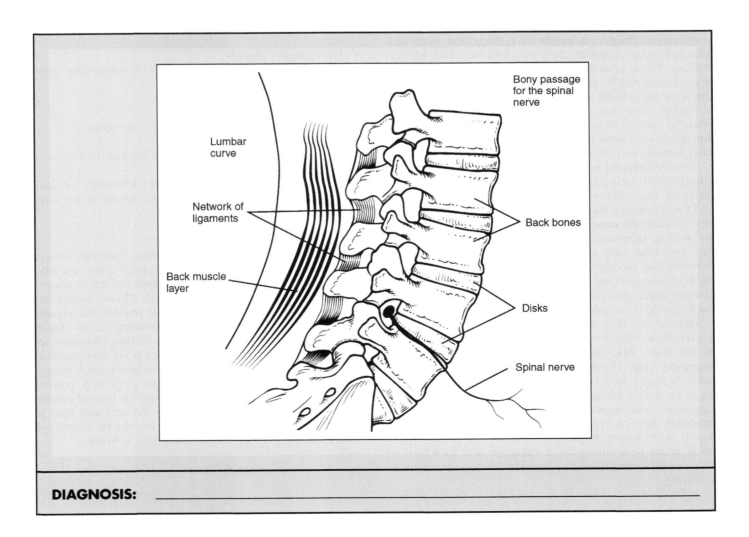

DIAGNOSIS: _____

should be performed while lying down in bed. As the pain and muscle spasms diminish, stretching can be performed in the standing position. Sets of 20 of each exercise are performed to the point of mild muscular aching. Any sharp pain or any electric shock–like or shooting pain down the leg may be a sign of nerve irritation or overstretching.

Ultrasound treatments are used in selected cases. A physical therapist or chiropractor must administer the treatments. The device causes a vibration-like feeling, but is actually heating the deep tissues. *Diathermy* is another special treatment that provides deep heating. Both are used for difficult-to-treat muscle spasms. A patient with a herniated disk should avoid these treatments.

Chiropractic manipulation is an effective alternative to home physical therapy. Realignment by adjustment of the spinal elements has been shown to provide temporary benefit for lumbar strain. It is not appropriate to consider chiropractic treatments if there has been or if there is a serious possibility of a compression fracture, a disk herniation, or disease directly involving the bones of the back.

Patients with severe symptoms unresponsive to the aforementioned treatments may require in-hospital *lumbar traction*. This type of treatment is rarely used today. Several days of pelvic traction at 20 to 25 lb are combined with intense use of a strong muscle relaxer and narcotic medications.

In the *recovery and rehabilitation phase*, greater emphasis is placed on progressive stretching exercises, muscle-toning exercises, aerobic exercises, and vertical traction. These treatments also are important for prevention. They typically are begun around 3 to 4 weeks after the acute symptoms have resolved.

Toning exercises of the abdominal and low back muscles consist of modified sit-ups, weighted side-bends, and gentle extension exercises. These are always performed after heating and stretching (see earlier).

Aerobic exercise is one of the best ways to prevent recurrent back strain. General toning of the body improves posture, muscular support, and flexibility. Swimming and cross-country ski machine workouts are probably the best overall exercises that do not aggravate the back. Swimming, in particular, is an excellent way to recover lost muscular tone and function after a herniated disk, compression fracture, or spinal surgery. Fast walking and light jogging also are acceptable forms of exercise. Exercise apparatus that places excessive bend or torque on the back should be avoided.

Vertical traction can be used at home as a part of a comprehensive back treatment program. The weight of the lower body and legs is used to pull the lumbar segments apart. Leaning on a countertop, suspending the body between two bar stools, or using inversion equipment for 1 to 3 minutes at a time allows the back bones, ligaments, and muscles to stretch apart and lengthen gradually. Several vertical stretches are performed each day. It is extremely important to relax the whole lower body when performing these exercises and to return to full weightbearing slowly by lowering down onto the legs gradually.

For chronic cases that do not respond to traditional physical therapy, a transcutaneous electric nerve stimulator can be prescribed to block or attenuate the persistent pain. This type of treatment should be combined with a thorough evaluation by a pain clinic.

Good Body Mechanics The positions and activities that follow are safest to perform, and over time they reduce the possibility of reinjury of the muscles and ligaments:

- Sitting and standing up straight
- Lifting by using the legs and knees
- Lifting and carrying weight close to the body
- Lifting using an external lumbar support
- Sleeping on a firm mattress, placing a pillow under the knees
- Maintaining ideal body weight
- Wearing seat belts and purchasing a car with an airbag
- Low-weight, high-repetition weightlifting
- Swimming, a cross-country ski machine (with low-tension arm setting to avoid back twisting or torque), a soft-platform treadmill, or fast walking

Activity Limitations The following positions and activities place excessive load or torque on the muscles, ligaments, and bones of the back:

- Lifting heavy objects
- Lifting objects away from the body (with the arms held out)
- Lifting in a twisted position
- Working in a stooped position
- Bending at the waist with excessive frequency
- Full sit-ups
- Bending over to touch the toes (at least in the recovery period)
- A rowing machine; heavy weightlifting; or any apparatus that puts too much bend, torque, or pressure onto the lower back

Precautions *Stretching and toning exercises* always should be increased gradually. If sharp pain, electric shock–like pain, or shooting pain down the leg develops, the exercises must be interrupted. These symptoms suggest nerve irritation. *Ultrasound treatments* should be avoided in patients with herniated disks. Deep heating may cause the disk to swell further. *Chiropractic manipulation* must be avoided with bony compression fractures, disk herniations, and disease of the back bones. *Vertical traction* must be used with caution. A patient must possess a strong upper body and be free of cardiovascular disease (blood can pool in the legs and lead to fainting). The health care provider should be contacted before this type of aggressive stretching is begun.

BACK-STRETCHING EXERCISES

Back-stretching exercises play a vital role in the treatment of lumbosacral muscle spasms. The lower back is heated for 15 to 20 minutes. Sets of 10 to 20 stretches, each held for 5 seconds, are performed on each side. The muscles are kept relaxed. Rest for 1 to 2 minutes between exercises. Mild muscle soreness is to be expected. Severe pain, electric shock–like sharp pain, or severe muscle spasms suggest overstretching.

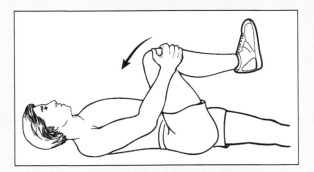

Knee-Chest Pulls

Bring your knee slowly up to your chest, holding it in place with your hands. Relax the buttock and back muscles. Do the left side, then the right side, and then both simultaneously (curling up in the fetal position).

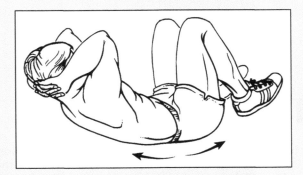

Pelvic Rocks

With knees bent, rotate your pelvis forward and then backward. The abdominal muscles do the work, as the back muscles are relaxed. *Caution:* Do not overextend when arching the back.

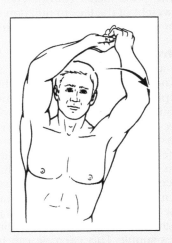

Side-Bends

While lying down, crawl your fingers down the side of your thigh. Hold in this tilted position for 5 seconds. Return to a neutral position. Repeat on the other side.

Initially, these exercises should be performed while lying down or while floating in the bath or hot tub. With improvement, these exercises can be performed standing or sitting. Follow these movements with exercises to strengthen the back.

PHYSICAL THERAPY SUMMARY

1. Cold applications for acute muscular spasm
2. Heating before stretching exercises
3. Stretching exercises of the back and side muscles
4. Aerobic exercises (e.g., walking, swimming, cross-country ski machine)
5. Strengthening exercises of the muscles of the back
6. Vertical stretching of the ligaments of the back
7. Ultrasound
8. Lumbar traction
9. Chiropractic manipulation

ADVANCED BACK-STRETCHING EXERCISES

This exercise is not appropriate for everyone. A strong upper body and a 2- to 4-week period of basic back exercises are prerequisites. The vertical stretch elongates the support ligaments, lengthens the back muscles, and allows the back bones to pull apart and realign. (I refer to this exercise as "the poor man's chiropractic adjustment.") Suspension between parallel bars is ideal, but any method to allow the weight of the legs to pull down on the back works (e.g., leaning on a countertop, using crutches, or supporting your weight between two bar stools).

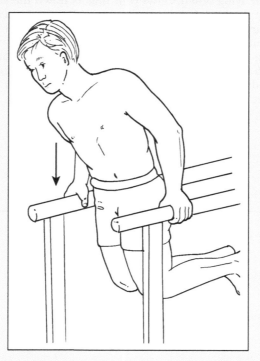

Vertical Stretching Exercise

Starting in a standing position, gradually shift the weight of your body to your outstretched arms. The toes are kept on the ground for balance. The back muscles should be relaxed. Allow the weight of your legs to draw out and pull out the lower back bones. Popping sensations or a gentle sensation of stretching should be felt in the lower back. Additional pulling occurs if you lean forward slowly. Hold this position for 30 to 60 seconds. Gradually shift your weight back to the legs, then stand up straight. Repeat once or twice. This exercise is especially helpful before going to bed.

This is a great way to keep the back limber and the back muscles supple. This exercise can be performed daily to prevent recurrent back strain.

BACK-STRENGTHENING EXERCISES

Before starting a strengthening program for the back, flexibility must be restored with 3 to 6 weeks of daily back stretching. Strengthening exercises should be performed when the body is well rested. First, the back muscles are stretched out for 5 to 10 minutes. Next, sets of 15 to 20 of the following exercises are performed daily for 6 weeks. As the strength of the back increases, the frequency can be reduced to three times a week.

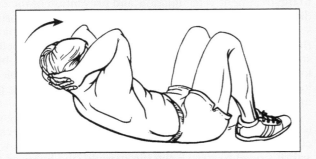

Modified Sit-ups

The knees are kept bent. The lower back is kept flush with the ground. The hands can be kept behind the neck or held over the chest. The head and neck are raised 3 to 4 inches and held for 5 seconds. The abdominal muscles gradually strengthen.

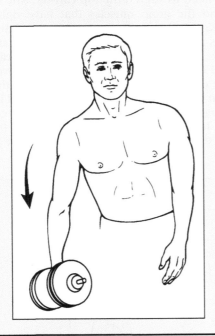

Weighted Side Bends

In a standing position, a 5- to 15-lb weight is held in the hand. The back is tilted to the weighted side and is brought back immediately to center. The back should be tilted only a few inches. The farther away from the body the weight is held, the greater is the amount of muscle work. After a set of 15 to 20, the weight is switched to the opposite side.

These specific exercises are complementary to a regular aerobic exercise program. No single exercise is better than another. If you are having problems doing any specific exercise, discuss it with your health care provider.

GENERAL CARE OF THE HIP

ANATOMY The hip is a *ball-and-socket joint* formed by the bony pelvis (the socket) and the end of the femur bone (the ball). Both bones are covered with a smooth layer of protective cartilage (articular cartilage). Loss of this cartilage from wear and tear, inflammation, or injury is called *arthritis*. The anatomy of the hip includes the following:

One main joint—the ball-and-socket joint

Five large lubricating bursal sacs—two at the outer hip, three surrounding the major muscles attached to the pelvis

Four major muscle groups—three buttock muscles and tendons, the top of the quadriceps muscle of the thigh, the tops of the hamstring muscles, and the large hip flexor muscle

One ligament—one thick capsule surrounding the joint to hold the hip in place and contain the lubricating fluid

CONDITIONS Bursitis is the most common cause of hip pain. It is an inflammation of one of the five lubricating sacs that surround the hip and ensure smooth motion. The two large outer bursal sacs become inflamed when the walking gait has been disturbed by any cause. Arthritis is the second most common problem affecting the hip. Damage to the normal protective layer of cartilage that covers the ball-and-socket joint can occur because of age,

wear and tear, injury, or rheumatism. Tendinitis is a rare problem at the hip. Some patients experience pain at the hip that has been referred from the back (sciatic nerve pain) or from impaired circulation in the abdominal and pelvic arteries.

PHYSICAL THERAPY Physical therapy is essential to the treatment, rehabilitation, and prevention of the conditions that affect the hip and its surrounding supporting structures. *Heating* the hip is necessary to stimulate blood flow deep in the tissues and to loosen the tissues before stretching. The hip is heated in a shower or warm bath for 10 to 15 minutes. Total body heating is preferable to local heat, which should come from a moist heating pad or a moist towel warmed in a microwave oven.

Stretching the supporting tendons (the outer and groin tendons) and the joint lining is the most important exercise for the conditions affecting the hip. Patients with arthritis need to stretch the hip capsule (the lining of the joint) and the groin muscles that have tightened from disuse. Knee-chest pulls, figure-of-four, and Indian sitting stretches are performed in sets of 15 to 20 after heating. Similarly, patients with bursitis should perform sets of 15 to 20 cross-leg pulls and side stretches to reduce the pressure of the large buttock tendons over the two large outer bursal sacs. Deep heating is performed before these stretching exercises. Some patients should combine the primary hip stretching exercises with the flexion exercises of the lower back. The hip and lower back are so

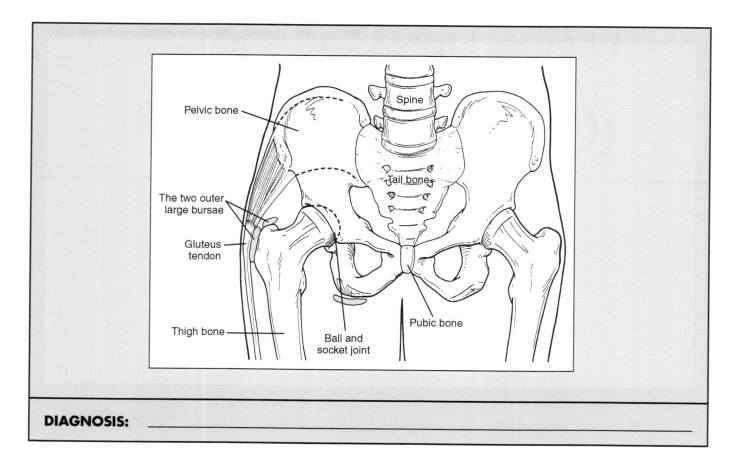

DIAGNOSIS: _____

STRETCHING EXERCISES FOR ARTHRITIS

Home physical therapy for hip arthritis consists of stretching and strengthening exercises. First, the hip is heated in a hot tub or bath or with moist heat for 20 minutes. Next, 15 to 20 knee-chest, figure-of-four, and Indian-style exercises are performed to stretch the muscles and ligaments around the hip. After relaxing for 5 minutes, weighted straight-leg raises and leg extensions are performed to strengthen the hip (see knee exercises).

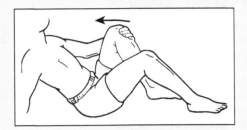

Knee-Chest Pulls

Bend the hip and knee to 90 degrees. Grasp the upper shin, and pull the knee onto the chest. Hold this position for 5 seconds, then relax back to 90 degrees. These exercises should be performed lying down.

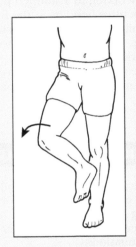

Figure-of-Four Stretch

The foot is placed over the knee. The leg is gently rocked outward. The higher the foot is raised on the leg, the greater is the stretch. Perform this exercise while lying down.

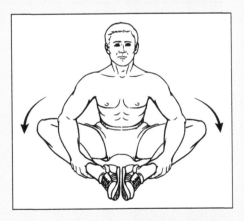

Indian Sitting Stretch

In a seated position, pull the feet up toward the buttocks. Lean forward gradually to increase the stretch.

intertwined that stiffness in either area contributes to problems in the other.

Ultrasound treatments are prescribed for patients who have recurrent or chronic bursitis. A physical therapist or chiropractor must administer such treatments. The ultrasound waves cause a vibration-like feeling but are actually heating the deep tissues. *Diathermy* is another specialized treatment that provides deep heating.

Muscle-toning exercises of the hip are rarely indicated. If deconditioning has occurred as a result of prolonged bed rest, cast immobilization, or lengthy inactivity, straight-leg-raising and leg-extension exercises can be performed.

Good Body Mechanics The following positions and activities are safest and reduce the possibility of reinjury to the hip joint and the bursal sacs that surround the hip:

- Sitting in a partially reclined position
- Sitting up straight with the leg turned out
- Standing with the weight equally distributed between the right and left legs
- Lifting and carrying weight close to the body
- Sleeping on the back with the legs spread apart
- Sleeping on the unaffected side with a large pillow between the knees
- Maintaining ideal body weight
- Low-weight, high-repetition weightlifting
- Swimming with the crawl kick (legs kept straight)
- Using a cross-country ski machine with low tension

Activity Limitations To reduce the chance of an arthritic flare of the hip joint, the extremes of motion should be avoided, and jarring and impact must be minimized. Limitations include the following:

- Avoiding running and jumping
- Limiting stop-and-go sports to reduce direct impact and jarring
- Not using a trampoline
- Avoiding any positions that cause a wide spreading of the legs

Patients with bursitis must reduce direct pressure over the outer hip and minimize repetitive bending. Limitations include the following:

- Avoiding direct pressure
- Avoiding prolonged sitting with the hip in a bent position
- Minimizing stair climbing
- Minimizing working in a stooped position
- Limiting repetitive bending at the hip
- Replacing full sit-ups with partial sit-ups
- Not bending over to touch the toes (at least in the recovery period)
- Avoiding the repetitive bending involved in the use of the rowing machine, stationary bicycle, stair-stepper, and glider

PHYSICAL THERAPY SUMMARY

1. Heat applications to the front and side of the joint
2. Stretching exercises of the supporting tendons and joint lining
3. Toning exercises of the buttock and flexor muscles
4. Activity limitations

STRETCH EXERCISES FOR HIP BURSITIS

The large buttock tendon over the outer hip has to be stretched to reduce the pressure over the bursal sac. First, the area is heated either in a tub or with moist heat. Sets of 15 to 20 stretches are performed daily. Begin these 2 to 4 weeks after the outer-hip pressure and pain have resolved.

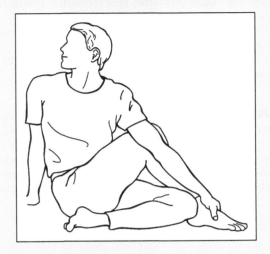

Cross-Leg Pulls

In a sitting position, either in a chair or on the floor, cross the affected leg over the other. Grasp the knee and pull the leg to the opposite side. Keep the buttocks flat and avoid twisting the back. A gentle pulling sensation should be felt in the outer buttocks or hip areas. Sharp pain suggests irritation of the bursa.

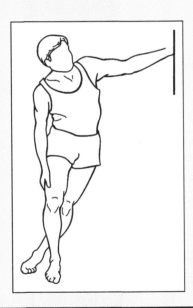

Outer Thigh Stretches

Stand an arm's length away from a wall, with the affected leg toward the wall. Cross the leg behind the outer leg. Carry all the weight on the good side. Lean into the wall, stretching the entire leg and lower side muscles. Perform sets of 15 to 20. The farther away from the wall you stand, the greater the stretch will be.

GENERAL CARE OF THE KNEE

ANATOMY   The knee is a *hinge joint* that connects the thigh bone (femur) and the lower leg bone (tibia). The knee cap (patella) sits in front of the joint, embedded in the large quadriceps tendon, providing protection and additional leverage to the quadriceps muscle. The hardest bone in the body (femur), the body's thickest and strongest tendon (quadriceps), and the body's largest and strongest muscle (quadriceps) require the greatest amount of lubrication. Surrounding the quadriceps mechanism are five large lubricating sacs. The knee joint is supported by the hinge ligaments (collateral ligaments), the crossing ligaments in the center of the joint (cruciates), and the large thigh muscles (quadriceps and hamstrings). The bones are covered with a thick layer of cartilage (articular cartilage) and are protected from the ravages of repetitive impact by the "shock-absorber cartilages" (meniscal, or football, cartilages).

In summary, the knee comprises the following parts:

Three joint compartments—the inner (medial), outer (lateral), and knee cap

Two major muscle groups—the quadriceps (front of the thigh) and hamstrings

Two hinge ligaments—the inner (medial collateral) and outer (lateral collateral)

Five lubricating bursal sacs—the prepatellar, infrapatellar, suprapatellar, anserine, and Baker's cyst

Two shock-absorber cartilages—the inner (medial) and outer (lateral) meniscus

CONDITIONS   Any part of the knee can wear out, experience injury, or become inflamed by overuse. Injury and irritation of the undersurface of the knee cap (painful knee caps) and wear-and-tear arthritis (degenerative arthritis) are the most common problems, accounting for nearly two thirds of all complaints. Twisting injuries most

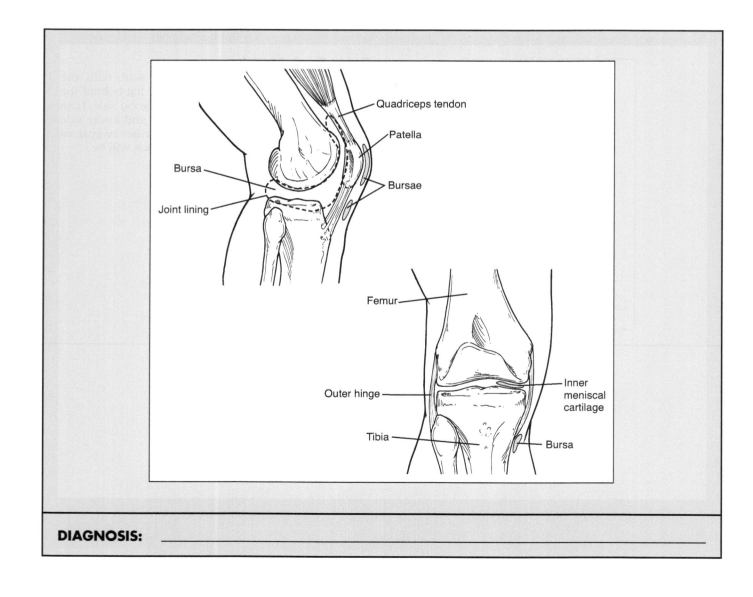

DIAGNOSIS: _____

often injure the inner hinge ligament and, less commonly, the inner meniscal cartilage. Any of the conditions that affect the joint can cause "water on the knee," the knee's response to injury.

PHYSICAL THERAPY   Physical therapy plays a vital role in the treatment of the variety of conditions that affect the knee and its supporting structures, and it is especially important in the rehabilitation of an injured knee. Specific exercises are fundamental to improving knee support and stability.

Ice is useful to control pain and swelling. Cold is applied for 15 to 20 minutes every 2 to 4 hours. A bag of ice, a bag of frozen corn, or an iced towel cooled in the freezer works well.

Ice and elevation are indicated for an acutely swollen knee. The knee should be kept above the level of the heart.

Rehabilitation of the knee begins with gentle toning exercises. *Straight-leg-raising* and *leg-extension* exercises are used to strengthen the quadriceps and hamstring muscles, to provide support to the joint, and to counteract the giving-out sensation caused by disuse or weakened ligaments. Begin with sets of 10 leg lifts and gradually work up to 20 to 25 lifts, each held 5 seconds. At first, these are performed without weight, but with improvement, weight is added to the ankle. Start with a 2-lb weight (e.g., a heavy shoe, fishing weights or coins in a sock, a purse with a large book in it) and gradually increase to a weight of 5 to 10 lb. Twisting and rotating the leg must be avoided. To secure the leg in the straight position, cock the ankle up.

If the straight-leg-raising exercises do not cause any aggravation of the underlying condition, weighted leg lifts with bended knee can be started. Initially, these should be performed at 30 degrees, using the same amount of weight and number of repetitions used with the straight-leg raises. The amount of bending is increased gradually as tolerated, in increments of 30 to 45 to 60 to 90 degrees of bending.

Activity limitations, proper exercises, and proper exercise equipment involve limiting exposure to repetitive impact, jarring, and bending (depending on the severity of the knee condition). Ideally, activities and exercises should maximize the toning of the thigh muscles, provide smooth motion to the knee, minimize impact, and emphasize the least amount of bending to accomplish the muscle toning.

Activity Limitations   The following positions and activities place excessive pressure on the knee joint and must be limited until the pain and swelling resolve:

- Squatting
- Kneeling
- Twisting and pivoting
- Repetitive bending (e.g., stairs, getting out of a seated position, clutch and pedal pushing)
- Jogging

KNEE-STRENGTHENING EXERCISES

Nearly all conditions that affect the knee cause loss of tone in the thigh muscles (quadriceps and hamstrings). The strength of these muscles must be restored to restore knee stability.

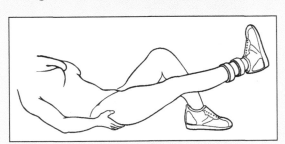

Straight-Leg Raises
While sitting on the edge of a chair or while lying down with the opposite leg bent, the leg is raised 3 to 4 inches off the ground. Sets of 15 to 20 leg raises (each held for 5 seconds) are performed daily. Bending the knee should be avoided. After 2 to 4 weeks, the exercises are performed with a 5- to 10-lb weight placed at the ankle (e.g., a sock with fishing weights, an old purse with a large book in it, Velcro ankle weights).

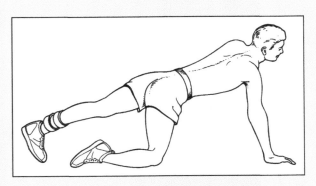

Leg Extensions
While lying on the stomach or while up on all fours, the leg is raised, perfectly straight, 3 to 4 inches off the ground. Sets of 15 to 20 extensions (each held 5 seconds) are performed daily. After 2 to 4 weeks, the exercise is performed with a 5- to 10-lb weight added to the ankle. *Note:* This exercise must be performed while lying flat if the kneecap is the source of knee irritation.

- Aerobic dance
- Playing stop-and-go sports (basketball and sports that require the use of rackets)
- Swimming using the frog or whip kick
- Bicycling

Equipment Limitations   The following types of exercise equipment place excessive pressure on the knee joint and must be limited until the pain and swelling resolve:

- Stair-stepper
- Stationary bicycle
- Rowing machine
- Universal gym using leg extensions

Acceptable Activities   The following activities place much less tension on the knee by limiting impact and repetitive bending:

- Fast walking
- Water aerobics

- Swimming, using the crawl stroke
- Cross-country ski glide machines
- Soft-platform treadmill
- Trampoline

Weight loss is always an important issue in retarding and preventing future problems of the knee.

PHYSICAL THERAPY SUMMARY

1. Direct applications of ice to the front and sides of the joint
2. Elevation to assist in the reabsorption of knee fluid
3. Toning exercises of the quadriceps and hamstring muscles to provide muscular support
4. Activity limitations
5. Exercises and exercise equipment that minimize repetitive impact and bending

GENERAL CARE OF THE ANKLE

ANATOMY   The ankle is a *hinge joint* that allows flexing up and down, but also allows the foot to turn in and out. It is held together by a network of ligaments along the sides of the joint (the "hinges") and is supported by four major tendons. To function normally, the ankle must be aligned properly with the lower leg, must have intact and strong ligaments, and must have flexible and well-toned tendons. The ankle comprises the following elements:

Two joint compartments—the main hinge joint (tibial-talar) and the swivel joint (subtalar)
Four major tendons—the Achilles (back), tibialis (inner), peroneus (outer), extensors (front)
Two hinge ligaments—the medial (inner) and lateral (outer)
Two lubricating bursal sacs—the heel bursa (pre-Achilles) and the ankle bursa (retrocalcaneal)
One thick arch ligament—the plantar fascia

CONDITIONS   The most common condition to affect the ankle is the common ankle sprain, which causes pain along the outer ankle joint. Twisting injuries and a violent turning of the ankle inward cause the supporting ligaments to split, partially separate, or completely tear. Pain below the ankle (heel pain) is often an inflammation of the origin of the arch ligament (plantar fasciitis). This inflammation often is associated with weak ankles (pronation) or loss of the strength of the arch (flat feet). Tendinitis at the ankle most commonly affects the Achilles tendon located behind the ankle. Arthritis almost always is caused by a previous injury (e.g., fracture, severe ankle sprain). Bursitis at the ankle is uncommon.

PHYSICAL THERAPY   Physical therapy does not play an active role in the treatment of acute ankle conditions. Stretching and toning exercises are vital, however, in the recovery, rehabilitation, and prevention of ankle conditions.

Ice is useful for the temporary control of pain and swelling of acute sprains, tendinitis, and the occasional case of ankle arthritis. Ice is applied for 15 to 20 minutes every 2 to 4 hours. A bag of ice, a bag of frozen corn, or an iced towel cooled in the freezer works well.

Heat commonly is recommended for recurrent or chronic ankle conditions that require stretching and toning

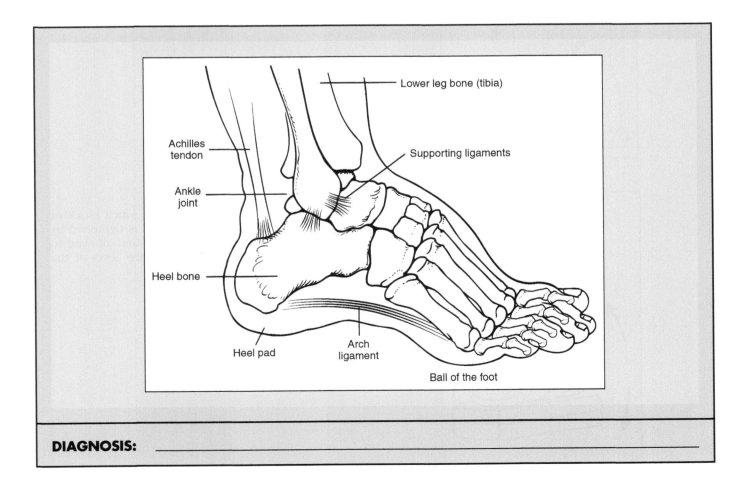

DIAGNOSIS: _____

exercises. Heating provides additional blood flow and facilitates stretching.

Stretching exercises commonly are used to treat and rehabilitate Achilles tendinitis and the inflammation of the arch ligament. These exercises always should be preceded by heating for 10 to 15 minutes. Stretching exercises should be carried out over many weeks to avoid aggravating the underlying condition. Successful stretching should improve gradually over weeks.

Isometric toning exercises are the most important means of improving ankle stability that has been weakened by disuse or injury. Large rubber tubing, a TheraBand, or large rubber bands are used to build up the tone and tension gradually in the lower leg muscles. Each direction of ankle motion (bending up and down and turning in and out) is toned individually. As the stability of the ankle improves, the ankle braces can be gradually withdrawn.

ACHILLES TENDON–STRETCHING EXERCISES

Rehabilitation for Achilles tendinitis involves a long period of protection and gradual stretching exercises. Four weeks after the swelling and inflammation have resolved, the tendon is gradually stretched. The ankles are heated in water for 15 to 20 minutes. For the first 5 to 7 days, the ankle is pulled up by hand in sets of 20. With progress, the following two active exercises are performed.

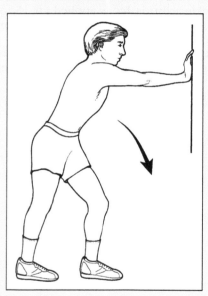

Wall Stretch
Face the wall and place your outstretched arms on the surface. Keep the affected leg in back. Partially flex the unaffected leg. While keeping the affected foot flat on the ground, gently lean forward. A pulling sensation should be felt in the calf, below the knee. Keep all of your body weight on the front leg.

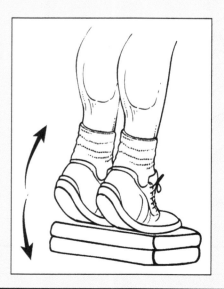

Toe-ups
The balls of the feet are placed on a 3-inch block or on the edge of the stairs. The muscle is tightened by tiptoeing. Then the muscle is relaxed and allowed to stretch when the heel drops below the level of the block. Do sets of 20 exercises.

Activity Limitations   The following activities place too much tension across the supporting ligaments and tendons of the ankle:

- Running and jogging
- Playing stop-and-go sports (racketball, tennis, basketball)
- Doing aerobics
- Jumping on a trampoline
- Using a stair-stepper
- Stair climbing with the ball of the foot
- Using pedals repetitively (e.g., a clutch, heavy equipment)

PHYSICAL THERAPY SUMMARY

1. Direct applications of ice to the front and sides of the joint
2. Heating before the stretching exercises
3. Stretching exercises of the ankle joint and the Achilles tendon
4. Toning exercises of the outer ankle tendons
5. Activity limitations
6. Exercises and exercise equipment that minimize repetitive impact and bending

ANKLE ISOMETRIC TONING EXERCISES

Isometric toning exercises of the ankle tendons are indicated for strengthening and stabilizing the ankle after disuse, injury, or immobilization. Large rubber tubing, a bungee cord, or large rubber bands are used to tone the lower leg muscles. Heating and stretching are performed before toning.

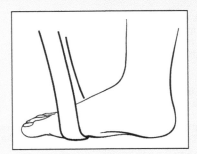

Achilles Tendon Toning
The rubber tubing is placed under the ball of the foot. The ankle is held steady at 90 degrees (a right angle). The rubber tubing is pulled up by hand pressure and held for 5 seconds. Sets of 20 are performed daily.

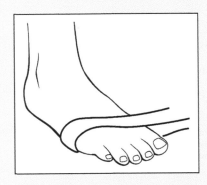

Peroneus Tendon Toning
The rubber tubing is placed around the outside of each foot, next to the little toes. The ankle is held steady at 90 degrees (a right angle). The legs are moved apart 2 to 3 inches while holding the ankle firm for 5 seconds. Sets of 20 are performed daily.

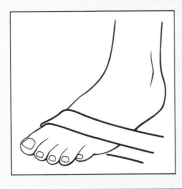

Posterior Tibialis Toning
The rubber tubing is placed around the inside of the foot next to the great toe and secured to a fixed object. The ankle is held steady at a 90-degree angle as the leg is pulled in toward the other. Sets of 20 (each held for 5 seconds) are performed daily.

FRACTURES THAT REQUIRE REFERRAL TO A SURGICAL ORTHOPEDIST

FRACTURE/DISLOCATION	REASON FOR ORTHOPEDIC REFERRAL
All compound fractures	Risk of infection and soft-tissue injury
Nearly all comminuted fractures	Unstable; risk of nonunion
Most intra-articular fractures	Risk of arthritis and poor joint function
Most spiral shaft fractures	Unstable; risk of shortening
Most displaced fractures	Unstable; risk of nonunion

Shoulder and Upper Arm

Clavicle	
Associated with rib fracture	Risk of lung or great vessel damage
Distal third associated with displacement	Risk of nonunion
Humerus	
Transverse shaft fusion	Risk of nonunion
Neck fracture with shoulder dislocation	Unstable; risk of arthritis
Fragment displacement >1 cm or angulation >45 degrees	Unstable
Supracondylar fracture with displacement	Risk of arthritis; brachial artery or median nerve injury

Elbow and Forearm

Displaced radial head fracture	Unstable
Displaced fracture of radius or ulna	Unstable; risk of compartment syndrome

Wrist

Displaced or intra-articular distal radius fracture	Unstable; risk of arthritis
Radius foreshortened by 5 mm or angulation	Risk of arthritis >20 degrees
Navicular fracture	Risk of avascular necrosis or nonunion
Perilunate dislocation	Referral for primary repair or fusion

Thumb

Gamekeeper's thumb, complete tear	Risk of poor function
Intra-articular metacarpal fracture of the thumb—Bennett fracture and Rolando fracture	Unstable; risk of arthritis
Dorsal dislocation of the metacarpal joint of the thumb	Single attempt at closed reduction; surgical referral if unsuccessful
Transverse fracture at the base or neck, spiral oblique, comminuted, and condylar fracture (intra-articular)	Unstable; risk of poor function and abnormal alignment

Hand

Metacarpal fracture (except the fifth)	Unstable
Boxer's fracture of the fifth metacarpal with angulation	Unstable; referral for pin fixation >40 degrees
Volar dislocation of the metacarpophalangeal joints with avulsion fragment >2-3 mm	Unstable; risk of arthritis
Volar subluxation of the distal interphalangeal joint >2-3 mm displacement, or involvement of >30% of the articular surface	Referral for primary repair
Rupture of the flexor digitorum profundus	Referral for primary repair tendon

Pelvis and Hip Joint

Pelvic/acetabular fracture	Multiple injuries; unstable; traction
Hip fracture	Unstable; internal fixation
Fracture of the femur	Unstable; traction; internal fixation

Knee

Supracondylar fracture	Unstable; internal fixation
Tibial plateau depressed >6-8 mm	Unstable; risk of arthritis; internal fixation
Rim fracture >10 degrees	Internal fixation
Bicondylar fracture	Skeletal traction; cast brace; internal fixation
Tibial spines	Molded long-leg cast for 4-6 weeks
Subcondylar fracture	Molded long-leg cast for 4-6 weeks
Patellar, displaced or comminuted	Cerclage or patellectomy
Osteochondritis dissecans, symptomatic with locking	Arthroscopy
Tibial and fibular fracture	Unstable; internal fixation

Ankle

Unstable bimalleolar fracture	Risk of arthritis; internal fixation
Trimalleolar fracture	Risk of arthritis; internal fixation
Fracture at or above the syndesmosis	Unstable; risk of arthritis
Displaced ankle fragments	Unstable; risk of arthritis

Continued

FRACTURES THAT REQUIRE REFERRAL TO A SURGICAL ORTHOPEDIST *(Continued)*

FRACTURE/DISLOCATION	**REASON FOR ORTHOPEDIC REFERRAL**
Calcaneus	
Intra-articular fracture	Risk of arthritis
Displaced posterior process fracture	Restore the integrity of the Achilles tendon
Nonunion of the anterior process	Internal fixation
Talus	
Displaced neck fracture	Risk of avascular necrosis
Navicular	
All displaced fractures	Unstable
Foot	
Neuropathic fracture	Risk of nonunion or malunion
Transverse fifth metatarsal fracture	Risk of nonunion or malunion
Displaced or comminuted proximal phalangeal fracture	Risk of nonunion or malunion

GLUCOSAMINE SULFATE AND CHONDROITIN

Cartilage is composed of chondrocytes sparsely spread through a matrix consisting of collagen, proteoglycans, inorganic salts, and water. The size and shape of cartilage are determined by the type II collagen that forms the fiber network. The proteoglycans and the glycoproteins determine the compressive properties of cartilage.

Glucosamine is a constituent of the glycosaminoglycans that combine to form hyaluronic acid and is altered to form the major organic constituent of the matrix—the proteoglycan molecule. These large polysaccharide molecules are composed of a hyaluronic acid backbone with chondroitin sulfate and keratin sulfate side chains. Glucosamine sulfate—the first over-the-counter disease-modifying medication—has been shown to retard the progression of osteoarthritis. Two randomized, placebo-controlled, double-blinded studies (Lancet 357:251–256, 2001; Arch Intern Med 162:2113–2123, 2002) have shown the ability of a daily dosage of 1500 mg of glucosamine sulfate to delay the progression of knee osteoarthritis. The Czech Republic study published in the *Archives of Internal Medicine* measured mid-tibiofemoral joint medial compartment widths on standing anteroposterior weightbearing radiographs of the knee in patients taking placebo and patients taking 1500 mg of glucosamine sulfate. Patients taking placebo lost 0.19 mm (190 µ) over 3 years. Patients treated with 1500 mg of glucosamine sulfate in a single daily dose experienced no average change. Similarly, patients taking placebo in the Belgium study published in *Lancet* lost 0.31 mm (310 µ) of articular cartilage width over 3 years. Patients treated with 1500 mg of glucosamine sulfate once a day had an insignificant loss of 0.06 mm on average. These two studies determined the natural rate of wear of articular cartilage in patients with mild to moderate knee osteoarthritis, averaging 1 mm every 8 to 16 years or 60 to 120 µ per year. The results of these studies also suggest that glucosamine sulfate taken every day can retard the natural progression of arthritis of the knee.

NONSTEROIDAL ANTI-INFLAMMATORY DRUGS

The effectiveness of oral nonsteroidal anti-inflammatory drugs (NSAIDs) in controlling the body's inflammatory response to irritation and injury depends on (1) the length of time of administration, (2) the penetration of the drug into the joint or inflamed tissue, and (3) the degree of local inflammation. To maximize the clinical response, these medications must be taken in full dose for a minimum of 10 to 14 days. The anti-inflammatory effect peaks at 7 to 10 days, as opposed to the analgesic or antipyretic effect, which occurs within 24 to 48 hours. If the inflammatory signs and symptoms have abated, the dose should be tapered gradually over the ensuing 1 to 2 weeks. In general, the inflammatory response must be suppressed for 3 to 4 weeks to allow the body to repair the injured joint or soft tissue.

Tissue penetration is the second most important factor determining the effectiveness of NSAIDs and the likely explanation of why conditions affecting the large joints have a much more predictable response to these drugs than conditions affecting the medium and small joints. Conditions that affect the shoulder, hip, and knee, such as rotator cuff tendinitis, trochanteric bursitis of the hip, and osteoarthritis of the knee, commonly respond to NSAIDs.

By contrast, lateral epicondylitis, trigger finger, and plantar fasciitis, conditions affecting the medium and small joints of the body, respond poorly. For this reason, the conditions affecting the wrist, hands, ankles, and feet are best treated with immobilization, local injection, or both rather than NSAIDs.

Not all conditions affecting the skeleton develop a measurable inflammatory response. Bony fractures rarely develop significant inflammation. Certain musculoskeletal conditions are purely mechanical in nature with little secondary inflammation, such as meniscal tear of the knee or the reactive muscle spasm of the neck and low back strain. This is not to say these drugs should not be used at all for these conditions. NSAIDs provide good pain control and are an excellent substitute for narcotic analgesics.

NSAIDs are contraindicated in patients diagnosed with active ulcer disease, uncontrolled reflux, bleeding disorders, or active renal disease; patients treated with warfarin (Coumadin); and patients who have had allergic reactions to the drugs. NSAIDs must be used with caution in diabetics with renal disease, patients with poorly controlled blood pressure, and patients with advanced congestive heart failure.

NONSTEROIDAL ANTI-INFLAMMATORY DRUGS

GENERIC NAME	TRADE NAME	DOSE (MG) (MAXIMUM DAILY)	COST PER 100 ($)
Acetaminophen	Tylenol	1000 (4 g)	3-5
Salicylates			
Acetylsalicylic acid*	Anacin, Ascriptin, Bufferin, Ecotrin	325, 500 (5-6 g)	4-5
Choline/magnesium*	Trilisate	0.5 g, 0.75 g, 1 g (3 g)	80-100
Diflunisal*	Dolobid	250, 500 (1500)	95-117
Salsalate*	Disalcid, Salsalate	500, 750 (3000)	25-30
Fenamates			
Meclofenamate*	Meclomen	50, 100 (400)	35-45
Oxicams			
Piroxicam	Feldene	10, 20 (20)	54-60
Pyrrolopyrrole			
Ketorolac	Toradol	15, 30, 60 (120-150)	117-120
Propionic Acids			
Fenoprofen calcium*	Nalfon	200, 300, 600 (3200)	57-87
Flurbiprofen*	Ansaid	50, 100 (300)	83-124
Ibuprofen*	Advil, Motrin, Nuprin, Rufen	200, 400, 600, 800 (3000)	15-18
Ketoprofen*	Orudis	25, 50, 75 (300)	90-120
Naproxen*	Naprosyn	250, 375, 500 (1500)	35-45
Naproxen sodium	Anaprox	275, 550 (1650)	100-141
Acetic Acids			
Diclofenac sodium*	Voltaren	25, 50, 75 (200)	54-116
Indomethacin*	Indomethacin	25, 50, 75 sustained release (200)	20-32
Nabumetone*	Relafen	500, 750 (2000)	99-120
Sulindac*	Clinoril	150, 200 (400)	35-45
Tolmetin*	Tolectin	200, 400 (1800)	22-61
Pyranocarboxylic Acid			
Etodolac	Lodine	200, 300 (1200)	73-84

NONSTEROIDAL ANTI-INFLAMMATORY DRUGS (continued)

GENERIC NAME	TRADE NAME	DOSE (MG) (MAXIMUM DAILY)	COST PER 100 ($)
COX-2 Inhibitors			
Celecoxib	Celebrex	100, 200 (200)	198-316
Rofecoxib	Vioxx	12.5, 25 (50)	250-331
Valdecoxib	Bextra	10	300-360

*The older NSAIDs are generally available only in generic form.

CORTICOSTEROIDS

TRADE NAME (ABBR) (GENERIC)	STRENGTH (MG/ML)	EQUIVALENT MG OF HYDROCORTISONE
Short-Acting Preparations (Soluble)		
Hydrocortisone (H) (hydrocortone phosphate)	25, 50	25, 50
Hydeltrasol (H20) (prednisolone)	20	80
Long-Acting Preparations (Depot or Time Released)		
Kenalog (K40) (triamcinolone acetonide)	40	200
Aristospan (A20) (triamcinolone hexacetonide)	20	100
Depo-Medrol (D80) (methylprednisolone acetate)	20, 40, 80	100-300
Decadron (Dex8) (dexamethasone phosphate)	4, 8	100, 200
Hydeltra T.B.A. (HTBA) (prednisolone tebutate)	20	80
Combination Preparations (Soluble and Depot)		
Celestone Soluspan (C6) (Betamethasone)	6	150

CALCIUM SUPPLEMENTATION

FOOD/SUPPLEMENT	AMOUNT	CALCIUM CONTENT (MG)	YEARLY COST ($)
Foods			
Milk (nonfat)	1 cup	290-300	200
Yogurt	1 cup	240-400	950
Cheese slice	1 oz	160-260	260
Cottage cheese	1/2 cup	80-100	960
Broccoli	1 cup	160-180	2000
Tofu	4 oz	145-155	1500
Salmon, canned	3 oz	170-200	3700
Supplements			
Calcium carbonate			
Oyster shell (generic)	625, 1250, 1500 mg	250, 500, 600	40
Os-Cal	625, 1250 mg	250, 500	108
Os-Cal + D	625, 1250 mg	250, 500	107
Tum-Ex	750 mg	300	55
Calcium-rich Rolaids	550 mg	220	53
Caltrate	1500 mg	600	108
Caltrate + D (125 IU)	1500 mg	600	108
Calcium phosphate			
Posture	1565 mg	600	115
Posture D (125 IU)	1565 mg	600	115
Calcium lactate	650 mg	85	350
Calcium gluconate	975 mg	90	522
Calcium citrate			
Citracal 950	950 mg	200	162
Citracal 1500 + D (200 IU)	1500 mg	315	162

LABORATORY TESTS IN RHEUMATOLOGY

RHEUMATOID FACTOR

"The most significant laboratory abnormality in rheumatoid arthritis"

Antibodies to the Fc portion of IgG

May take 6 months to become positive (it is *insensitive* as a "screening test")

75% to 80% of adults with rheumatoid arthritis have significant titers (i.e., >1:160), and 20% to 25% are "seronegative"; only 20% of children with juvenile rheumatoid arthritis are "seropositive"; seropositivity correlates with HLA-DR4 haplotype

IgM rheumatoid factor is most common

High titers are associated with more severe disease, active joint disease, presence of nodules, and poorer prognosis

IgG rheumatoid factor is associated with more severe disease

IgA rheumatoid factor is associated with bony erosions

Positive rheumatoid factor can occur in normal individuals and patients with tuberculosis, bacterial endocarditis, syphilis, pulmonary fibrosis, chronic active hepatitis, infectious hepatitis, Sjögren's syndrome, systemic lupus erythematosus (SLE), progressive systemic sclerosis, and polymyositis (i.e., there are many false positives)

CRYSTALS

Best identified using a polarizing microscope

Monosodium urate crystals—needle-shaped, negatively birefringent, gout

Calcium pyrophosphate dihydrate crystals—polygonal shaped, positive birefringent, pseudogout

Calcium hydroxyapatite crystals—glossy globules that stain with alizarin red S stain on light microscopy, electron microscopy for specific chemical content, calcium hydroxyapatite crystal deposition disease

ANTINUCLEAR ANTIBODIES

ANA

Homogeneous—reacts against deoxynucleoprotein and histone DNA; the *most common* pattern of ANA; least specific for SLE (many false positives)

Rimmed or membranous—reacts against double stranded DNA and native DNA; uncommon; far more specific for SLE than homogeneous

Speckled—reacts against ENAs (extractable nuclear antigens); 30% of patients with SLE

Nucleolar—reacts against RNP (ribonucleoprotein); unusual pattern; more suggestive of progressive systemic sclerosis than of SLE

Centromeric—reacts against topoisomerase I; two thirds of CREST syndrome

DNA

Anti-DNA—reacts against double-stranded DNA; diagnostic of SLE; correlates with disease activity in most patients

ENA

Anti-RNP—reacts against antigen susceptible to RNase digestion; 50% of SLE patients and all patients with mixed connective tissue disease

Anti-Sm—also called anti-Smith; the only ENA that is specific for SLE; only15% to 30% of SLE (low sensitivity)

Anti-Ro—also called anti-SSA; reacts against RNA-protein antigen; 25% to 40% of SLE patients; 70% of Sjögren's syndrome patients

Anti-La—also called anti-SSB; reacts against RNA-protein antigen; 10% to 15% of SLE patients; 50% of Sjögren's syndrome patients

Interpretation

The testing for autoantibodies (ANA testing) should *not* be used as a screen for rheumatic disease. The ANA test should be used to confirm the clinical diagnosis of a patient with symptoms compatible with SLE.

Positive ANA: consider the clinical setting; titers <1:160 with few clinical criteria for SLE are probably false positives. Moderate titers >1:320 to1:5120 warrant further evaluation (a high titer is >1:5120); moderate or high titers warrant anti-DNA and anti-ENA testing for confirmation of SLE or other rheumatic conditions

Positive ANA from drugs: often a homogeneous pattern; procainamide, hydralazine, and isoniazid

Positive ANAs and diseases: common in patients >50 years old with chronic inflammatory conditions, such as chronic active hepatitis, chronic pulmonary fibrosis, chronic infections, and malignancy, particularly lymphoma; usually titers are <1:640

Positive ANA with age: 5% to 10% of 50-year-olds have positive ANAs; 20% of 70-year-olds have a positive ANA

CLINICAL CRITERIA FOR SYSTEMIC LUPUS ERYTHEMATOSUS

Malar rash; discoid rash; photosensitivity; oral ulcers; arthritis; serositis; renal disease of proteinuria and cellular casts; neurologic disorders of seizures or psychosis; hematologic disorders of hemolytic anemia or leukopenia or lymphopenia or thrombocytopenia; positive lupus erythematosus preparation, anti-DNA, anti-SM, or false-positive Venereal Disease Research Laboratory; and positive ANA

SYNOVIAL FLUID ANALYSIS

	NORMAL SYNOVIAL FLUID	NONINFLAMMATORY FLUID (GROUP I)	INFLAMMATORY FLUID (GROUP II)	INFECTIOUS FLUID (GROUP III)
Appearance	Clear	Clear or slightly turbid, bloody	Turbid	Very turbid
Color	Colorless or slightly yellow	Yellow	Yellow-white	White-yellow
Viscosity	Normal	Decreased	Decreased	Decreased
Total WBC per mm³	>200	<2500	2500-25,000	>50,000
Differential % PMLs	7	13-20	50-70	90
Blood versus Fluid Glucose Difference (mg/dL)	0	5	0-30	70-90
Clinical Examples		Osteoarthritis, patellofemoral syndrome, mechanical derangement, SLE, hyperparathyroidism	Rheumatoid arthritis, pseudogout, gout, Reiter's syndrome, gonococcus, rheumatic fever, tuberculosis, SLE	Septic arthritis, tuberculosis

PMLs, polymorphonuclear leukocytes; SLE, systemic lupus erythematosus; WBC, white blood cells.

GENERAL

Anderson BC. Stretching. Bolinas, Calif, Shelter Publications, 1980.

Cyriax J. Textbook of Orthopedic Medicine, 8th ed. London, Baillière Tindall, 1982.

Ellis RM, Hollingworth GR, MacCollum MS. Comparison of injection techniques for shoulder pain: results of a double-blind, randomized study. BMJ 287:1339-1341, 1983.

Gray RG, Tenebaum J, Gottlieb NL. Local corticosteroid injection treatment in rheumatic disorders. Semin Arthritis Rheum 10:231-253, 1981.

Hill JJ, Trapp RG, Colliver JA. Survey on the use of corticosteroid injections by orthopedists. Contemp Orthop 18:39-45, 1989.

Hollander JL, Brown EM, Jessar RA, Brown CY. Hydrocortisone and cortisone injection into arthritic joints: comparative effects of and use of hydrocortisone as a local antiarthritic agent. JAMA 147:1629-1631, 1951.

Hoppenfeld S. Physical Examination of the Spine and Extremities. New York, Appleton-Century-Crofts, 1976.

Lapidus PW, Guidotti FP. Local injections of hydrocortisone in 495 orthopedic patients. Industr Med Surg 26:234-244, 1957.

Rockwood CA, Green DP, Bucholz RW. Fractures, 3rd ed. Philadelphia, JB Lippincott, 1991.

Scott DB. Techniques of Regional Anesthesia. Norwalk, Conn, Appleton & Lange, 1989.

Simon RR, Koenigsknecht SJ, Stevens C. Emergency Orthopedics, 2nd ed. East Norwalk, Conn, Appleton & Lange, 1987.

Sivananda Yoga Vedanta Center. Yoga Mind and Body. New York, Dorling Kindersley Publishing, 1996.

NECK

Cervical Strain

Frost FA, Jessen B, Siggaard-Andersen J. A controlled double-blind comparison of mepivacaine injection versus saline injection for myofascial pain. Lancet 1:499-500, 1980.

Goldenberg DL, Felson DT, Dinerman H. A randomized controlled trial of amitriptyline and Naprosyn in the treatment of patients with fibromyalgia. Arthritis Rheum 29:1371-1377, 1986.

Radanov BP, Sturzennegger M, Stefano GD. Long-term outcome after whiplash injury. Medicine 74:281-297, 1995.

Cervical Radiculopathy

Dillin W, Booth R, et al. Cervical radiculopathy: a review. Spine 11:988-991, 1986.

Honet JC, Puri K. Cervical radiculitis: treatment and results in 82 patients. Arch Phys Med Rehabil 57:12-16, 1976.

Kelly TR. Thoracic outlet syndrome: current concepts of treatment. Ann Surg 190:657-662, 1979.

Saal JS, Saal JA, Yurth EF. Nonoperative management of herniated cervical intervertebral disc with radiculopathy. Spine 21:1877-1883, 1996.

Tsairis P, Dyck PJ, Mulder DW. Natural history of brachial plexus neuropathy: report on 99 patients. Arch Neurol 27:109-117, 1972.

Greater Occipital Neuritis

Hecht JS. Occipital nerve block in postconcussive headaches: a retrospective review and report of ten cases. J Head Trauma Rehabil 19:58-71, 2004.

Inan N, Ceyhan A, Inan LK, et al. C2-C3 nerve blocks and greater occipital nerve block in cervicogenic headache treatment. Funct Neurol 16:239-243, 2001.

Mosser SW, Guyuron B, Janis JE, Rohrich RJ. The anatomy of the greater occipital nerve: implications for the etiology of migraine headaches. Plast Reconstr Surg 113:293-297, 2004.

Peres MF, Stiles MA, Siow HC, et al. Greater occipital nerve blockade for cluster headache. Cephalalgia 22:520-522, 2002.

Vijayan N. Greater occipital nerve blockade for cluster headache. Cephalalgia 23:323, 2003.

Ward JB. Greater occipital nerve block. Semin Neurol 23:59-62, 2003.

Temporomandibular Joint

Ahlqvist J, Legrell PE. A technique for the accurate administration of corticosteroids in the temporomandibular joint. Dentomaxillofac Radiol 22:211-213, 1993.

Alpaslan GH, Alpaslan C. Efficacy of temporomandibular joint arthrocentesis with and without injection of sodium hyaluronate in treatment of internal derangements. J Oral Maxillofac Surg 59:613-618, 2001.

Boering G. Temporomandibular Joint Arthrosis: An Analysis of 400 Cases. Leiden, Stafleu, 1996.

DeLeeuw R, Boering G, Stengenga B, et al. Clinical signs of TMJ osteoarthrosis and internal derangement 30 years after nonsurgical treatment. J Orofac Pain 8:18-24, 1994.

Dolwick MF. Temporomandibular disorders. *In* Koopman WJ (ed): Arthritis and Allied Conditions. Philadelphia, Lippincott Williams & Wilkins, 2001, pp 2019-2025.

Hepguler S, Akhoc YS, Pehlivan M, et al. The efficacy of intra-articular sodium hyaluronate in patients with reducing displaced disc of the temporomandibular joint. J Oral Rehabil 29:60-80, 2002.

Kopp S, Wenneberg B, Haraldson T, Carlsson GE. The short term effect of intra-articular injections of sodium hyaluronate and corticosteroid on the temporomandibular joint pain and dysfunction. J Oral Maxillofac Surg 43:429-435, 1985.

Nyberg J, Adell R, Svensson B. Temporomandibular joint discectomy for treatment of unilateral internal derangement—a 5 year follow-up evaluation. Int J Oral Maxillofac Surg 33:8-12, 2004.

Suarex OF, Ourique SA. An alternate technique for management of acute closed locks. Cranio 18:233-234, 2000.

Toller P. Use and misuse of intra-articular corticosteroids in treatment of temporomandibular joint pain. Proc R Soc Med 70:461–463, 1977.

Vallon D, Akerman S, Nilner M, Peterson A. Long-term follow-up of intra-articular injections into the temporomandibular joint in patients with rheumatoid arthritis. Swed Dent J 26:149–158, 2002.

Yura S, Totsuka Y, Yoshikawa T, Inoue N. Can arthrocentesis release intracapsular adhesions? Arthroscopic findings before and after irrigation under sufficient hydraulic pressure. J Oral Maxillofac Surg 61:1253–1256, 2003.

Fibromyalgia

Felson DT, Goldenberg DL. The natural history of fibromyalgia. Arthritis Rheum 29:1522–1526, 1986.

Simms RW, Goldenberg DL, Felson DT, et al. Tenderness in 75 anatomical sites: distinguishing fibromyalgia patients from controls. Arthritis Rheum 31:182–187, 1988.

Wolfe F. Fibromyalgia: the clinical syndrome. Rheum Dis Clin North Am 15:1–17, 1989.

SHOULDER

Anderson BC, Kaye S. Shoulder pain: Differential diagnosis. West J Med 138:268, 1983.

Chuang TY, Hunder GG, Ilstrup DM, et al. Polymyalgia rheumatica: a 10-year epidemiologic and clinical study. Ann Intern Med 97:672–680, 1982.

Codman EA. The Shoulder. Boston, Thomas Todd, 1934.

Fiddian NJ, King RJ. The winged scapula. Clin Orthop 185:228–236, 1984.

Impingement Syndrome

Brox JI, Staff PH, Ljunggren AE, Brevik JI. Arthroscopic surgery compared with supervised exercises in patients with rotator cuff disease (stage II impingement syndrome). BMJ 307:899–903, 1993.

Lozman PR, Hechtman KS, Uribe JW. Combined arthroscopic management of impingement syndrome and acromioclavicular joint arthritis. J South Orthop Assoc 4:177–181, 1995.

Neer CS II. Anterior acromioplasty for the chronic impingement syndrome in the shoulder: a preliminary report. J Bone Joint Surg Am 54A:41–50, 1972.

Neer CS. Impingement syndromes. Clin Orthop 173:70–77, 1983.

Neer CS. Anterior acromioplasty for the chronic impingement syndrome of the shoulder. J Bone Joint Surg Am 73A:707–715, 1991.

Rotator Cuff Tendinitis/Bursitis

Bosworth BM. Calcium deposits in the shoulder and subacromial bursitis: a survey of 12,222 shoulders. JAMA 116:2477–2482, 1941.

Chard MD, Sattelle MD, Hazleman BL. The long-term outcome of rotator cuff tendonitis: a review study. Br J Rheumatol 27:385–389, 1988.

Crisp EJ, Kendall PH. Treatment of periarthritis of the shoulder with hydrocortisone. BMJ 1:1500–1501, 1955.

Ellis RM, Hollingworth GR, MacCollum MS. Comparison of injection techniques for shoulder pain: results of a double-blind, randomized study. BMJ 287:1339–1341, 1983.

Fearnley M, Vadasz I. Factors influencing the response of lesions of the rotator cuff of the shoulder to local steroid injection. Ann Phys Med 10:53–63, 1969.

Petri M, Dobrow R, Neiman R, et al. Randomized, double-blind placebo-controlled study of the treatment of the painful shoulder. Arthritis Rheum 30:1040–1045, 1987.

Valtonen EJ. Double-acting betamethasone (Celestone Chronodose) in the treatment of supraspinatus tendonitis. J Intern Med 6:463–467, 1978.

White RH, Paull DM, Fleming KW. Rotator cuff tendonitis: comparison of subacromial injection of a long-acting corticosteroid versus oral indomethacin therapy. J Rheumatol 13:608–613, 1986.

Rotator Cuff Tendon Rupture

Ahovuo J, Paavolainen P, Slatis P. The diagnostic value of arthrography and plain radiography in rotator cuff tears. Acta Orthop Scand 55:220–223, 1984.

Codman EA, Akerson IV. The pathology associated with rupture of the supraspinatus tendon. Ann Surg 93:348–359, 1931.

Darlington LG, Coomes EN. The effects of local steroid injection for supraspinatus tears. Rheumatol Rehabil 16:172–179, 1977.

Samilson RL, Binder WF. Symptomatic full-thickness tears of the rotator cuff. Orthop Clin North Am 6:449–466, 1975.

Watson M. Major ruptures of the rotator cuff: the results of surgical repair in 89 patients. J Bone Joint Surg Br 67B:618–624, 1985.

Biceps Tendinitis/Tear

Mariani EM, Cofield RH, Askew LJ, et al. Rupture of the tendon of the long head of the biceps brachii: surgical versus nonsurgical treatment. Clin Orthop 228:233–239, 1988.

Soto-Hall R, Stroot JH. Treatment of ruptures of the long head of the biceps brachii. Am J Orthop 2:192–193, 1960.

Frozen Shoulder

Andren L, Lundbery BJ. Treatment of rigid shoulders by joint distension during arthrography. Acta Orthop Scand 36:45–53, 1965.

Bulgren DY, Binder AI, Hazleman BL, et al. Frozen shoulder: a prospective clinical study with an evaluation of three treatment regimens. Ann Rheumatol Dis 43:353–360, 1984.

Jacobs LGH, Barton MAJ, Wallace WA, et al. Intra-articular distension and steroids in the management of capsulitis of the shoulder. BMJ 302:1498–1501, 1991.

Rizk TE, Pinals RS. Frozen shoulder. Semin Arthritis Rheum 11:440–452, 1982.

Steinbocker O, Argyros TG. Frozen shoulder: treatment by

local injection of depot corticosteroids. Arch Phys Med Rehabil 55:209-212, 1974.

Weiss JJ. Arthrography-assisted intra-articular injection of steroids in treatment of adhesive capsulitis. Arch Phys Med Rehabil 59:285-287, 1978.

Acromioclavicular Disorders

Weinstein DM, McCann PD, McIlveen SJ, et al. Surgical treatment of complete acromioclavicular dislocations. Am J Sports Med 23:324-331, 1995.

ELBOW

Lateral Epicondylitis

Boyd HB, McLeod AC. Tennis elbow. J Bone Joint Surg Am 55A:1183-1197, 1973.

Day BH, Gavindasamy N. Corticosteroid injection in the treatment of tennis elbow. Pract Med 220:459-462, 1978.

Fillion PL. Treatment of lateral epicondylitis. Am J Occup Ther 45:340-343, 1991.

Nirschl RP, Pettrone FA. Tennis elbow: the surgical treatment of lateral epicondylitis. J Bone Joint Surg Am 61A:832-839, 1979.

Potter HG, Hannafin JA, Morsessel RM, et al. Lateral epicondylitis: correlation with MR imaging, surgical and histopathologic findings. Radiology 196:43-46, 1995.

Olecranon Bursitis

Hassell AB, Fowler PD, Dawes PT. Intra-bursal tetracycline in the treatment of olecranon bursitis in patients with rheumatoid arthritis. Br J Rheumatol 33:859-860, 1994.

Knight JM, Thomas JC, Maurer RC. Treatment of septic olecranon and prepatellar bursitis with percutaneous placement of a suction-irrigation system: a report of 12 cases. Clin Orthop 206:90-93, 1986.

Smith DL, McAfee JH, Lucas LM, et al. Treatment of nonseptic olecranon bursitis: a controlled blinded prospective trial. Arch Intern Med 149:2527-2530, 1989.

Weinstein PS, Canosos JJ. Long-term follow-up of corticosteroid injection for traumatic olecranon bursitis. Ann Rheum Dis 43:44-46, 1984.

Elbow Arthritis

Doherty M, Preston B. Primary osteoarthritis of the elbow. Ann Rheum Dis 48:743-747, 1989.

WRIST

Allan CH, Joshi A, Lichtman DM. Kienböck's disease: diagnosis and treatment. J Am Acad Orthop Surg 9:128-136, 2001.

Wrist Sprain

Adelaar RS. Traumatic wrist instabilities. Contemp Orthop 4:309-324, 1982.

Dorsal and Volar Wrist Ganglia

Angelides AC, Wallace PF. The dorsal ganglion of the wrist: its pathogenesis, gross and microscopic anatomy and surgical treatment. J Hand Surg 1:228-235, 1978.

Crock HV. Large ganglia occurring in tendons. Br J Surg 47:319-321, 1959.

Jacobs LGH, Govaers KJM. The volar wrist ganglion: just a simple cyst? J Hand Surg 15B:342-346, 1990.

Kozin SH, Urban MA, Bishop AT, Dobyns JH. Wrist ganglia: diagnosis and treatment of a bothersome problem. J Musculoskel Med 10:21-44, 1993.

Ogino T, Minami A, Fukada K, et al. The dorsal occult ganglion of the wrist and ultrasonography. J Bone Joint Surg Br 13B:181-183, 1988.

Richman JA, Gelberman RH, Engber WD, et al. Ganglions of the wrist and digits: results of treatment by aspiration and cyst wall puncture. J Hand Surg 123A:1041-1043, 1987.

Carpometacarpal Osteoarthritis

Berggren M, Joost-Davidsson A, Lindstrand J, et al. Reduction in the need for operation after conservative treatment of osteoarthritis of the first carpometacarpal joint: a seven year prospective study. Scand J Plast Reconstr Surg Hand Surg 35:415-417, 2001.

Damen A, Dijkstra T, van der Lei B, et al. Long-term results of arthrodesis of the carpometacarpal joint of the thumb. Scand J Plast Reconstr Surg Hand Surg 35:407-413, 2001.

Hartigan BJ, Stern PJ, Kiefhaber TR. Thumb carpometacarpal osteoarthritis: arthrodesis compared with ligament reconstruction and tendon interposition. J Bone Joint Surg Am 83A:1470-1478, 2001.

Kriegs-Au G, Petje G, Fojti E. Ligament reconstruction with or without tendon interposition to treat primary thumb carpometacarpal osteoarthritis: a prospective randomized study. J Bone Joint Surg Am 86A:209-218, 2004.

Sachle T, Sande S, Finsen V. Abductor pollicis longus tendon interposition for arthrosis in the first carpometacarpal joint: 55 thumbs reviewed after 3 (1-5) years. Acta Orthop Scand 73:674-677, 2002.

Schroder J, Kerkhoffs GM, Voerman HJ, Marti RK. Surgical treatment of basal joint disease of the thumb: comparison between resection-interposition arthroplasty and trapezio-metacarpal arthrodesis. Arch Orthop Trauma Surg 122:35-38, 2002.

Carpal Tunnel Syndrome

Armstrong T, Devor W, Borschel L, Contreras R. Intracarpal steroid injection is safe and effective for short-term management of carpal tunnel syndrome. Muscle Nerve 29:82-88, 2004.

Braun RM, Rechnic M, Fowler E. Complications related to carpal tunnel release. Hand Clin 18:347-357, 2002.

Demirci S, Kutluhan S, Koyuncuoglu HR, et al. Comparison of open carpal tunnel release and local steroid treatment outcomes in idiopathic carpal tunnel syndrome. Rheumatol Int 22:33-37, 2002.

Ellis J. Clinical results of a cross-over treatment with

pyridoxine and placebo of the carpal tunnel syndrome. Am J Clin Nutr 32:2040-2046, 1979.

Foster JB, Goodman HV. The effect of local corticosteroid injection on median nerve conduction in carpal tunnel syndrome. Ann Phys Med 6:287-294, 1962.

Gelberman RH, Aronson D, Weisman MH. Carpal-tunnel syndrome: results of a prospective trial of steroid injection and splinting. J Bone Joint Surg Am 62A:1181-1184, 1980.

Graham RG, Hudson DA, Solomons M, Singer M. A prospective study to assess the outcome of steroid injections and wrist splinting for the treatment of carpal tunnel syndrome. Plast Reconstr Surg 113:550-556, 2004.

Hagebeuk EE, de Weerd AW. Clinical and electrophysiological follow-up after local steroid injection in the carpal tunnel syndrome. Clin Neurophysiol 115:1464-1468, 2004.

Jimenez DF, Gibbs SR, Clapper AT. Endoscopic treatment of carpal tunnel syndrome: a critical review. Neurosurg Focus 3:e6, 1997.

MacDonald RI, Lichtman DM, Hanon JJ: Complications of surgical release of carpal tunnel syndrome. J Hand Surg 7:70-76, 1978.

Marshall S, Tardif G, Ashworth N. Local corticosteroid injection for carpal tunnel syndrome. Cochrane Database Syst Rev 4:CD001554, 2002.

Phalen GS. Carpal tunnel syndrome: 17 years of experience in diagnosis and treatment. J Bone Joint Surg Am 48A:211-228, 1966.

Phalen GS. The carpal tunnel syndrome: clinical evaluation of 598 hands. Clin Orthop 83:29, 1972.

Sevim S, Dogu O, Camdeviren H, et al. Long-term effectiveness of steroid injections and splinting in mild and moderate carpal tunnel syndrome. Neurol Sci 25:48-52, 2004.

Shapiro S. Microsurgical carpal tunnel release. Neurosurgery 37:66-70, 1995.

DeQuervain's Tenosynovitis

Anderson C, Manthey R, Brouns MC. Treatment of DeQuervain's tenosynovitis with corticosteroids. Arthritis Rheum 34:793-798, 1991.

Arons MS. De Quervain's release in working women: a report of failures, complications, and associated diagnoses. J Hand Surg 12:540-544, 1987.

Clark DD, Ricker JH, MacCollum MS. The efficacy of local steroid injection in the treatment of stenosing tenovaginitis. Plast Reconstr Surg 49:179-180, 1973.

Faithful DK, Lamb DW: De Quervain's disease: A clinical review. Hand 3:23-30, 1971.

Harvey FJ, Harvey PM, Horsly MW. DeQuervain's disease: surgical or nonsurgical treatment. J Hand Surg 15A:83-87, 1990.

Distal Radius Fractures

Cooney WP 3rd, Dobyns JH, Linscheld RI. Complications of Colles' fractures. J Bone Joint Surg Am 62A:613-619, 1980.

Dias JJ, Wray CC, Jones JM, Gregg PH. The value of early

mobilization in the treatment of Colles' fractures. J Bone Joint Surg Br 69B:463-467, 1987.

Ladd AL, Pliam NB. The role of bone graft and alternatives in unstable distal radius fracture treatment. Orthop Clin North Am 32:337-351, 2001.

Markiewitz AD, Gellman H. Five-pin external fixation and early range of motion for distal radius fractures. Orthop Clin North Am 32:329-335, 2001.

Ring D, Jupiter JB. Percutaneous and limited open fixation of fractures of the distal radius. Clin Orthop 375:105-115, 2000.

Simic PM, Weiland AJ. Fractures of the distal aspect of the radius: changes in treatment over the past two decades. J Bone Joint Surg Am 85A:552-564, 2003.

Navicular Fracture

Bhat M, McCarthy M, Davis TR, et al. MRI and plain radiography in the assessment of displaced fractures of the waist of the carpal scaphoid. J Bone Joint Surg Br 86B:705-713, 2004.

Bohler L, Trojan E, Jahna H. The results of treatment of 734 fresh, simple fractures of the scaphoid. J Hand Surg 28:319-331, 2003.

Magelvoort RW, Kon M, Schurman AH. Proximal row carpectomy: a worthwhile salvage procedure. Scand J Plast Reconstr Hand Surg 36:289-299, 2002.

McAdams TR, Spisak S, Beaulieu CF, Ladd AL. The effect of pronation and supination on the minimally displaced scaphoid fracture. Clin Orthop 411:255-259, 2003.

Merrell GA, Wikfe SW, Slade JF 3rd. Treatment of scaphoid nonunions: quantitative meta-analysis of the literature. J Hand Surg 27:685-691, 2002.

Saeden B, Tornkvist H, Ponzer S, Hoglund M. Fracture of the carpal scaphoid: a prospective, randomized 12-year follow-up comparing operative and conservative treatment. J Bone Joint Surg Br 83B:230-234, 2001.

Trumble TE, Salas P, Barthel T, et al. Management of scaphoid nonunions. J Am Acad Orthop Surg 12:33A, 2004.

HAND

General

Belsky MR, Feldon P, Millender LH, et al. Hand involvement in psoriatic arthritis. J Hand Surg 7:203-207, 1982.

Reginato AJ, Ferreiro JL, O'Connor CR, et al. Clinical and pathologic studies of twenty-six patients with penetrating foreign body injury to the joint, bursae, and tendon sheath. Arthritis Rheum 33:1753-1762, 1990.

Trigger Finger

Anderson BC, Kaye S. Treatment of flexor tenosynovitis of the hand ("trigger finger") with corticosteroids. Arch Intern Med 151:153-156, 1991.

Gray RG, Kiem IM, Gottlieb NL. Intratendon sheath corticosteroid treatment of rheumatoid arthritis-associated and idiopathic flexor tenosynovitis. Arthritis Rheum 21:92-96, 1978.

Lyu SR. Closed division of the flexor tendon sheath for trigger finger. J Bone Joint Surg Br 74:418-420, 1992.

Murphy D, Failla JM, Koniuch MP. Steroid versus placebo injection for trigger finger. J Hand Surg 20:628-631, 1995.

Stothard J, Kumar A. A safe percutaneous procedure for trigger finger release. J R Coll Surg 39:116-117, 1994.

Dupuytren's Contracture

Abe Y, Rokkaku T, Ofuchi S, et al. Dupuytren's disease on the radial aspect of the hand: report on 135 hands in Japanese patients. J Hand Surg 29:359-362, 2004.

Beltran JE, Jimeno-Urban F, Yunta A. The open palm and digital technique in the treatment of Dupuytren's contracture. Hand 8:73-77, 1976.

Beyermann K, Prommersberger KJ, Jacobs C, Lanz UB. Severe contracture of the proximal interphalangeal joint in Dupuytren's disease: does capsuloligamentous release improve outcome? J Hand Surg 29B:240-243, 2004.

Khan AA, Rider OJ, Jayadex CU, et al. The role of manual occupation in the aetiology of Dupuytren's disease in men in England and Wales. J Hand Surg 29:12-14, 2004.

Larsen S, Frederiksen H. Genetic and environmental influence in Dupuytren's disease among 6,105 males. J Hand Surg 28(Suppl 1):13, 2003.

Leclereq C, Fernandez H. Complications following fasciectomy with primary closure in Dupuytren's disease. J Hand Surg 28(Suppl 1):12, 2003.

Meek RM, McLellan S, Reilly J, Crossen JF. The effect of steroids on Dupuytren's disease: role of programmed cell death. J Hand Surg 27:270-273, 2002.

Rowley DI, Couch M, Chesney RB, Norris SH. Assessment of percutaneous fasciotomy in the management of Dupuytren's contracture. J Hand Surg 9B:163-164, 1984.

Skoff HD. The surgical treatment of Dupuytren's contracture: a synthesis of techniques. Plast Reconstr Surg 113:540-544, 2004.

Tonkin MA, Burke FD, Varian JPW. Dupuytren's contracture: a comparative study of fasciectomy and dermofasciectomy in one hundred patients. J Hand Surg [Br] 9:156-162, 1984.

Rheumatoid Arthritis

Arnett FC, Edworthy SM, Bloch DA, et al. The American Rheumatism Association 1987 revised criteria for the classification of rheumatoid arthritis. Arthritis Rheum 31:315-324, 1988.

Fehlauer SC, Carson CW, Cannon GW. Two year follow up of treatment of rheumatoid arthritis with methotrexate: clinical experience in 124 patients. J Rheumatol 16:307-312, 1989.

Fries JF, Spitz PW, Williams CA, et al. A toxicity for comparison of side effects among different drugs. Arthritis Rheum 31:121-130, 1990.

Goemaere S, Ackerman C, Goethals K, et al. Onset of symptoms of rheumatoid arthritis in relation to age, sex, and menopausal transition. J Rheumatol 17:1620-1622, 1990.

Kovarsky J. Intermediate-dose intramuscular methylprednisolone acetate in the treatment of rheumatic disease. Ann Rheumatol Dis 42:308-310, 1983.

Kushner O. Does aggressive therapy of rheumatoid arthritis affect outcome? J Rheumatol 16:1-5, 1989.

Schumacher HR. Palindromic onset of rheumatoid arthritis. Arthritis Rheum 31:519-525, 1992.

Steere AC. Lyme disease. N Engl J Med 321:586-596, 1989.

Steere AC, Bartenhagen NH, Craft JE, et al. The early clinical manifestations of Lyme disease. Ann Intern Med 99:76-82, 1983.

Weiss MM. Corticosteroids in rheumatoid arthritis. Semin Arthritis Rheum 19:9-21, 1989.

Williams HJ, Willkens RF, Samuelson CO Jr, et al. Comparison of low-dose oral pulse methotrexate and placebo in the treatment of rheumatoid arthritis. Arthritis Rheum 28:721-730, 1985.

Zuckner J, Uddin J, Ramsey RH. Intramuscular administration of steroids in treatment of rheumatoid arthritis. Ann Rheum Dis 23:456-462, 1964.

Complex Regional Pain Syndrome (Reflex Sympathetic Dystrophy)

Adebajo A, Hazleman B. Shoulder pain and reflex sympathetic dystrophy. Curr Opin Rheumatol 2:270-275, 1990.

Christensen K, Jensen EM, Noer I. The reflex dystrophy syndrome response to treatment with systemic corticosteroids. Acta Chir Scand 148:653-655, 1982.

Crozier F, Champsaur P, Pham T, et al. Magnetic resonance imaging in reflex sympathetic dystrophy syndrome of the foot. Joint Bone Spine 70:503-508, 2003.

Grabow TS, Tella PK, Raja SN. Spinal cord stimulation for complex regional pain syndrome: an evidence-based medicine review of the literature. Clin J Pain 19:371-383, 2003.

Karacan I, Aydin T, Ozaras N. Bone loss in the contralateral asymptomatic hand in patients with complex regional pain syndrome type 1. J Bone Miner Metab 22:44-47, 2004.

Kemler MA, De Vet HX, Barendse GA, et al. The effect of spinal cord stimulation in patients with chronic reflex sympathetic dystrophy: two years' follow-up of the randomized controlled trial. Ann Neurol 55:13-18, 2004.

Kozin F, McCarty DJ, Dims J, Genant H. The reflex sympathetic dystrophy syndrome: I. clinical and histologic studies: evidence for bilaterality, response to corticosteroids and articular involvement. Am J Med 60:321-331, 1976.

Kozin F, Ryan LM, Carerra GF, et al. The reflex sympathetic dystrophy syndrome (RSDS): III. scintigraphic studies, further evidence for the therapeutic efficacy of systemic corticosteroids, and proposed diagnostic criteria. Am J Med 70:23-30, 1981.

Macinnon SE, Holden LE: The use of three-phase radionuclide bone scanning in the diagnosis of reflex sympathetic dystrophy syndrome. J Hand Surg 9A:556-563, 1984.

Mallis A, Furlan A. Sympathectomy for neuropathic pain. Cochrane Database Syst Rev 2:CD002918, 2003.

Sandroni P, Benrud-Larson LM, McClelland RL, Low PA. Complex regional pain syndrome type I: incidence and prevalence in Olmsted county, a population-based study. Pain 103:199-207, 2003.

Wasner G, Schattschneider J, Binder A, Baron R. Complex

regional pain syndrome—diagnostic, mechanisms, CNS involvement and therapy. Spinal Cord 41:61–75, 2003.

Zyluk A. Results of the treatment of posttraumatic reflex sympathetic dystrophy of the upper extremity with regional intravenous blocks of methylprednisolone and lidocaine. Acta Orthop Belg 64:452–456, 1998.

Zyluk A. Scoring system in the assessment of the clinical severity of reflex sympathetic dystrophy of the hand. Hand Clin 19:517–521, 2003.

CHEST WALL

Costochondritis

Kamel M, Kotob H. Ultrasonographic assessment of local steroid injection in Tietz's syndrome. Br J Rheumatol 36:547–550, 1997.

Mendelson G, Mendelson H, Horowitz SF, et al. Can (99m) technetium methylene diphosphonate bone scans objectively document costochondritis? Chest 111:1600–1602, 1997.

Wise CM, Semble L, Dalton CB. Musculoskeletal chest wall syndromes in patients with noncardiac chest pain, a study of 100 patients. Arch Phys Med Rehabil 72:147–149, 1992.

Sternoclavicular Arthritis

Benitez CL, Mintz DN, Potter HG. MR imaging of the sternoclavicular joint following trauma. Clin Imaging 28:59–63, 2004.

Ernberg LA, Potter HG. Radiographic evaluation of the acromioclavicular and sternoclavicular joints. Clin Sports Med 22:255–275, 2003.

Hiramuro-Shoji F, Wirth MA, Rockwood CA Jr. Atraumatic conditions of the sternoclavicular joint. J Shoulder Elbow Surg 12:79–88, 2003.

Noble JS. Degenerative sternoclavicular arthritis and hyperostosis. Clin Sports Med 22:407–422, 2003.

Pingsmann A, Patsalis T, Michiels I. Resection arthroplasty of the sternoclavicular joint for the treatment of primary degenerative sternoclavicular arthritis. J Bone Joint Surg 84:513–517, 2002.

Ross JJ, Shamsuddin H. Sternoclavicular septic arthritis: review of 180 cases. Medicine 83:139–148, 2004.

BACK

Carette S, Graham DC, Little HA, et al. The natural disease course of ankylosing spondylitis. Arthritis Rheum 26:186–190, 1983.

Khan MA, Khan MK. Diagnostic value of HLA-B27 testing in ankylosing spondylitis and Reiter's syndrome. Ann Intern Med 96:70–76, 1982.

Stroebel RJ, Ginsburg WW, McLeod RA. Sacral insufficiency fractures: an often unsuspected cause of low back pain. J Rheumatol 18:117–119, 1991.

Low Back Strain

Akinpelu AO, Adeyemi AI. Range of lumbar flexion in chronic low back pain. Cent Afr J Med 35:430–432, 1989.

Basmajian JV. Acute back pain and spasm: a controlled multicenter trial of combined analgesic and antispasm agents. Spine 14:438–439, 1989.

Benzon HT. Epidural steroid injections for low back pain and lumbosacral radiculopathy. Pain 24:277–295, 1986.

Bogduk N, Cherry D. Epidural corticosteroid agents for sciatica. Med J Aust 143:402–406, 1985.

Carette S, Marcoux S, Truchon R, et al. A controlled trial of corticosteroid injection into facet joints for chronic low back pain. N Engl J Med 325:1002–1007, 1991.

Cullen AP. Carisoprodol (Soma) in acute back conditions: a double-blind, randomized, placebo controlled study. Curr Ther Res 20:557–562, 1976.

Deyo RA, Diehl AK, Rosenthal M. How many days of bed rest for acute low back pain? A randomized clinical trial. N Engl J Med 315:1064–1070, 1986.

Deyo RA, Walsh NE, Martin DC, et al. A controlled trial of transcutaneous electrical nerve stimulation (TENS) and exercise for chronic low back pain. N Engl J Med 322:1627–1634, 1990.

Garvey RA, Marks MR, Wiesel SW. A prospective, randomized, double-blind evaluation of trigger-point injection therapy for low-back pain. Spine 14:962–964, 1989.

Jackson RP, Jacobs RR, Montesano PX. Facet joint injection in low back pain: a prospective statistical study. Spine 13:966–971, 1988.

Kepes ER, Duncalf D. Treatment of back ache with spinal injections of local anesthetics, spinal and systemic steroids: a review. Pain 22:33–47, 1985.

Macrai IF, Wright V. Measurement of back movement. Ann Rheum Dis 28:584–589, 1969.

Rollings HE, Glassman JM, Joyka JP. Management of acute musculoskeletal conditions—thoracolumbar strain or sprain: a double-blind evaluation comparing the efficacy and safety of carisoprodol with cyclobenzaprine hydrochloride. Curr Ther Res 34:917–928, 1983.

Vad VB, Bhat AL, Lutz GE, Cammisa F. Transforaminal epidural steroid injection in lumbosacral radiculopathy: a prospective randomized study. Spine 27:11–16, 2002.

Wang JC, Lin E, Brodke DS, Youssef JA. Epidural injections for the treatment of symptomatic lumbar discs. J Spinal Disord Tech 15:269–272, 2002.

Westbrook L, Cicala RJ, Wright H. Effectiveness of alprazolam in the treatment of chronic pain: results of a preliminary study. Clin J Pain 6:32–36, 1990.

Lumbosacral Disk Disease

Cucler JM, Bernini PA, Wiesel SW, et al. The use of epidural steroids in the treatment of lumbar radicular pain: a prospective, randomized, double blind study. J Bone Joint Surg Am 67A:63–66, 1985.

Wiesel SW, Tsourmas N, Feffer HL, et al. A study of computer-assisted tomography: 1. the incidence of positive CAT scans in an asymptomatic group of patients. Spine 9:549–551, 1984.

Cauda Equina

Kostuik JP, Harrington I, Alexander D, et al. Cauda equina syndrome and lumbar disc herniation. J Bone Joint Surg Am 68:386–391, 1986.

Tussous MW, Skerhut HE, Story JL, et al. Cauda equina syndrome of long-standing ankylosing spondylitis: case report and review of the literature. J Neurosurg 73:441–447, 1990.

Sacroiliac Disease

Ahlstrom H, Feltelius N, Nyman R, et al. Magnetic resonance imaging of sacroiliac joint inflammation. Arthritis Rheum 33:1763–1769, 1990.

Arneet F. Seronegative spondyloarthropathies. Bull Rheum Dis 37:1–12, 1987.

Burgos-Vargas R, Pineda C. New clinical and radiographic features of the seronegative spondyloarthropathies. Curr Opin Rheum 3:562–574, 1991.

Klein RG, Ech BC, DeLong WB, et al. A randomized double blind trial of dextrose-glycerine-phenol injections for chronic low back pain. J Spinal Disord 6:23–33, 1993.

Coccygodynia

Hodges SD, Eck JC, Humphreys SC. A treatment and outcomes analysis of patients with coccydynia. Spine J 4:138–140, 2004.

Malgne JY, Doursounian L, Chatellier G. Causes and mechanisms of common coccydynia: role of body mass index and coccygeal trauma. Spine 25:3072–3079, 2000.

Perkins R, Schofferman J, Reynolds J. Coccygectomy for refractory sacrococcygeal joint pain. J Spinal Discord Tech 16:100–103, 2003.

HIP

General

Carney BT, Weinstein SL, Noble J. Long-term follow-up of slipped capital femoral epiphysis. J Bone Joint Surg Am 73:667–674, 1991.

Lakhandpal S, Ginsberg WW, Luthra HS, Handen GG. Transient regional osteoporosis: a study of 56 cases and a review of the literature. Ann Intern Med 106:444–450, 1987.

Smith RG, Appel SH. The Lambert-Eaton syndrome. Hosp Pract 27:101–114, 1992.

Soubrier M, Dubost JJ, Bolsgard S, et al. Insufficiency fracture: a survey of 60 cases and review of the literature. Joint Bone Spine 70:209–218, 2003.

Trochanteric Bursitis/Piriformis Syndrome

Barton PM. Piriformis syndrome: a rational approach to management. Pain 47:345–352, 1991.

Brooker AF Jr. The surgical approach to refractory trochanteric bursitis. Johns Hopkins Med J 145:98–100, 1979.

Ege-Rasmussen KJ, Fano N. Trochanteric bursitis: treatment by corticosteroid injection. Scand J Rheumatol 14:417–420, 1985.

Fishman LM, Zyber PA. Electrophysiologic evidence of piriformis syndrome. Arch Phys Med Rehabil 73:359–364, 1992.

Rothenberg RJ. Rheumatic disease aspects of leg length inequality. Semin Arthritis Rheum 17:196–205, 1988.

Hip Arthritis

Keener JD, Callaghan JJ, Goetz DD, et al. Twenty-five-year results after Charnley total hip arthroplasty in patients less than fifty years old. J Bone Joint Surg Am 85:1066–1072, 2003.

Margules KR. Fluoroscopically directed steroid instillation in the treatment of hip osteoarthritis: safety and efficacy in 510 cases. Arthritis Rheum 44:2449–2450, 2001.

Santos-Ocampo AS, Santos-Ocampo RS. Non-contrast computed tomography-guided intra-articular corticosteroid injections of severe bilateral hip arthritis in a patient with ankylosing spondylitis. Clin Exp Rheumatol 21:239–240, 2003.

Meralgia Paresthetica

Lee CC. Entrapment syndromes of peripheral nerve injuries. In Winn HR (ed). Youman's Neurological Surgery, 5th ed. Philadelphia, Elsevier, 2004, pp 3923–3939.

Avascular Necrosis of the Hip

Chan TW, Dalinka MK, Steinberg ME, et al. MRI appearance of femoral head osteonecrosis following core decompression and bone grafting. Skeletal Radiol 20:103–107, 1991.

Colwell CW Jr. The controversy of core decompression of the femoral head for osteonecrosis. Arthritis Rheum 32:797–800, 1989.

Ficat RP. Idiopathic bone necrosis of the femoral head: early diagnosis and treatment. J Bone Joint Surg Br 67:3–9, 1985.

Mitchell DG, Rao VM, Dalinka MK, et al. Femoral head avascular necrosis: correlation of MR imaging, radiographic staging, radionuclide imaging, and clinical findings. Radiology 162:709–715, 1987.

Zizic TM, Marcoux C, Hungerford DS, et al. Corticosteroid therapy associated with ischemic necrosis of bone in systemic lupus erythematosus. Am J Med 79:586–604, 1985.

Zizic TM, Marcoux C, Hungerford DS, et al. The early diagnosis of ischemic necrosis of bone. Arthritis Rheum 29:1177–1186, 1986.

Osteitis Pubis

Holt MA, Keene JS, Graf BK, Helwig DC. Treatment of osteitis pubis in athletes: results of corticosteroid injection. Am J Sports Med 23:601–606, 1995.

KNEE

General

Berman A, Espinoza LR, Diaz JD, et al. Rheumatic manifestations of human immunodeficiency virus infection. Am J Med 85:59–64, 1988.

Espinoza LR, Aguilar JL, Berman A, et al. Rheumatic

manifestations associated with human immunodeficiency virus infection. Arthritis Rheum 32:1615-1622, 1989.

Fischer SP, Fox JM, Del Pizzo W, et al. Accuracy of diagnosis from MRI of the knee: a multicenter analysis of one thousand and fourteen patients. J Bone Joint Surg Am 73A:2-10, 1991.

Krause BL, Williams JP, Catterall A. Natural history of Osgood-Schlatter's disease. J Pediatr Orthop 10:65-68, 1990.

Pritchard MH, Jessop JD. Chondrocalcinosis in primary hyperparathyroidism. Ann Rheum Dis 36:146-151, 1977.

Patellofemoral Syndrome

Cox JS. Chondromalacia of the patella: a review and update—part I. Contemp Orthop 6:17-31, 1983.

Insall J. Current concepts review: patellar pain. J Bone Joint Surg Am 64A:147, 1982.

Osteoarthritis of the Knee

Balch HW, Gibson JM, Eighorbarev AF, et al. Repeated corticosteroid injections into knee joints. Rheumatol Rehabil 19:62-66, 1970.

Bhattacharyya T, Gale D, Dewire P, et al. The clinical importance of meniscal tears demonstrated by magnetic resonance imaging in osteoarthritis of the knee. J Bone Joint Surg Am 85A:4-9, 2003.

Chang RW, Falconer J, Stulberg SD, et al. A randomized, controlled trial of arthroscopic surgery versus closed-needle joint lavage for patients with osteoarthritis of the knee. Arthritis Rheum 36:289-296, 1993.

Friedman DM, Moore ME. The efficacy of intra-articular steroids in osteoarthritis: A double-blind study. J Rheumatol 7:850-855, 1980.

Hernborg J, Nilsson BE. The relationship between osteophytes in the knee joints, osteoarthritis and aging. Acta Orthop Scand 44:69-74, 1973.

Hollander JL. Intra-articular hydrocortisone in arthritis and allied conditions: a summary of two years' clinical experience. J Bone Joint Surg 35:983-990, 1953.

Kehr MJ. Comparison of intra-articular cortisone analogues in osteoarthritis of the knee. Ann Rheum Dis 18:325-328, 1959.

Lane NE, Block D, Jones A, et al. Running and osteoarthritis: a controlled study: long distance running, bone density, and osteoarthritis. JAMA 255:1147-1151, 1986.

Miller JH, White J, Norton TH. The value of intra-articular injections in osteoarthritis of the knee. J Bone Joint Surg Br 40B:636-643, 1958.

Nakhostine M, Friedrich NF, Muller W, Kentsch A. A special high tibial osteotomy technique for treatment of unicompartmental osteoarthritis of the knee. Orthopedics 16:1255-1258, 1993.

Panush RS, Schmidt C, Caldwell JR, et al. Is running associated with degenerative joint disease? JAMA 255:1152-1154, 1986.

Zitnan D, Sitaj S. Natural course of articular chondrocalcinosis. Arthritis Rheum 19(Suppl):363-390, 1976.

Hemarthrosis

Adalberth T, Roos H, Lauren M, et al. Magnetic resonance imaging, scintigraphy, and arthroscopic evaluation of traumatic hemarthrosis of the knee. Am J Sports Med 25:231-237, 1997.

Calmback WL, Hutchens M. Evaluation of patients presenting with knee pain: Part II. differential diagnosis. Am Fam Physician 68:917-922, 2003.

Casteleyn PP, Handelberg F, Opdecam P. Traumatic haemarthrosis of the knee. J Bone Joint Surg Br 70B:404-406, 1988.

Kocher MS, Micheli LJ, Zurakowski D, Luke A. Partial tears of the anterior cruciate ligament in children and adolescents. Am J Sports Med 30:697-703, 2002.

Maffulli N, Binfield PM, King JB, Good CJ. Acute haemarthrosis of the knee in athletes: a prospective study of 106 cases. J Bone Joint Surg Br 75B:945-949, 1993.

Sarimo J, Rantanen J, Heikkila J, et al. Acute traumatic hemarthrosis of the knee: is routine arthroscopic examination necessary? A study of 320 consecutive patients. Scand J Surg 91:361-364, 2002.

Shepard L, Abdollahi K, Lee J, et al. The prevalence of soft tissue injuries in nonoperative tibial plateau fractures as determined by magnetic resonance imaging. J Orthop Trauma 16:628-631, 2002.

Anserinus Bursitis

Forbes JR, Helms CA, Janzen DL. Acute pes anserinus bursitis: MR imaging. Radiology 194:525-527, 1995.

Prepatellar Bursitis

Bellon EM, Sacco DC, Steiger DA, Coleman PE. Magnetic resonance imaging in "housemaid's knee." Magn Reson Imaging 5:175-177, 1987.

Kerr DR. Prepatellar and olecranon arthroscopic bursectomy. Clin Sports Med 12:137-142, 1993.

Knight JM, Thomas JC, Maurer RC. Treatment of septic olecranon and prepatellar bursitis with percutaneous placement of a suction-irrigation system: a report of 12 cases. Clin Orthop 206:90-93, 1986.

McAfee JH, Smith DL. Olecranon and prepatellar bursitis: diagnosis and treatment. West J Med 149:607-610, 1988.

Meniscal Tears

Boyd KT, Myers PT. Meniscus preservation: rationale, repair techniques and results. Knee 10:1-11, 2003.

Englund M. Meniscal tear—a feature of osteoarthritis. Acta Orthop Scand 75(Suppl):1-45, 2004.

Pearse EO, Craig DM. Partial meniscectomy in the presence of severe osteoarthritis does not hasten the symptomatic progression of osteoarthritis. Arthroscopy 19:963-968, 2003.

Sethi PM, Cooper A, Jokl P. Technical tips in orthopaedics: meniscal repair with use of an in situ fibrin clot. Arthroscopy 19:E44, 2003.

Zanetti M, Pfirrmann CW, Schmid MR, et al. Patients with suspected meniscal tears: prevalence of abnormalities seen on MRI of 100 symptomatic and 100 contralateral asymptomatic knees. AJR Am J Roentgenol 181:635-641, 2003.

Iliotibial Band Syndrome

Barber FA, Sutker AN. Iliotibial band syndrome. Sports Med 14:144-148, 1992.

Ekman EF, Pope T, Martin DF, Curl WW. Magnetic resonance imaging of iliotibial band syndrome. Am J Sports Med 22:851-854, 1994.

Faraj AA, Moulton A, Sirivastava VM. Snapping iliotibial band: report of ten cases and review of the literature. Acta Orthop Belg 67:19-23, 2001.

Fredericson M, White JJ, Macmahon JM, Andriacchi TP. Quantitative analysis of the relative effectiveness of 3 iliotibial band stretches. Arch Phys Med Rehabil 83:589-592, 2002.

Puniello MS. Iliotibial band tightness and medial patellar glide in patients with patellofemoral syndrome. J Orthop Sports Phys Ther 17:144-148, 1993.

Richards DP, Alan Barber F, Troop RL. Iliotibial band Z-lengthening. Arthroscopy 19:326-329, 2003.

Anterior Cruciate Ligament Injuries

Fithian DC, Paxton LW, Goltz DH. Fate of the anterior cruciate ligament-injured knee. Orthop Clin North Am 33:621-636, 2002.

Osteochondritis Dissecans

Cahill BR. Current concepts review: osteochondritis dissecans. J Bone Joint Surg Am 79A:471-472, 1997.

Cahill BR, Phillips MR, Navarro R. The results of conservative management of juvenile osteochondritis dissecans using joint scintigraphy: a prospective study. Am J Sports Med 17:601-606, 1989.

Linden B. Osteochondritis dissecans of the femoral condyles: a long-term follow-up study. J Bone Joint Surg 59:769-776, 1977.

Peterson L, Minas T, Brittberg M, Lindahl A. Treatment of osteochondritis dissecans of the knee with autologous chondrocyte transplantation. J Bone Joint Surg Am 85A:17-24, 2003.

Septic Arthritis

Blackburn WD, Alarcon GS. Prosthetic joint infections: a role for prophylaxis. Arthritis Rheum 34:110-117, 1991.

Gardner GR, Weisman MH. Pyarthrosis in patients with rheumatoid arthritis: a report of 13 years and a review of the literature from the past 40 years. Am J Med 88:503-510, 1990.

Goldenberg DL, Reed JI. Bacterial arthritis. N Engl J Med 312:764-771, 1985.

Vincent GM, Amirault JD. Septic arthritis in the elderly. Clin Orthop 251:241-245, 1990.

Von Essen R. Bacterial infections following intra-articular injection. Scand J Rheumatol 10:7-13, 1989.

LOWER LEG

General

Pineda C, Fonseca C, Martinez-Lavin M. The spectrum of soft tissue and skeletal abnormalities of hypertrophic osteoarthropathy. J Rheumatol 17:773-778, 1990.

Tibial Fracture

Aoki Y, Yasuda K, Tohyama H, et al. Magnetic resonance imaging in stress fracture and shin splints. Clin Orthop 421:260-267, 2004.

Boniotti V, Del Giudice E, Fengoni E, et al. Imaging of bone micro-injuries. Radiol Med (Torino) 105:425-435, 2003.

Iwamoto J, Takeda T. Stress fractures in athletes: review of 196 cases. J Orthop Sci 8:273-278, 2003.

Migrom C, Finestone A, Segev S, et al. Are overground or treadmill runners more likely to sustain tibial stress fractures? Br J Sports Med 37:160-163, 2003.

Sonoda N, Chosa E, Totoribe K, Tajima N. Biomechanical analysis for stress fractures of the anterior middle third of the tibia in athletes: nonlinear analysis using a three-dimensional finite element method. J Orthop Sci 8:505-513, 2003.

ANKLE

General

Abramowitz Y, Wollstein R, Barzilay Y, et al. Outcome of resection of a symptomatic os trigonum. J Bone Joint Surg Am 85A:1051-1057, 2003.

Horton WA, Collins DL, DeSmet AA, et al. Familial joint instability syndrome. Am J Med Genet 6:221-228, 1980.

Oloff LM, Schulhofer SD, Cocko AP. Subtalar joint arthroscopy for sinus tarsi syndrome: a review of 29 cases. J Foot Ankle Surg 40:152-157, 2001.

Ankle Sprain

Cetti R. Conservative treatment of injury to the fibular ligaments of the ankle. Br J Sports Med 16:47-52, 1982.

Kerkhoffs GM, Handoll HH, de Bie R, et al. Surgical versus conservative treatment for acute injuries of the lateral ligament complex of the ankle in adults. Cochrane Database Syst Rev 3:CD000380, 2002.

Kerkhoffs GM, Rowe BH, Assendelft WJ, et al. Immobilisation for acute ankle sprain: a systematic review. Arch Orthop Trauma Surg 121:462-471, 2001.

Kitsoaka HB, Lee MD, Morrey BF, Cass JR. Acute repair and delayed reconstruction for lateral ankle instability: twenty-year follow-up study. J Orthop Trauma 11:530-535, 1997.

Konradsen L, Bech L, Ehrenbjerg M, Nickelsen T. Seven years follow-up after ankle inversion trauma. Scand J Med Sci Sports 12:129-135, 2002.

Konradsen L, Holmer P, Sondergaard L. Early mobilizing

treatment for grade III ankle ligament injuries. Foot Ankle Int 12:69-73, 1991.

Lynch SA, Renstrom PA. Treatment of acute lateral ankle ligament rupture in the athlete: conservative versus surgical treatment. Sports Med 27:61-71, 1999.

Moller-Larsen F, Withelund JO, Jurik AG, et al. Comparison of three different treatments for ruptured lateral ankle ligaments. Acta Orthop Scand 59:564-566, 1988.

Niedermann B, Andersen A, Andersen SB, et al. Ruptures of the lateral ligaments of the ankle: operation or plaster cast? Acta Orthop Scand 52:579-587, 1981.

Pijnenburg AC, Bogaard K, Krips R, et al. Operative and functional treatment of rupture of the lateral ligament of the ankle: a randomized, prospective trial. J Bone Joint Surg Br 85B:525-530, 2003.

Stiell IG, McKnight RD, Greenberg GH. Implementation of the Ottawa ankle rules. JAMA 271:827-832, 1994.

Achilles Tendinitis/Rupture

Astrom M. Partial rupture in chronic Achilles tendinopathy: a retrospective analysis of 342 cases. Acta Orthop Scand 69:404-407, 1998.

Cowan MA, Alexander S. Simultaneous bilateral rupture of Achilles tendons due to triamcinolone. Br Med J 5240:1658, 1961.

DaCruz DJ, Geeson M, Allen MJ, Phair L. Achilles paratendonitis: an evaluation of steroid injection. Br J Sports Med 22:64-65, 1988.

Fox JM, Blazina ME, Jobe FW, et al. Degeneration and rupture of the Achilles tendon. Clin Orthop 107:221-224, 1975.

Fredberg U, Bolvig L, Pfeiffer-Jensen M, et al. Ultrasonography as a tool for diagnosis, guidance of local steroid injection and, together with pressure algometry, monitoring of the treatment of athletes with chronic jumper's knee and Achilles tendonitis: a randomized, double-blind, placebo-controlled study. Scand J Rheumatol 33:94-101, 2004.

Gilcrest EL. Ruptures and tears of muscles and tendons of the lower extremity. JAMA 100:153-160, 1933.

Gill SS, Gelbke MK, Mattson SL, et al. Fluoroscopically guided low-volume peritendinous corticosteroid injection for Achilles tendinopathy: a safety study. J Bone Joint Surg Am 86A:802-806, 2004.

Hugate R, Pennypacker J, Saunders M, Juliano P. The effects of intratendinous and retrocalcaneal intrabursal injections of corticosteroid on the biomechanical properties of rabbit Achilles tendons. J Bone Joint Surg Am 86A:794-800, 2004.

Khan KM, Forster BB, Robinson J, et al. Are ultrasound and magnetic resonance imaging of value in the assessment of Achilles tendon disorders? A two year prospective study. Br J Sports Med 37:149-153, 2003.

Melmed SP. Spontaneous bilateral rupture of the calcaneal tendon during steroid therapy. J Bone Joint Surg Br 47:104-105, 1965.

Read MT. Safe relief of rest pain that eases with activity in achillodynia by intrabursal or peritendinous steroid injection: the rupture rate was not increased by these steroid injections. Br J Sports Med 33:134-135, 1999.

Weber M, Nieman M, Lanz R, Muller T. Nonoperative treatment of acute rupture of the Achilles tendon: results of a new protocol and comparison with operative treatment. Am J Sports Med 31:685-691, 2003.

Pre-Achilles Bursitis

Calder JD, Saxby TS. Surgical treatment of insertional Achilles tendinosis. Foot Ankle Int 24:119-121, 2003.

Cozen L. Bursitis of the heel. Am J Orthop 3:372-374, 1961.

Gerster JC, Piccinin P. Enthesopathy of the heels in juvenile onset seronegative B-27 positive spondyloarthropathy. J Rheumatol 12:310-314, 1985.

Ohberg L, Alfredson H. Sclerosing therapy in chronic Achilles tendon insertional pain—results of a pilot study. Knee Surg Sports Traumatol Arthrosc 11:339-343, 2003.

Posterior Tibialis Tendinitis

Bare AA, Haddad SL. Tenosynovitis of the posterior tibial tendon. Foot Ankle Clin 6:37-66, 2001.

Plantar Fasciitis

Acevedo JI, Beskin JL. Complication of plantar fascia rupture associated with corticosteroid injection. Foot Ankle Int 19:91, 1998.

Barrett SL, Day SV. Endoscopic plantar fasciotomy for chronic plantar fasciitis/heel spur syndrome: surgical technique—early clinical results. J Foot Surg 30:568-570, 1991.

Blockey NJ. The painful heel: a controlled trial of the value of hydrocortisone. BMJ 1:1277-1278, 1956.

Buchbinder R. Clinical practice: plantar fasciitis. N Engl J Med 350:2159-2166, 2004.

Daly PJ, Kitaoka HB, Chao EY. Plantar fasciotomy for intractable plantar fasciitis. Foot Ankle Int 13:188-195, 1992.

DiGiovanni BF, Nawoczenski DA, Lintal ME. Tissue-specific plantar fascia-stretching exercises enhance outcomes in patients with chronic heel pain. J Bone Joint Surg Am 85:1270-1277, 2003.

Furey JG. Plantar fasciitis: the painful heel syndrome. J Bone Joint Surg Am 57A:672-673, 1975.

Gould EA. Three generations of exostoses of heel inherited from father to son. J Hered 33:228, 1942.

Jerosch J, Schunck J, Liebach D, Filler T. Indication, surgical technique and results of endoscopic fascial release in plantar fasciitis. Knee Surg Sports Traumatol Arthrosc 12:471-477, 2004.

Lapidus PW, Guidotti FP. Painful heel: report of 323 patients with 364 painful heels. Clin Orthop 39:178-186, 1959.

Newell SG, Miller SJ. Conservative treatment of plantar fascial strain. Physician Sports Med 5:68-73, 1977.

Riddle DL, Pulisic M, Pidcoe P, Johnson RE. Risk factors for plantar fasciitis: a matched case-control study. J Bone Joint Surg Am 85A:872-877, 2003.

Sellman JR. Plantar fascia rupture associated with corticosteroid injections. Foot Ankle Int 15:376, 1994.

Wapner KL, Sharkey PF. The use of night splints for treatment of recalcitrant plantar fasciitis. Foot Ankle Int 12:135, 1991.

Wolgin M, Dook D, Graham C, Mauldin D. Conservative treatment of plantar heel pain: long-term follow-up. Foot Ankle Int 15:97–102, 1994.

Tarsal Tunnel Syndrome

Gondring WH, Shields B, Wenger S. An outcomes analysis of surgical treatment of tarsal tunnel syndrome. Foot Ankle Int 24:545–550, 2003.

Kim DH, Ryn S, Tiel RI, Kline DG. Surgical management and results of 135 tibial nerve lesions at the Louisiana State University Health Sciences Center. Neurosurgery 53:1114–1124, 2003.

Lau JT, Stavrou P. Posterior tibial nerve—primary. Foot Ankle Clin 9:271–285, 2004.

McGuigan L, Burke D, Fleming A. Tarsal tunnel syndrome and peripheral neuropathy in rheumatoid arthritis. Ann Rheum Dis 42:128–131, 1983.

Mondelli M, Morana P, Padua L. An electophysiological severity scale in tarsal tunnel syndrome. Acta Neurol Scand 109:284–289, 2004.

Sammarco GJ, Chang L. Outcome of surgical treatment of tarsal tunnel syndrome. Foot Ankle Int 24:125–131, 2003.

Ankle Arthritis

Thomas RH, Daniels TR. Current concepts review: ankle arthritis. J Bone Joint Surg Am 85A:923–936, 2003.

FOOT

Bunions

Ferrari J, Higgins JP, Prior TD. Interventions for treating hallux valgus (abductovalgus) and bunions. Cochrane Database Syst Rev 1:CD000964, 2004.

Piggott H. The natural history of hallux valgus in adolescence and early adult life. J Bone Joint Surg 42:749–760, 1960.

Vanore JV, Christensen JC, Kravitz SR, et al. Diagnosis and treatment of first metatarsophalangeal joint disorders: Section 5: hallux valgus. J Foot Ankle Surg 42:148–151, 2003.

Hallux Rigidus and Limitus

Coughlin MJ, Shurnas PS. Hallux rigidus: demographics, etiology, and radiographic assessment. Foot Ankle Int 24:731–743, 2003.

Foukis TS, Jacobs PM, Dawson DM, et al. A prospective comparison of clinical, radiographic, and intraoperative features of hallux rigidus: short-term follow-up and analysis. J Foot Ankle Surg 41:158–165, 2002.

Grady JF, Axe TM, Zager EJ, Sheldon LA. A retrospective analysis of 772 patients with hallux limitus. J Am Podiatr Med Assoc 92:102–108, 2002.

Hammer Toes

Cahill BR, Connor DE. A long-term follow-up on proximal phalangectomy for hammer toes. Clin Orthop 86:191–192, 1972.

Caterini R, Farsetti P, Tarantino U, et al. Arthrodesis of the toe joints with an intramedullary cannulated screw for correction of hammertoe deformity. Foot Ankle Int 25:256–261, 2004.

Myerson MS, Shereff MJ. The pathological anatomy of claw and hammer toes. J Bone Joint Surg Am 71A:45–49, 1989.

Newman RJ, Fitton JM. An evaluation of operative procedures in the treatment of hammer toe. Acta Orthop Scand 50:709–712, 1979.

Sorto LA Jr. Surgical correction of hammer toes: a 5-year postoperative study. J Am Podiatry Assoc 64:930–934, 1974.

Morton's Neuroma

Basadonna PT, Rucco V, Gasparini D, Onorato A. Plantar fat pad atrophy after corticosteroid injection for an interdigital neuroma: a case report. Am J Phys Med Rehabil 78:283–285, 1999.

Diebold PF, Daum B, Dang-Vu V, Litchinko M. True epineural neurolysis in Morton's neuroma: a 5-year follow up. Orthopedics 19:397–400, 1996.

Fanucci E, Masala S, Fabiano S, et al. Treatment of intermetatarsal Morton's neuroma with alcohol injection under US guide: 10-month follow-up. Eur Radiol 14:514–518, 2004.

Nashi M, Venkatachalam A, Muddu BN. Surgery of Morton's neuroma: dorsal or plantar approach. J R Coll Surg Edinb 423:36–37, 1997.

Okafor B, Shergill G, Angel J. Treatment of Morton's neuroma by neurolysis. Foot Ankle Int 18:284–287, 1997.

Ruushkanen MM, Niinimaki T, Jalovaara P. Results of the surgical treatment of Morton's neuroma in 58 operated intermetatarsal spaces followed over 6 (2-12) years. Arch Orthop Trauma Surg 113:78–80, 1994.

Sharp RJ, Wade CM, Hennessy MS, Saxby TS. The role of MRI and ultrasound imaging in Morton's neuroma and the effect of size of lesion on symptoms. J Bone Joint Surg Br 85B:999–1005, 2003.

Strong G, Thomas PS. Conservative treatment of Morton's neuroma. Orthop Rev 16:343–345, 1987.

Thomson C, Gibson J, Martin D. Interventions for the treatment of Morton's neuroma. Cochrane Database Syst Rev 3:CD003118, 2004.

Vito GR, Talarico LM. A modified technique for Morton's neuroma: decompression with relocation. J Am Podiatr Med Assoc 93:190–194, 2003.

Wolfort SF, Dellon AL. Treatment of recurrent neuroma of the interdigital nerve by implantation of the proximal nerve into muscle in the arch of the foot. J Foot Ankle Surg 40:404–410, 2001.

Younger AS, Claridge RJ. The role of diagnostic block in the management of Morton's neuroma. Can J Surg 41:127–130, 1998.

Gout

Agudelo CA, Weinberger A, Schumacher HR, et al. Definite diagnosis of gouty arthritis by identification of urate crystals in asymptomatic metatarsophalangeal joints. Arthritis Rheum 22:559–560, 1979.

Campion EW, Glynn RJ, DeLabry LO. Asymptomatic hyperuricemia: risk and consequences in the normative aging process. Am J Med 82:421–426, 1987.

Emmerson BT. The management of gout. N Engl J Med 334:445–451, 1996.

Fernandez C, Noguera R, Gonzalez JA, Pascual E. Treatment of acute attacks of gout with a small dose of intraarticular triamcinolone acetonide. J Rheumatol 26:2285–2286, 1999.

Grahame R, Scott JT. Clinical survey of 354 patients with gout. Ann Rheum Dis 29:461–470, 1970.

Taylor CT, Brooks NC, Kelley KW. Corticotropin for acute management of gout. Ann Pharmacother 35:365–368, 2001.

Werlen D, Gabay C, Vischer TL. Corticosteroid therapy for the treatment of acute attacks of crystal-induced arthritis: an effective alternative to nonsteroidal anti-inflammatory drugs. Rev Rhum Engl Educ 63:248–254, 1996.

Sesamoiditis

Biedert R, Hintermann B. Stress fractures of the medial great toe sesamoids in athletes. Foot Ankle Int 24:137–141, 2003.

Vanore JV, Christensen JC, Kravitz SR, et al. Diagnosis and treatment of first metatarsophalangeal joint disorders: Section 4. sesamoid disorders. J Foot Ankle Surg 42:143–147, 2003.

MEDICAL DIAGNOSES, SUPPLEMENTS, MEDICATIONS

Osteoporosis

Barzel US. Estrogens in the prevention and treatment of postmenopausal osteoporosis: a review. Am J Med 85:847–850, 1988.

Dawson-Hughes B, Dallal GE, Krall EA, et al. A controlled trial of the effect of calcium supplementation on bone density in postmenopausal women. N Engl J Med 323:878–883, 1990.

Hui SL, Siemenda CW, Johnston CC. Age and bone mass as predictors of fractures in a prospective study. J Clin Invest 81:1804–1809, 1988.

Lindsay R, Gallagher JC, Kleerekoper M, Pickar JH. Effect of lower doses of conjugated equine estrogens with and without medroxyprogesterone acetate on bone in early postmenopausal women. JAMA 287:2668–2676, 2002.

Lukert BP, Raisz LG. Glucocorticoid-induced osteoporosis: pathogenesis and management. Ann Intern Med 112:352, 1990.

NIH Consensus Development Panel. Osteoporosis prevention, diagnosis, and therapy. JAMA 285:785–795, 2001.

Raisz LG. Local and systemic factors in the pathogenesis of osteoporosis. N Engl J Med 318:818, 1988.

Reid IR, Ames RW, Evans MC, et al. Effect of calcium supplementation on bone loss in postmenopausal women. N Engl J Med 328:460–464, 1993.

Speroff L, Rowan J, Symons J, et al. The comparative effect on bone density, endometrium, and lipids of continuous hormones as replacement therapy (CHART study): a randomized controlled trial. JAMA 276:1397–1403, 1996.

Tilyard MW, Spears GFS, Thomson J, et al. Treatment of postmenopausal osteoporosis with calcitriol or calcium. N Engl J Med 326:357–362, 1992.

Corticosteroid Injection Side Effects

Bedi SS, Ellis W. Spontaneous rupture of the calcaneal tendon in rheumatoid arthritis after steroid injection. Ann Rheum Dis 29:494–495, 1970.

Halpern AA, Horowitz BG, Nagel DA. Tendon ruptures associated with corticosteroid therapy. West J Med 127:378–382, 1977.

Hedner P, Persson G. Suppression of the hypothalamic-pituitary-adrenal axis after a single intramuscular injection of methylprednisolone acetate. Ann Allergy 47:176–179, 1981.

Hollander JL, Jessar RA, Brown EM. Intra-synovial corticosteroid therapy: a decade of use. Bull Rheum Dis 11:239–240, 1961.

Ismail AM, Balakrishnan R, Rajakumar MK. Rupture of patellar ligament after steroid infiltration: report of a case. J Bone Joint Surg Br 51B:503–505, 1969.

Kendall PH. Untoward effects following local hydrocortisone injection. Ann Phys Med 4:170–175, 1961.

Kleinman M, Gross AE. Achilles tendon rupture following steroid injection. J Bone Joint Surg Am 65A:1345–1347, 1983.

Libanati CR, Baylink DJ. Prevention and treatment of glucocorticoid-induced osteoporosis: a pathogenetic perspective. Chest 102:1426–1435, 1992.

Roseff R, Canoso JJ. Femoral osteonecrosis following several hundred soft tissue corticosteroid infiltrations. Am J Med 77:1119–1120, 1984.

Rostron PKM, Calver RF. Subcutaneous atrophy following methylprednisolone injection in Osgood-Schlatter epiphysitis. J Bone Joint Surg Am 61A:627–628, 1979.

Glucosamine Sulfate

Bruyere O, Honore A, Ethgen O, et al. Correlation between radiographic severity of knee osteoarthritis and future disease progression: results from a 3-year prospective, placebo-controlled study evaluating the effect of glucosamine sulfate. Osteoarthritis Cartilage 11:1-5, 2003.

McAlindon T. Glucosamine for osteoarthritis: dawn of a new era. Lancet 357:247–248, 2001.

Muller-Fassbender H, Bach GL, Haase W, et al. Glucosamine sulfate compared to ibuprofen in osteoarthritis of the knee. Osteoarthritis Cartilage 2:61–69, 1994.

Noyszewski EA, Wriblewski K, Dodge GR, et al. Preferential incorporation of glucosamine into the galactosamine moieties of chondroitin sulfates in articular cartilage explants. Arthritis Rheum 44:1089–1095, 2001.

Pavelka MD, Gatterova J, Olejarova M, et al. Glucosamine sulfate use and delay of progression of knee osteoarthritis: a 3-year, randomized, placebo-controlled, double-blind study. Arch Intern Med 162:2113–2123, 2002.

Seroggie DA, Albright A, Harris MD. The effect of glucosamine-chondroitin supplementation on glycosylated hemoglobin levels in patients with type 2 diabetes mellitus: a placebo-controlled, double-blinded, randomized clinical trial. Arch Intern Med 163:1587–1590, 2003.

Hyaluronic Acid Injections

Dahlberg L, Lohmander LS, Ryd L. Intraarticular injections of hyaluronan in patients with cartilage abnormalities and knee pain: a one-year double-blind, placebo-controlled study. Arthritis Rheum 37:521–528, 1994.

Evanich JD, Evanich CJ, Wright CA, et al. Efficacy of intra-articular hyaluronic acid injections in knee osteoarthritis. Clin Orthop 390:173–181, 2001.

Leopold SS, Brigham BR, Winston J, et al. Corticosteroid compared with hyaluronic acid injections for the treatment of osteoarthritis of the knee. J Bone Joint Surg Am 85A:1197–1203, 2003.

Prolotherapy

Yelland MJ, Mar C, Pirozzo S, et al. Prolotherapy injection for chronic low-back pain. Cochrane Database Syst Rev 2:CD004059, 2004.

Laboratory Testing

Barland P, Lipstein E. Selection and use of laboratory tests in the rheumatic diseases. Am J Med 100:16S–23S, 1996.

Cohen PL. What antinuclear antibodies can tell you. J Musculoskeletal Med 10:37–46, 1993.

Sox HC, Liang MH. The erythrocyte sedimentation rate: guidelines for rational use. Ann Intern Med 104:515–523, 1986.

White RH, Robbins DL. Clinical significance and interpretation of antinuclear antibodies. West J Med 147:210, 1987.

Young B, Gleeson M, Cripps AW. C-reactive protein: a critical review. Pathology 23:2417–2420, 1992.

Synovial Fluid Analysis

Cohen AS, Brandt KD, Krey PR. Synovial fluid. *In* Cohen AS (ed): Laboratory Diagnostic Procedures in the Rheumatoid Diseases, 2nd ed. Boston, Little, Brown, 1975, pp 1–62.

Goldenberg DL, Reed JI. Bacterial arthritis. N Engl J Med 312:764–771, 1985.

James MJ, Cleland LG, Rofe AM, Leslie AL. Intra-articular pressure and the relationship between synovial perfusion and metabolic demand. J Rheumatol 17:521–527, 1990.

Krey PR, Bailen DA. Synovial fluid leukocytosis: a study of extremes. Am J Med 67:436–442, 1979.

Ropes MW, Bauer W. Synovial Changes in Joint Disease. Cambridge, Harvard University Press, 1953.

Nonsteroidal Anti-inflammatory Drugs

Rashad S, Revell P, Hemmingway A, et al. Effect of nonsteroidal anti-inflammatory drugs on the course of osteoarthritis. Lancet 2:519–522, 1989.

Edwards Brothers Malloy
Ann Arbor MI. USA
February 29, 2016